THE ANTIBODIES
Volume 3

THE ANTIBODIES
Volume 3

Edited by

Maurizio Zanetti, MD

University of California
San Diego

and

J. Donald Capra, MD

University of Texas
Southwestern Medical Center, Dallas

harwood academic publishers

Australia • Canada • China • France • Germany • India •
Japan • Luxembourg • Malaysia • The Netherlands • Russia •
Singapore • Switzerland • Thailand • United Kingdom

Amsteldijk 166
1st Floor
1079 LH Amsterdam
The Netherlands

British Library Cataloguing in Publication Data

The antibodies
  Vol. 3
  1.Immunoglobulins 2.Immunology
  I.Zanetti, Maurizio II.Capra, J. Donald, 1937–
  616'.0793

  ISBN 90-5702-523-X

CONTENTS

PREFACE

Immunology is a discipline just over a century old that has played a central role in medicine and, more recently, in the biomedical sciences. Immunology has often been referred to as "imperialistic" for its tendency to spread to other biomedical fields like no other discipline. A myriad of publications have continually documented the incredible series of discoveries in this field. During times when many areas of immunology have undergone a formidable revolution, antibodies have always been central to any major progress in the field. From the pioneering work of von Behring and Kisatato at the end of the last century through the seminal experiments of Bordet, Ehrlich, Landsteiner, Oudin and Kunkel, just to name a few, and the conceptualizations of Burnet and Jerne, antibodies have dominated the scene. During the last two decades such major breakthroughs as the advent of monoclonal antibodies and the development of new techniques of antibody engineering have kept antibodies in the forefront of immunology and medical science. From diagnostic tools to vehicles for modern therapy against cancer, infections and autoimmune diseases, the study of antibodies has attracted a multitude of scientists.

While the race for better molecules for diagnosis and therapy is still on, it is evident that our knowledge of antibodies — their properties and structural characteristics — is still incomplete. Antibody genes and their regulation, intracellular assembly and secretion, antigen binding properties, effector function and immunity represent just a few of the topics that continue to be investigated using the tools of molecular biology, cell biology, immunochemistry, X-ray crystallography and computer-aided three-dimensional modeling. New technological developments now afford exploration of new areas of study and medical application for antibodies.

With *The Antibodies*, it is our intent to provide the scientific community with its first platform for a comprehensive review of topics of contemporary interest for specialists in this area. At the same time, we will take the opportunity to revisit more traditional aspects of the field so that relevant information and concepts are maintained in parallel with the more modern aspects. While the work ahead can be viewed with a sense of optimism and excitement, we do not underestimate the task that it will take to cover all areas of interest.

We extend our gratitude and thanks to all our colleagues who accepted our invitation to contribute their views and work, and who have made this volume a reality. We hope this collective effort will continue, contributing to keeping the field alive and exciting, and finding a legitimate identity in the immunological literature.

Maurizio Zanetti, MD
University of California
San Diego

J. Donald Capra, MD
University of Texas
Southwestern Medical Center
Dallas

PREFACE

Volume 3

Although antibodies were first described over a century ago, they still remain a focus of intense scrutiny by scientists throughout the world. As we appreciate more and more the extraordinary machinery involved in the production of an antibody molecule, we continue to be puzzled by the mechanisms of antibody diversification. As *The Antibodies: Volume 3* goes to press, there are exciting developments in all aspects of antibody structure and function, particularly in areas that involve the recombinational machinery that participates in the initial production of the first rearranged immunoglobulin genes in B cells.

In chapter 1 David Weaver reviews his work, as well as the field of VDJ recombination. Enormous progress has been made since the discovery of the RAG1 and RAG2 genes in 1989. We now know that the process of VDJ recombination is exquisitely regulated and that RAG1 and RAG2 are but the beginning of the process. Dr. Weaver's review is timely and complete.

Westley Reeves and his associates provide an exhaustive review of the Ku autoantigen in chapter 2. Ku is known to bind any double-stranded DNA end regardless of its sequence. However, as Dr. Reeves et al. point out, as Ku interacts with other molecules, exquisite specificity is provided in the VDJ recombination reaction.

Kathy Meek and her colleagues (chapter 3) describe the differential effects of DNA-PK expression in both equine and murine SCID. Both of these represent diseases that impact on VDJ recombination, and the distinction between murine and equine SCID cells provides rare insights into the recombination process.

Gary Litman has long been a major contributor to our understanding of the molecular genetics of antigen-binding molecules from widely divergent species, particularly cartilaginous and bony fishes. His most recent work provides new insights on the evolution of antigen-recognition molecules. In chapter 4 he, Michele Anderson, and Jonathan Rast provide a new model for the evolutionary origin of these genes and the mechanisms driving their divergence.

Chapter 5 was contributed by Drs. Michel Kazatchkine and Srini Kaveri. Dr. Kazatchkine has been among the major driving forces in the use of intravenous immunoglobulin in human immunotherapy. In particular, his laboratory has provided key insights into the molecular mechanisms that explain the efficacy of intravenous immunoglobulins as powerful therapeutic modalities in various pathological conditions. Intravenous immunoglobulins are among the most used biotechnological products in humans.

Finally, Jacob Natvig, who has contributed to the literature on rheumatoid factors for nearly three decades, summarizes his most recent work in chapter 6. He and his colleagues review the field and address the issue as to whether any features of rheumatoid factors produced in rheumatoid arthritis patients can be identified as predisposing them to a pathogenetic role. Their extensive analysis of V region structures among rheumatoid factors isolated from the synovial tissue of patients

with rheumatoid arthritis has provided important insights into the origin of rheumatoid factors as an antigen-driven process. In addition, their three-dimensional
model of these molecules provides important information concerning the structure
of the binding site itself.

We join in thanking our colleagues for delivering their manuscripts in a most
timely fashion.

Maurizio Zanetti, MD   *J. Donald Capra, MD*
University of California   University of Texas
San Diego   Southwestern Medical Center
                                                                    Dallas

CONTRIBUTORS

Ajay K. Ajmani, University of North Carolina, Chapel Hill

Michele K. Anderson, California Institute of Technology, Pasadena

Vincent Bonagura, Long Island Jewish Medical Center, New York

Marie Børretzen, Oslo Sanitetsforenings Rheumatism Hospital, Norway

Srini V. Kaveri, Hôpital Broussais, Paris, France

Michel D. Kazatchkine, Hôpital Broussais, Paris, France

Ray Leber, University of Texas Southwestern Medical Center, Dallas

Gary W. Litman, University of South Florida, St. Petersburg

Katheryn Meek, University of Texas Southwestern Medical Center, Dallas

Jacob B. Natvig, Oslo Sanitetsforenings Rheumatism Hospital, Norway

Jonathan P. Rast, University of South Florida, St. Petersburg

Westley H. Reeves, University of North Carolina, Chapel Hill

Minoru Satoh, University of North Carolina, Chapel Hill

Euy Kyun Shin, University of Texas Southwestern Medical Center, Dallas

Lovorka Stojanov, University of North Carolina, Chapel Hill

Keith M. Thompson, Oslo Sanitetsforenings Rheumatism Hospital, Norway

Jingsong Wang, University of North Carolina, Chapel Hill

David T. Weaver, Harvard Medical School, Boston

Rhonda Wiler, University of Texas Southwestern Medical Center, Dallas

Chapter

ONE

V(D)J Recombination: From Beginning to End

DAVID T. WEAVER

Division of Tumor Immunology, Dana-Farber Cancer Institute
and Department of Microbiology and Molecular Genetics,
Harvard Medical School, Boston, MA 02115, USA

Antigen recognition proteins of the immune system, immunoglobulin (Ig) and T-cell receptors (TCR) are created by a complex DNA recombination pathway in developing lymphocytes. The molecular mechanism, termed V(D)J recombination, takes place at chromosomal regions where the V, D, and J gene segments of these extensive gene families reside. In 1996, V(D)J recombination needs little introduction to immunology and molecular biology audiences. Here I will summarize recently published data highlighting a series of breakthrough discoveries that reveal new information on the pathway.

Each V, D, and J gene segment participating in the VDJ pathway is flanked by recognition DNA elements that dictate the positioning of rearrangement events. The elements, termed recombination signal sequences (RSS) are the essential DNA identifiers for rearrangement sites. Because extensive arrays of V, D, and J elements are tandemly located on the same chromosome, RSS elements alone do not control the accessibility of chromosome regions for rearrangements, although they certainly may influence the frequency of utilization of particular elements. RSS are found as two principle types (Figure 1A). RSS(12) elements contain a highly conserved heptamer flanked by a spacer of 12 nucleotides from a nonamer sequence. RSS(23) elements also contain the heptamer and nonamer sequences, but they are separated by approximately 23 nucleotides as a spacer. The heptamer generally fits the consensus CACAGTG whereas the nonamer consensus is ACAAAAACC. A key principle of the V(D)J recombination reaction that transcends the Ig and TCR gene families is the use of pairs of opposite type RSS elements in single step recombination cycles. Thus, RSS(12) and RSS(23) are partners in single rearrange-

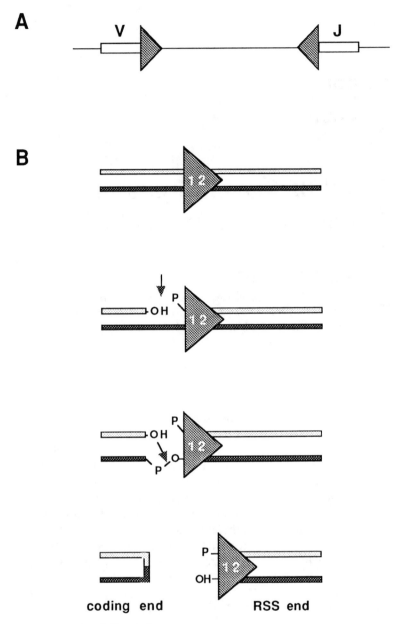

Figure 1 (see COLOR PLATE 1). Model for the V(D)J recombination cleavage steps.
A: DNA substrates for V(D)J recombination are pairs of Recombination Signal Sequences (RSS, blue and red triangles) containing opposite spacer lengths of 12 and 23 bp. Ig and T cell receptor coding sequences are adjoined to these RSS. **B**: The cleavage reactions of V(D)J recombination initiation. A two step reaction has been formulated for this process (McBlane et al., 1995; van Gent et al., 1996). Single-strand cleavage of the phosphodiester bond flanking the RSS element (top strand in the orientation shown, XXX'CACAGTG) is followed by hairpin generation by intramolecular nucleophilic attack. Red arrows denote cleavage positions on both strands. Both steps require RAG1 and RAG2. Coordination of the cleavage reactions between RSS(12) and RSS(23) elements obeys the 12/23 spacer rule (Eastman et al., 1996).

ment events. The evolutionary placement of RSS(12) or RSS(23) in particular gene segment groups is less significant than the establishment of an order between the groups, so that the joining of opposite RSS types are achieved.

I. INITIATION OF THE REACTION-MOVING IN VITRO

Since the discoveries of the *RAG1* and *RAG2* genes in 1989 and 1990 (Oettinger et al., 1990; Schatz et al., 1989), a significant effort has been directed at identifying the role that these two gene products perform in the V(D)J recombination mechanism. Based on the ability to stimulate V(D)J recombination of extrachromosomal DNA substrates in non-lymphoid cells, *RAG1* and *RAG2* were hypothesized to initiate gene rearrangement. However, the demonstration of this function required evidence of biochemical activities for one or both proteins that would be relevant to a DNA recombination assay, because RAG1/RAG2 might act by stimulating the transcription of other lymphoid-restricted genes that would be more directly involved in gene rearrangement. Fulfillment of the hypothesis of a direct role for RAG1 and RAG2 has been achieved recently by associating DNA recombination enzymatic properties to the RAG1/RAG2 complex.

Hairpins as DNA Intermediates

The backdrop for understanding the role of RAG1 and RAG2 in V(D)J recombination is the findings of several laboratories about the DNA steps of the reaction mechanism. In turn, the identification of the DNA products of V(D)J recombination was instrumental in developing ideas about what intermediates might form during the reaction. The formulation of putative DNA intermediates in V(D)J recombination has previously been reviewed (Gellert, 1992a, 1992b; Lewis, 1994; Weaver, 1995), but will be briefly restated here.

Coding junctions of V(D)J recombination are heterogeneous in DNA sequence. Inspection of hundreds of reaction products from the same V and J gene segments illustrates that the recombination process itself is variable, creating many different junctional outcomes, and lending to the diversity in the immune response by forming subtle differences in amino acid selection at the hypervariable regions of Ig and TCR products (Tonegawa, 1983). Usually, the V(D)J coding junctions are processed to generate small deletions of 1–5 bp per coding segment (Figure 2A). Occasionally the products have added nucleotides in the junction (Alt and Baltimore, 1982; Lafaille et al., 1989; McCormack et al., 1989). These added nucleotide residues are subdivided into two mechanistically distinct groups: N and P residues. N bases are new nucleotides that are not encoded by the DNA surrounding the junction. In other words, N residues are untemplated, and must be added during the processing steps prior to ligation. It is now well-established that N residues are added by an enzymatic process catalyzed by the product of the terminal deoxynucleotidyl transferase (*TDT*) gene. Mice lacking *TDT* are able to undergo V(D)J recombination, but both Ig and TCR gene rearrangement products completely lack N regions in VDJ junctions (Gilfillan et al., 1993; Komori et al., 1993). The sole function of *TDT* may be to generate increased junctional diversity of Ig and TCR gene products.

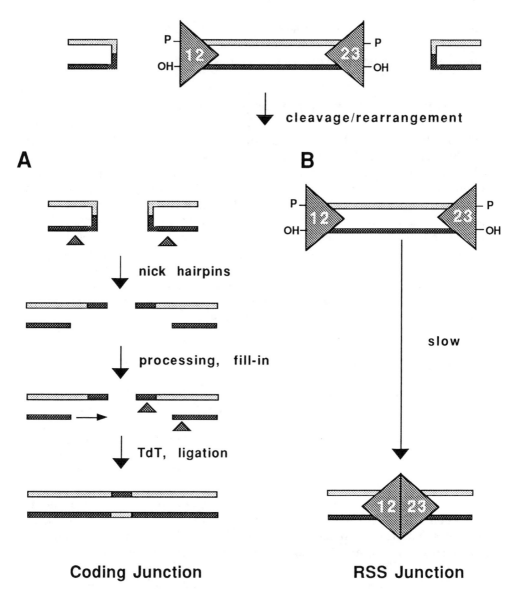

Coding Junction   **RSS Junction**

Figure 2 (see COLOR PLATE 2). Model for the rearrangement and joining steps of V(D)J recombination. The products of the initiation steps of V(D)J recombination are two covalently sealed coding DNA ends (hairpins) and two blunt-ended RSS elements displayed in the linear array consistent with a chromosomal deletional event. Gene rearrangement involves the rejoining of strands from the two cleavages as shown in Part A and B. The relationship between cleavages and rearrangement strand selection are poorly understood. **A**: Coding end joining may be viewed as being started by the terminal endonucleolytic scission of hairpins (red arrows), generating a variety of DNA overlaps. Processing of these structures includes the deletion and addition of nucleotides in the novel junctions formed. P nucleotides arise from asymmetric cleavage of hairpins (indicated by portions of the bottom strand appended to top strand ends) and filling in. Additional red arrows denote mismatch correction of coding ends prior to ligation. N nucleotides are added in an untemplated fashion. **B**: Blunt-end cleaved RSS ends are joined in a separable reaction, producing RSS-RSS fusions that are precise.

The other category of newly added nucleotides in V(D)J recombination junctions, P nucleotides, were discovered from rearrangement products of Ig and TCR genes of limited diversity (Lafaille et al., 1989; McCormack et al., 1989). P nucleotides are templated residues from the coding strands undergoing the V(D)J joining step (Figure 2A). In specific joining events where there is no or limited deletion of coding V, D, or J DNA, it was demonstrated that non-random nucleotides consistently appeared in the junctional products. These P regions of junctions were usually a single residue or templated dinucleotides although larger P stretches are also observed less frequently.

A model consistent with the occasional appearance of P nucleotides and junctional deletion most of the time is the formation of a specific coding DNA intermediate. Such an intermediate is hypothesized to be the V, D, or J coding DNA with no free ends, but DNA that is completely covalently closed in a hairpin configuration (Gellert, 1992b) (Figure 2A). By the utilization of hairpin-ended coding DNA as a template for later steps, a number of different molecular outcomes can emerge depending on the variable processing of these structures.

Experimental verification of the hairpin model was first developed by Roth and Gellert and coworkers (Roth et al., 1992a, 1992b). Examining TCR δ gene rearrangements from neonatal thymocytes, they noticed that DJδ chromosomal DNA fragments were stably produced consistent with unrepaired DSBs (Roth et al., 1992a). Importantly, hairpins were found in a surprisingly large fraction of the total cleavage events when neonatal *scid* thymocytes were evaluated (Roth et al., 1992b). These intriguing observations were consistent with a hairpin model in the V(D)J recombination cleavage reaction, although did not prove this pathway as an intermediate in the mechanism (see below). Since *scid* was demonstrated to be deficient in coding junction formation steps of V(D)J recombination, potentially blocking the pathway at the stage where the SCID protein would be utilized may lead to the accumulation of DNA intermediates. A discussion of the SCID factor is also found in later sections.

The rules governing the processing of coding sequence hairpins are not understood. In theory, V(D)J recombination hairpins may be cleaved at different positions by endonucleolytic steps. Since hairpin ended DNAs are not thermodynamically stable with the terminal residues being base-paired, a more reasonable view of these structures is terminal bubbles of single-stranded DNA. If hairpin cleavages occur on the 3' or bottom strand as shown, the DNA end generated by cleavage would contain 3' overhangs of the top strand. As DNA polymerases are able to polymerize only in the 5' to 3' direction, these DNA fragments may be non-ligatable without nucleolytic processing. Likewise, if hairpin digestion would occur along the 5' or top strand as shown, 5' overhangs of the bottom strand (and recessed 3'-OH ends of the top strand) would be formed. Such a template would be available for a combination of nucleolytic and polymerization steps. Considering such a model of differential cleavages, the processing of hairpins might be expected to have some DNA sequence dependence. Appropriately, studies investigating the influences of DNA sequence composition on V(D)J recombination are supportive of this mechanism as well (Boubnov et al., 1993; Meier and Lewis, 1993). Particular coding DNA sequences flanking RSS elements were observed to form P nucleotides at much higher incidence.

RSS DNA Ends in V(D)J Recombination

RSS products form with precision in V(D)J recombination. The vast majority of V(D)J joining RSS products exactly fuse the two RSS elements at the external borders of both heptamer elements as shown (Figure 2B). This product is not known to have an immune system function being deleted from the rearranging chromosome in most V(D)J recombination reactions that are most often deletional. Therefore, RSS product formation may serve to drive the reaction mechanism forward, as its main role.

Roth and coworkers and Schlissel and coworkers developed a sensitive assay for detecting broken DNA arising during the progress of V(D)J recombination in developing lymphocytes (Roth et al., 1993; Schlissel et al., 1993). Ligation-mediated PCR (LMPCR) is a method that can detect DNA breaks by coupling the ligation of specific primers to the ends of these DNA fragments with the ability to stimulate PCR with added primers. Using LMPCR, DSBs occurring during V(D)J recombination that are possible intermediates and thus available only at low frequency, can be studied. Both laboratories discovered that Ig and TCR gene segment RSS DNA ends were detectable by LMPCR. Further, the RSS ends were blunt-ended and contained 5'-phosphate residues at RSS heptamers (Figure 2). These DNA structures did not appear in cells from *RAG1*-deficient knockout mice, also suggesting that the RSS ends were formed during V(D)J recombination.

To summarize, these data developed a picture of the early stages of V(D)J recombination where cleavages occur at the outside borders of RSS heptamer elements, creating coding DNA hairpins and blunt RSS ends. However, because these products could only be demonstrated under specific conditions (i.e., the *scid* mutant background for hairpins) the establishment of the structures as true intermediates in gene rearrangement was not complete.

RAG1/RAG2-Mediated Cleavages During V(D)J Recombination

The *RAG1* and *RAG2* genes are co-localized in the genome and co-expressed during the progenitor stages of lymphoid differentiation (Oettinger, 1992; Schatz et al., 1992). Relative to the timing of V(D)J recombination, RAG1 and RAG2 levels are produced appropriately. Since their definition by functional induction of V(D)J recombination in non-rearranging cells in culture, these proteins have been hypothesized to initiate V(D)J recombination.

The minimal regions of functionally active RAG1 and RAG2 has been defined by mutagenesis studies using the transient transfection of these modified genes and induced V(D)J recombination as a readout (Cuomo and Oettinger, 1994; Sadofsky et al., 1994; Sadofsky et al., 1993; Silver et al., 1993). Truncated RAG1 and RAG2 proteins in combination are active in generating both products of the V(D)J recombination mechanism in cell transfections. These regions can be considered a core protein retaining RAG activity that undoubtedly are missing additional epitopes that may be relevant to the regulation of RAG functioning in lymphocytes. For example, the minimal RAG2 protein that is active for the V(D)J recombination reaction is truncated at the C-terminus, removing phosphorylation sites demonstrated to be significant in effecting RAG2 stability at the G1/S cell cycle transition (Lin and Desiderio, 1993; Lin and Desiderio, 1994).

Gellert and colleagues were the first to succeed in inducing V(D)J recombination-specific cleavages in a cell-free system. They formed nuclear extracts from cells overproducing RAG1 and RAG2, and then added a truncated RAG1 protein that was purified separately (aa 384-1008) (van Gent et al., 1995). Cleavages in DNA substrates containing RSS(12) and/or RSS(23) were detected by using LMPCR as previously developed in their laboratory (Roth et al., 1992a, 1992b, 1993; Schlissel et al., 1993). Broken DNA at RSS elements was shown to be dependent on the added RAG1 and on the presence of induced levels of RAG2 from the cell extracts. In the absence of either of these conditions, no DNA modifications were detected. These observations are completely consistent with the absence of any V(D)J recombination products or DSB intermediates in RAG1 −/− or RAG2 −/− knockout mice (Mombaerts et al., 1992; Shinkai et al., 1992). Importantly, the DNA breaks characterized were consistent with the previously observed DNA breaks at the borders of RSS formed in the midst of V(D)J recombination in whole cells (Roth et al., 1992a, 1992b, 1993; Schlissel et al., 1993; Zhu and Roth, 1995). van Gent et al. demonstrated RAG-dependent hairpin formation at the broken coding sequences flanking RSS elements (van Gent et al., 1995). Likewise, the application of the LMPCR technology showed that the newly formed RSS ends were blunt-ended and 5'-phosphorylated in structure.

An important suggestion from these studies was that RAG1 and RAG2 protein may alone be capable of inducing the DNA cleavages consistent with initiation of V(D)J recombination (van Gent et al., 1995). This model was testable when biochemically purified RAG1 and RAG2 proteins were produced. Preparation of soluble RAG1 and RAG2 proteins was accomplished by overproduction of truncated versions of each polypeptide in baculovirus and vaccinia vectors, where the fusion proteins could be readily be purified utilizing epitope tags (McBlane et al., 1995). Significantly, the preparations of RAG1 and RAG2 protein mixed together stimulated cleavages of RSS(12) or RSS(23)-containing DNA substrates (McBlane et al., 1995). Any cleavage of DNA was dependent on addition of both proteins. Furthermore, both covalently sealed coding ends (hairpins) and RSS blunt ends were formed in the RAG1/RAG2-dependent reaction. Utilizing double-stranded oligonucleotides as the substrates for cleavage, it was established that both nicking of the phosphodiester bond flanking the RSS heptamer or a DSB at this position were detectable. In time course reactions, nicks at the position XXX'CACAGTG-spacer-nonamer appeared prior to the formation of hairpins and RSS ends, arguing that a single-stranded nick in the template might be the first DNA cleavage step in the reaction. Also, preformed nicks in the substrate could be efficiently converted to hairpins by adding RAG1 and RAG2, and this reaction was dependent on an RSS element in the template. In contrast, if a nick is constructed on the opposite strand at the same position YYY'GTGTCAC, only a doubly nicked product was found, and no hairpin. Since hairpin-ended products accumulate to a much greater extent than nicks with increasing time, it suggests that the RAG1/RAG2-dependent cleavages proceed in two steps. The striking conclusion of these valuable studies is that the RAG1 and RAG2 proteins are directly required for the cleavage steps initiating V(D)J recombination. Also, these two proteins alone are able to form the previously identified broken DNAs of specific structures: hairpins and RSS ends.

Supporting genetic evidence for the specificity of these proteins in the cleavage reactions was the determination that particular RAG1 mutations alters the efficiency of the complete reaction in cell transfection experiments in an interesting way (Sadofsky et al., 1995). The RAG1 D32 mutant consists of the previously characterized RAG1 core protein (aa 384-1008) (Sadofsky et al., 1993), with the substitution (aa 606-607 SE changed to VD) and deletion (aa 608-611). The RAG1 D32 mutant works poorly in stimulating V(D)J recombination for some of the standard plasmid templates for measuring coding junction, RSS junction, and inversional recombination designed by the Gellert laboratory, but not for others (Sadofsky et al., 1995). It was shown that this mutant RAG-1 protein had a dramatic preference in the coding DNA sequence flanking the RSS. Construction of a family of nearby mutations to the changes in D32 RAG1 did not recapitulate these findings indicating that the mutant protein may possess a relatively unique configuration allowing it to show such sequence preferences. Although the full meaning of these structural changes is not yet discerned, clearly mutations such as D32 demonstrate that RAG1 is sensing the DNA sequence in the vicinity of RSS elements undergoing V(D)J recombination.

These mechanistic data were sufficient to suggest that the relatively unique hairpin formation of this reaction likely occurs by an intramolecular attack of the phosphodiester bond by the other strand 3'-OH following the nicking step. This second step of the reaction, that is also catalyzed by RAG1 and RAG2, could be accomplished by a number of reaction mechanisms. Gellert and colleagues recently showed that the reaction proceeds by a direct transesterification path, similar to other recombination mechanisms, such as retroviral integration (van Gent et al., 1996). By using oligonucleotides possessing Rp or Sp stereoisomers at the lower strand phosphate in pre-nicked substrates, they showed that the second step of the reaction only occurs with the molecules in the Sp configuration. Thus, RAG1 and/or RAG2-DNA intermediates are not necessary for the reaction mechanism.

An important issue in the formation of cleavages dependent on RAG1 and RAG2 is the regulation of these events in the immune system. Since Ig and TCR genes are built from tandemly placed gene segments each possessing flanking RSS elements available for recombination, additional controls must be in place in vivo to ensure that cleavages are coordinated with rearrangement and joining processes. Recent progress has suggested that a coupling of the cleavage steps may be in part responsible for this level of regulation. Characterization of V(D)J recombination products led to the development of rules governing the rearrangement process. Central to the efficient execution of the reaction is the observation that pairs of RSS elements possessing opposite spacer lengths are most efficiently recombined in the chromosome and for episomal templates (Gellert, 1992a; Tonegawa, 1983). The spacer rule may place a constraint on the activation of the first steps of V(D)J recombination in vivo.

The stringency of the spacer rule was tested recently using the recently developed in vitro system (Eastman et al., 1996). Similar to the cell-free extracts of Gellert and coworkers, Eastman et al. developed extracts stimulating RSS-dependent DNA cleavages because of the overproduction of RAG1 and RAG2 core proteins (Eastman et al., 1996). Linear DNA substrates containing single RSS(12) and RSS(23) elements were constructed. Incubation of these templates with RAG1/ RAG2-containing cell extracts led to cleavages at the appropriate positions flanking the RSS elements and the formation of covalently sealed or hairpin-ended coding sequences (Figure 1 and 2). Importantly, the cleavages were dependent on an unmutated RSS(12) and RSS(23) together on the same DNA strand. The efficiency of the reaction was observed to be dependent on the choice of divalent cation. Eastman et al. showed that Mn^{2+} stimulated approximately a 10-fold greater reaction cleavage efficiency than Mg^{2+}, that was used in the previous studies (McBlane et al., 1995). On the other hand, the use of truncated versions of RAG1 and RAG2 in these studies, had little impact on the spacer rule. These intriguing findings offer a clue to the control of V(D)J recombination in vivo. Possibly RAG1 and RAG2 complexes are essential in directing coupled cleavages. Additional proteins or cofactors present in cell-free extracts that are absent in the purified RAG1/RAG2-dependent cleavages may direct the execution of cleavage efficiency.

The 12/23 spacer rule also implies that multiprotein complexes forming at each RSS may be significant in the efficiency and the regulation of V(D)J recombination initiation complexes. These complexes now would be expected, if not required, to contain both the RAG1 and RAG2 proteins in some stoichiometric order. Some RAG1 and RAG2 protein associations have already been described, suggesting that these proteins do form higher order complexes with each other (Leu and Schatz, 1995). Additional protein cofactors may be significant, and RAG1 has been described to associate with additional proteins in two-hybrid assays (Cortes et al., 1994; Cuomo et al., 1994). The significance of SRP1 and RCH1 for V(D)J recombination is yet to be determined.

The combination of the biochemical findings reveal a clear picture of the importance of RAG1 and RAG2 in directing the initiation events of V(D)J recombination. Future studies will better specify the reaction mechanism, distinguishing the means by which RAG1 and RAG2 have coordinated and possibly separable functions in accomplishing the process. Comprehensive structural and genetic studies of RAG1 and RAG2 will undoubtedly be pursued to better understand the roles of these fascinating proteins. As yet, little information is available to distinguish them with individualized functions.

II. JOINING STEPS OF V(D)J RECOMBINATION AND THE RELEVANCE OF DNA REPAIR PROTEINS

Ku Genes

The abundant nuclear DNA binding protein complex, Ku, is necessary for V(D)J recombination. The evidence that the Ku complex is relevant has come from the contributions of many laboratories from a number of different experimental directions. The recent history of Ku leads to a compelling picture of its direct role in V(D)J recombination and DSB repair. Although much of the information regarding Ku has been reviewed, I will highlight salient points that demonstrate the significance of this intriguing protein complex.

Ku was discovered as an autoantigen (Mimori et al., 1981; Mimori and Hardin, 1986), and antisera to Ku is commonly observed with systemic lupus erythematosus and mixed connective tissue disease patients (Reeves, 1985). Thus, the early phase of research on Ku was an interesting example of having a protein and antibodies recognizing the protein without knowledge of its function. The term Ku has come to refer to a biochemically distinct nuclear heterodimer of 70 and 80 kDa subunits (termed Ku70 and Ku80). Perhaps the key to Ku function is its ability to avidly bind to double-stranded DNA. In particular, Ku associates with DNA ends in an apparently sequence nonspecific manner (deVries et al., 1989; Falzon et al., 1993; Mimori et al., 1986; Mimori et al., 1986; Paillard and Strauss, 1991; Reeves, 1985). Ku binds to "altered" DNA structures, such as partially denatured or partially annealed single-stranded DNA, and to unusual variations in double-stranded DNA, including hairpins (Falzon et al., 1993; Paillard et al., 1991). Ku also bind to nicks and gaps in DNA (Blier et al., 1993). With these molecular properties, Ku might directly play a role in V(D)J recombination.

The connection between Ku and V(D)J recombination emerged from studies directed at identifying gene products relevant to V(D)J recombination and DNA repair. Following the discovery of the *scid* mutation leading to dual mutant phenotypes: errors in VDJ joining and IR sensitivity, it was conjectured that additional genes may play a part in both mechanisms like SCID. The evaluation of V(D)J recombination defects in the small set of IR sensitive cell lines has been instrumental in uncovering additional types of mutations for analysis (Weaver et al., 1995; Weaver, 1995). Included in this group are the *XRCC5* and *XR-1* IR sensitive cell lines that were originally identified to be deficient in both DNA products of V(D)J recombination by Taccioli et al. (Taccioli et al., 1993) (Figure 3).

Purified Ku stably associates with small DNA fragments. Thus, DNA end binding (DEB) coupled with mobility gel shift analysis has been widely used to characterize Ku-DNA interactions and as a monitor of active Ku complexes in cell extracts (Falzon et al., 1993; Ono et al., 1994; Paillard et al., 1991; Rathmell and Chu, 1994a). Using the above assay, the *XRCC5* mammalian cell mutants were demonstrated to be devoid of Ku DEB (Boubnov et al., 1995; Getts and Stamato, 1994; Rathmell and Chu, 1994a, 1994b; Taccioli et al., 1994a). *XRCC5* group cell lines thus far have been derived from Chinese hamster ovary or lung cell lines (Jeggo and Kemp, 1983; Lee et al., 1995; Zdzienicka and Simons, 1987). These lines have been shown to be in the same complementation group by a number of criteria, but particularly by the use of somatic cell hybrid analysis (Boubnov et al., 1995). The DNA repair defects of *XRCC5* mutants are discussed in other reviews (Jeggo, 1990; Weaver et al., 1995).

In addition to loss of Ku function, the *XRCC5* mutants can be complemented by reintroducing Ku genes by DNA transfection. Either mouse or human Ku80 genes introduced into *XRCC5* cells restored V(D)J recombination defects, IR sensitivity, and Ku DEB (Boubnov et al., 1995; Smider et al., 1994; Taccioli et al., 1994a). In addition, XRCC5 and Ku80 map to the same region on human chromosome 2 (Cai et al., 1994; Taccioli et al., 1994a). Also, Ku80 mutations have been documented for several of the *XRCC5* mutants. For example, the *sxi-3* and *sxi-2* mutants fail to produce Ku80 mRNA (Boubnov et al., 1995). More recently, the *xrs6* mutant allele has been shown to contain an internal deletion of Ku80, producing a truncated and unstable protein (Errami et al., 1996).

The small Ku subunit, Ku70, has been more problematic in mutational analysis. To date, no specific Ku70 mutants are available. One cell line, *sxi-1*, has the expected phenotypes: VDJ recombination-deficient, IR sensitive and Ku DEB deficient (Lee et al., 1995). The *sxi-1* IR sensitivity and DEB defects are complemented by fusion with *XRCC5*, *scid*, *V-3*, and *XR-1* mutants, suggesting that *sxi-1* is in a distinct complementation group from the other IR repair mutants. However, Ku80

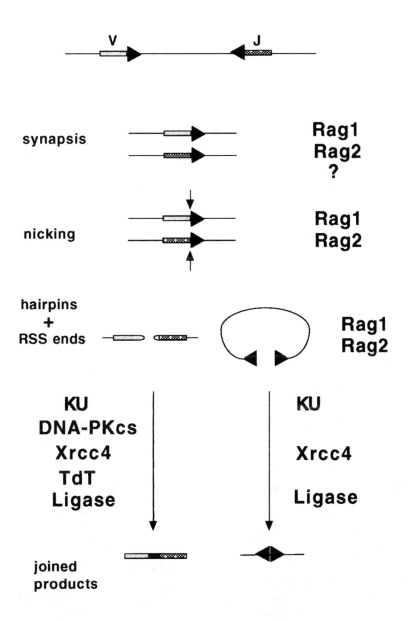

Figure 3 (see COLOR PLATE 3). Protein requirements for V(D)J recombination. Two lymphoid specific proteins, RAG1 and RAG2, are essential for the initiation reactions of V(D)J recombination. Both proteins are needed for the two steps involved in making double strand breaks at each RSS. A group of DNA repair proteins are important for the product formation steps of V(D)J recombination as shown. The Ku heterodimer and Xrcc4 protein are necessary for both RSS and coding end joining. In contrast, the DNA-dependent protein kinase catalytic subunit, which associates with Ku, is primarily needed only for coding end joining. Processing enzymes, including factors that cleave hairpins, fill-in or excise DNA ends, and ligate products have not been identified.

RNA levels are reduced in *sxi-1* cells, and either transfection of either human Ku70 or Ku80 reconstitutes the mutant defects. Even though the complexity of the *sxi-1* mutation has not been resolved, Ku deficiency strongly correlates with lack of biological functions in recombination and repair.

Prior to the observations that the initiation of the V(D)J recombination cleavages could occur without Ku, it was difficult to discern whether this protein may have influenced initiation of the reaction as well as joining steps. Since both joining products are impacted in Ku-deficient cells, models where Ku association influenced cleavages were possible. Considering the connection of Ku mutations and DSB repair defects of Ku-deficient cells, and the ability of RAG1 + RAG2 alone to produce RSS DS ends and coding sequence hairpins, a role in initiation and cleavage steps of V(D)J recombination is highly unlikely. Rather, the importance of Ku for this reaction probably begins by the recruitment of the protein complex to the sites of V(D)J joining once cleavages have initiated. To understand the mechanism by which a general DNA repair protein may be involved in these later steps of V(D)J recombination, several laboratories have examined Ku functions in other eukaryotes.

Structural Comparisons of Ku Genes

Ku is expressed widely in the eukaryotic world. DNA end binding, consistent with Ku complexes have been observed in diverse species from *Saccharomyces cerevisiae* to humans (Beall et al., 1994; Feldmann and Winnacker, 1993; Jacoby and Wensink, 1994; Rathmell and Chu, 1994a). Many of the species where Ku is present do not undergo V(D)J recombination, and thus it is very likely that the evolutionarily recent VDJ joining mechanism appeared in the biological context of Ku being used for other cell functions.

Ku DEB activity and a Ku heterodimer have been characterized in *Saccharomyces cerevisiae* (ScKu) and *Drosophila melanogaster* (DmKu). ScKu was purified by the DEB activity observed in yeast extracts (Feldmann et al., 1993). From purified protein, a homolog to mammalian Ku70 was cloned, and a knockout mutation of this gene, HDF1, was generated. *hdf1* cells lose DEB activity. Also, HDF1 was identified by complementation of an unusual phenotype uncovered in a screen for the *nes24-1* mutation sensitive to neomycin and temperature-sensitive growth (Shimma and Uno, 1990; Yoshida et al., 1994). *Drosophila melanogaster* Ku70 was isolated by two groups based on its binding to specific DNA sequences (Beall et al., 1994; Jacoby et al., 1994). A Ku70 homolog was cloned following peptide sequencing by both groups and named *Irbp* (Beall et al., 1994) or *ypf1* (Jacoby et al., 1994) respectively. *Irbp* and *ypf1* encode the same gene (DmKu70). The other Ku subunit was not identified in any of these studies but both organisms have a Ku heterodimer. An ScKu80 homolog was recently identified by inspecting the yeast genome database for homologs to Ku80 (Milne et al., 1996). Knockout mutation of ScKu80 leads to loss of DEB activity. Also, by using epitope-tagged versions of Ku80 and Hdf1 it was shown that these proteins associate to form the major DEB complex of yeast. Therefore, the yeast Ku heterodimer consists of a Ku70 homolog (HDF1) and a Ku80 homolog (ScKu80).

Important structural components of Ku may be identified by contrasting the Ku genes isolated from different species. The mammalian, yeast and Drosophila Ku70 homologs are similar across the length of Ku70 (Figure 4). DmKu70 is 27% identical and 34% (Beall et al., 1994). ScKu70 has reduced similarity throughout (Feldmann et al., 1993), particularly at the N- and C-termini. The greatest similarity amongst Ku70 homologs is found in an internal region (aa 226-578 of ScKu70 and aa 213-556 of human Ku70) where there is approximately 22% identity. The internal region may reflect the core properties of Ku associated with DNA end binding. There is not yet any experimental verification of the significance of these Ku70 regions for associations with the other subunit or with DNA.

Mouse and human Ku80 genes are slightly more divergent (77% identity) than Ku70 genes, but human Ku80 is still able to complement *XRCC5* mutants, arguing that the biological functions of Ku are conserved (Boubnov et al., 1995). The yeast Ku80 homolog, ScKu80, is 21% and 20.5% homologous and 45.9% and 43.8% similar to human and murine Ku80 proteins respectively (Figure 5). As for Ku70, the similarity between yeast and mammalian Ku80 homologs spans most of the length of the genes. Because of the requirement of both proteins for DEB complexes, it may be that the structural requirements of Ku80 and Ku70 are interrelated so that the combination of these proteins creates the DNA binding properties of Ku. To date, mutational analysis that may separate epitopes required for Ku subunit association from DNA binding functions have not been identified. The implications for V(D)J recombination are several fold. First, regions not conserved in the evolution of Ku may be essential for V(D)J recombination not used for DNA repair. For example, the association of other proteins to Ku complexes may be species specific (see below). Second, the extensive similarity for both subunits of Ku across the protein lengths is supportive of the notion that a central function is also conserved, and that this function is incorporated into the V(D)J joining pathway.

The scid Mutation and the DNA-Dependent Protein Kinase

The molecular basis of the mouse *scid* mutation has been the subject of intense research activity recently. Following the demonstration of DSB repair defects of *scid* cells, it was hypothesized that the Scid protein, like Ku, would be involved in the dual processes of V(D)J recombination and DSB repair. A strong candidate for the identity of the Scid factor was another protein that was known to associate with Ku in cells. The DNA-dependent protein kinase (DNA-PK), identified first in rabbit reticulocyte lysates (Walker et al., 1985), has been found in extracts from several vertebrates (Human, mouse, hamster, rat, cow, monkey), marine animals such as Xenopus, Spisula, sea urchin, and insects including Drosophila (reviewed in Carter and Anderson, 1991). DNA-PK is a serine/threonine-type kinase that requires DNA for activation of the enzyme (reviewed in Anderson, 1993). The key to DNA-PK activity appears to be its association with Ku that provides the DNA binding functions. Here I will review recent data building the association between DNA-PK and *scid*, and speculate on the role of this protein complex in V(D)J recombination.

DNA-PK is a trimeric protein complex, composed of a catalytic subunit (DNA-PK$_{cs}$) and the two Ku subunits (reviewed in Anderson, 1993; Anderson and Lees-Miller, 1992). Purification of DNA-PK first showed that a large protein of >350 kDa

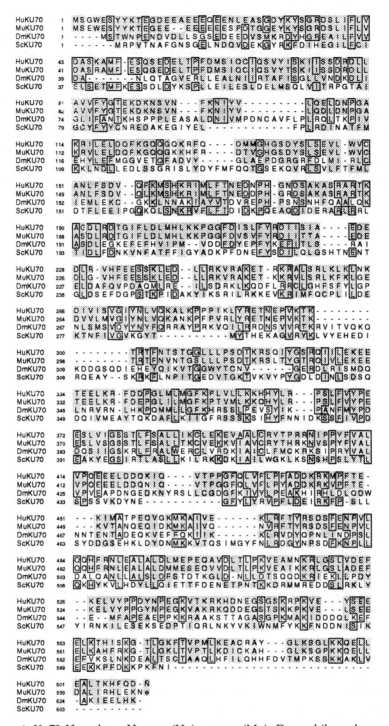

Figure 4. Ku70 Homologs. Human (Hu), mouse (Mu), Drosophila melanogaster (Dm), and *S. cerevisiae* (Sc) homologs of Ku70 have been determined. Alignment of these projected translation product indicates widespread homology across the lengths of these proteins. Boxes, identity; shading, similarity based on Pileup computational analysis.

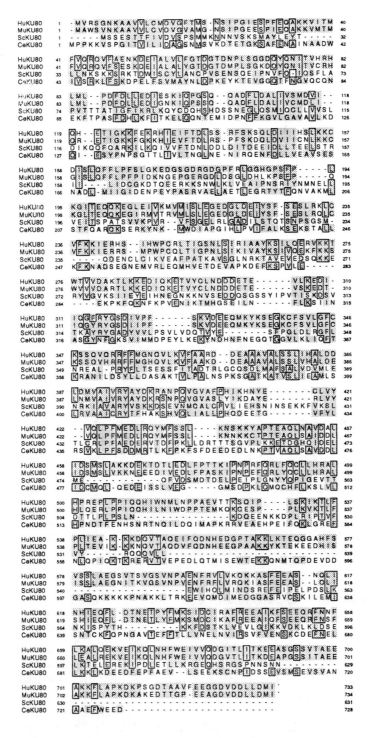

Figure 5. Ku80 Homologs. Mammalian, *S. cerevisiae*, and a potential *Caennorhabditis elegans* Ku80 homolog genes have been identified. Boxes, identity; shading, similarity based on Pileup computational analysis.

was likely to be the kinase subunit (Lees-Miller et al., 1990). It was found that the most active protein fraction always contained smaller molecular weight proteins at the sizes of Ku subunits. Precipitation with anti-Ku antisera show that Ku and DNA-PK$_{cs}$ are associated (Lees-Miller et al., 1990; Suwa et al., 1994). Also, DNA crosslinking studies display >350 kDa, 70 and 80 kDa polypeptides (Lees-Miller et al., 1990), suggesting that all three subunits are in contact with DNA. Additional evidence that Ku is the DNA binding subunit of DNA-PK came from the observations that Ku DEB is required for DNA-PK activity in assays where phosphorylation of a protein substrate is examined on linear DNA templates (Gottlieb and Jackson, 1993). Furthermore, in vitro extracts from XRCC4 mutants have reduced DNA-PK activity (Finnie et al., 1995). These Ku-deficient extracts can be reactivated for DNA-PK activity by the addition of Ku protein indicating that DNA-PK$_{cs}$ is stable in the absence of Ku. Therefore, "active" DNA-PK is minimally a four component system, requiring DNA-PK$_{cs}$ catalytic protein, the two Ku subunits and DNA ends. Even though Ku may activate DNA-PK$_{cs}$ by its binding, a substantial fraction of DNA-PK$_{cs}$ does not appear to be associated with Ku normally. Thus, additional mechanisms may be possible for activating DNA-PK$_{cs}$.

With the biochemical connection between Ku and DNA-PK$_{cs}$, an intriguing possibility was that the scid mutant V(D)J joining and DSB repair defects may be due to loss of DNA-PK$_{cs}$ functions. It is now very likely that the mouse scid gene encodes the DNA-PK$_{cs}$, although the mouse scid mutation has not yet been found. First, human chromosome 8 complements the mouse scid mutation V(D)J recombination and IR sensitivity defects (Banga et al., 1994; Kirchgessner et al., 1993; Komatsu et al., 1993; Kurimasa et al., 1993). In attempts to clone scid complementing functions, several laboratories tried unsuccessfully to restore V(D)J recombination potential or IR resistant phenotypes by introduction of mammalian cell genomic DNA or cDNAs. Importantly, yeast artificial chromosomes (YACs) containing human chromosome 8q11 genomic fragments were identified that were able to complement the dual defects of the V-3 mutant cell line, a member of the scid complementation group (Blunt et al., 1995) (Figure 3). V-3 had previously been demonstrated to have identical V(D)J recombination and IR-sensitive and DSB repair defects as scid cells (Taccioli et al., 1994b). Supportive evidence of the connection has emerged from the analysis of partial cDNA clones of DNA-PK$_{cs}$ that map to 8q11 by in situ hybridization (Sipley et al., 1995). Likewise, human chromosome 8-complemented V-3 and scid mutants are immunoreactive with human DNA-PK$_{cs}$ protein and reconstitute in vitro DNA-PK activity (Blunt et al., 1995; Boubnov and Weaver, 1995; Kirchgessner et al., 1995; Peterson et al., 1995).

In addition to the complementation of scid mutational defects, a corresponding alteration in DNA-PK biochemical activity has been detected for each of the members of the XRCC7 complementation group (Blunt et al., 1995; Boubnov and Weaver, 1995; Lees-Miller et al., 1995; Peterson et al., 1995). Because rodent cells have lower levels of DNA-PK, a more sensitive assay has been adapted by several groups to compare DNA-PK activity for mutant cell lines. In these assays, termed "pull-down" experiments by Finnie et al., the affinity of Ku to DNA and DNA-PK is exploited to concentrate DNA-PK from extracts to DNA beads. This methodology is DNA end-specific (Boubnov and Weaver, 1995). XRCC7 mouse and hamster mutants were shown to be deficient in DNA-PK activity in vitro by monitoring consensus site phosphorylation of peptides, Ku phosphorylation, or HSP90 phosphorylation (Blunt et al., 1995; Boubnov and Weaver, 1995; Peterson et al., 1995). Complementation of the *XRCC7* mutants by human chromosome 8 or YACs reconstitutes the DNA-PK deficiencies to wild-type levels. Likewise, addition of purified human DNA-PK$_{cs}$ is able to restore DNA-PK activity to *XRCC7* mutants (Blunt et al., 1995). No DNA-PK$_{cs}$ RNA, protein, or DNA-PK activity is observed in a human glioblastoma tumor cell line, M059J (Lees-Miller et al., 1995), even though human whole cell extracts generally have readily detectable DNA-PK activity. M059J cells produce normal levels of Ku and addition of purified DNA-PK$_{cs}$ to these extracts will reconstitute DNA-PK activity. Thus, three separate mutant alleles from *scid*, *V-3*, and M059J cells are deficient in DNA-PK biochemical activity.

What is the nature of DNA-PK$_{cs}$ mutations in the *XRCC7* mutants where DNA-PK activity is affected? For the two mutants where V(D)J recombination data is available, *scid* and *V-3*, DNA-PK$_{cs}$ protein levels are substantially reduced to approximately 1–10% of the wildtype level (Kirchgessner et al., 1995; Peterson et al., 1995). These decreases in protein levels may be sufficient to account for the loss of DNA-PK activity although the sensitivity of the activity assays is not so great. Similarly, UV-crosslinking of *scid* and *V-3* whole cell extracts indicates that there is significantly less DNA-PK$_{cs}$ protein associating with DNA, that is complemented by addition of YACs in the case of *V-3* (Blunt et al., 1995). In each of these assays some protein of the same high molecular weight is detectable immunoblots, consistent with a non-null mutant allele (Kirchgessner et al., 1995). Thus, defects caused by decreased protein levels can not yet be distinguished from a specific loss of kinase activity, and the issue of whether DNA-PK is used as a structural component or not in V(D)J recombination and DSB repair will have to await a more comprehensive mutational analysis using reverse genetics.

Starting from information derived from peptide sequencing of purified DNA-PK$_{cs}$ protein, the DNA-PK$_{cs}$ human gene was cloned (Hartley et al., 1995). DNA-PK$_{cs}$ is a ubiquitously expressed 13 kB mRNA. The DNA-PK$_{cs}$ ORF encodes a 460 kDa protein that is considerably larger than the estimated size from biochemical analysis. Strikingly, DNA-PK$_{cs}$ has a C-terminal protein kinase domain that places this gene into a family of related serine, threonine protein kinases (Figure 6). Based on the kinase homology, DNA-PK$_{cs}$ is a PI-3-related kinase, but has no demonstrated lipid kinase activity (Hartley et al., 1995). Instead, DNA-PK protein kinase activity is observed with numerous in vitro substrates (Anderson, 1993).

Recently, a group of protein kinases with related structure to DNA-PK$_{cs}$ have been identified from several organisms (reviewed in Keith and Schreiber, 1995; Zakian, 1995) (Figure 6). Additional kinases in this group include the yeast genes TOR2, TOR1, DRR1, ESR1/MEC1, TEL1, the Drosophila MEI41 gene, and the human genes ATM FRAP, p110α,β and γ PI-3 kinase, VPS34 (Greenwell et al., 1995; Hari et al., 1995; Hartley et al., 1995; Morrow et al., 1995; Savitsky et al., 1995). Interestingly, many of these proteins have been implicated in signal transduction pathways for growth control and DNA repair pathways. Homology in the kinase domains of the above genes ranks DNA-PK$_{cs}$ as being most closely related to the PIK-related kinases including *TOR2, TOR1, FRAP, ATM, TEL1*, MEI41, and *MEC1* (Keith et al., 1995; Zakian, 1995). Homologs between species probably fall into the groups (*TOR1, TOR2, FRAP*) (*TEL1* and *ATM*) (*MEC1* and *MEI41*) and no DNA-PK$_{cs}$ homologs are known (Figure 6). Several of the related kinases are more closely aligned with the ATM kinase domain than DNA-PK$_{cs}$. An additional motif in the

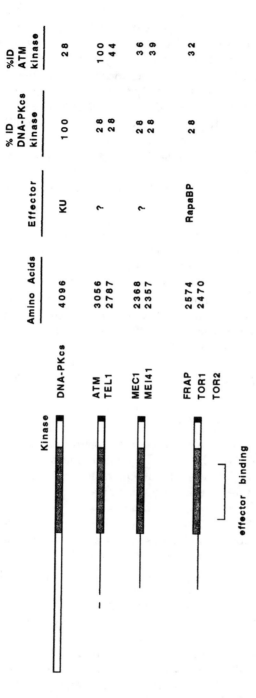

Kinase	Amino Acids	Effector	% ID DNA-PKcs kinase	%ID ATM kinase
DNA-PKcs	4096	KU	100	28
ATM	3056	?	28	100
TEL1	2787		28	44
MEC1	2368	?	28	36
MEI41	2357		28	39
FRAP	2574	RapaBP	28	32
TOR1	2470			
TOR2				

effector binding

Figure 6 (see COLOR PLATE 4). Homology between DNA-PK$_{cs}$-related gene products. The DNA-dependent protein kinase catalytic subunit is a member of the PI-3 type kinase family. The other related protein kinases in this group also have C-terminal protein kinase domains as shown. Identity relative to DNA-PK$_{cs}$ and ATM kinase domains are illustrated, and the homology groups are ordered as previously (Hartley et al., 1995; Jackson, 1996; Keith et al., 1995). DNA-PK$_{cs}$ and FRAP are the only members of this group for which protein cofactors (the Ku heterodimer and Rapamycin binding protein) have been identified. Yellow = kinase homology; green = family-specific homology in the COOH terminus; blue = homology regions that may mediate effector binding.

C-terminal 30 residues of PIK-related genes has been noted for these kinases ($LN_9LN_4AN_5LN_5GWNP/AW/FN$-COOH; Figure 6), but its significance is not yet understood (Keith et al., 1995). It is interesting that some of the PI-3-type kinase family members are more closely related to DNA-PK than others based on protein structure (Jackson, 1996). In particular, the product of the *ATM* gene, and its *S. cerevisiae* homolog, *TEL1*, are slightly more similar to DNA-PK$_{cs}$ across the lengths of the proteins (Greenwell et al., 1995; Morrow et al., 1995; Savitsky et al., 1995; Zakian, 1995). A large region flanking the C-terminal kinase domain may be a domain for protein effectors to bind to these protein kinases (Figure 6). The protein binding region for one of the family members, FRAP, has been localized to this region (Keith et al., 1995).

ATM encodes the protein that is mutated in patients with *ataxia telangiectasia*, a complex human disease consisting of cerebellar degeneration, immunodeficiency, DNA repair defects, and a greatly elevated frequency of cancer (Gatti et al., 1994). Some of the *ATM* mutations are likely to be null mutations (Savitsky et al., 1995). The immunodeficiency defects are not related to direct effects on V(D)J recombination (Hsieh et al., 1993). Instead, AT cells are deficient in a variety of responses to IR damage, indicating a requirement of the protein in signalling DNA damage events. Included in these effects is a non-responsiveness to IR damage in interrupting cell cycle progression (Kastan et al., 1992; Painter and Young, 1980). Notably, accumulation of the tumor suppressor, p53, following IR damage is retarded in AT cells (Kastan et al., 1992; Lu and Lane, 1993). AT cells also have an unstable chromosome content indicating that although the gene is not essential, genome stability may be dependent on its functioning. *TEL1* mutations were isolated based on a telomere shortening defect, but otherwise show no significant growth or DNA repair defects (Lustig and Petes, 1986). However, *tel1Δ* and *mec1Δ* strains are severely IR-sensitive and show many DNA repair defects (Greenwell et al., 1995; Morrow et al., 1995). These observations suggest that TEL1 and *MEC1* may be functionally redundant for some DNA repair functions, and introduces the notion that similar effects may be observed in conjunction with DNA-PK mutations. In yeast, the Ku-deficient *hdf1Δ* strains have an additional mutant phenotype that is intriguing regarding the interplay of PI-type kinases in the nucleus. *hdf1Δ* strains were found to have a telomere shortening defect in a manner not epistatic to *tel1Δ* (Porter et al., 1996). This finding is consistent with a role for Ku in telomere and chromosome stability. Possibly Ku associates with *TEL1* in yeast, and *ATM* and DNA-PK$_{cs}$ may both be able to associate with Ku in mammalian cells. Perhaps the role of DNA-PK in V(D)J recombination is fairly specific and can not be replaced by the ATM or MEC1 kinases. The interrelationship and regulation of these kinases is fruitful ground for future studies.

III. MECHANISTIC IMPLICATIONS OF Ku AND DNA-PK IN V(D)J JOINING

Ku-Mediated Product Formation

Identification of mutant cells that are DNA-PK deficient and unable to complete VDJ joining steps has provided a new level of insight into the requirements of DNA end joining during gene rearrangement. The properties of DNA-PK-deficient cell lines are consistent with Ku and DNA-PK$_{cs}$ having separable functions for the two joining steps in V(D)J recombination. Both product steps in the reaction are Ku-dependent, whereas only coding junction formation may be DNA-PK-dependent (Figure 3). Because Ku has the features of associating with DNA ends, a possible model is that Ku is loaded at sites of V(D)J joining following the RAG1/RAG2 cleavages of the reaction. Since RAG1/RAG2 complexes are able to form coding hairpins, Ku may be targeted to these DNA structures by higher Ku binding affinity. Hairpin ends created by RAG1/RAG2 would be expected to partially denature at their termini once formed due to thermodynamic instability of a complete duplex structure. Hairpin substrates for Ku binding have been shown to have as high of a binding affinity as double-stranded ends of DNA (Falzon et al., 1993).

Ku70 and Ku80 complex formation is expected to be essential for Ku function because neither subunit is stable without the other (Boubnov et al., 1995; Mimori et al., 1986; Satoh et al., 1995; Wang et al., 1994). All *XRCC5* mutants have a reduced steady state level of the Ku70 protein (Rathmell and Chu, 1994a), that can be stabilized by transfection of a complementing Ku80 gene (Boubnov et al., 1995; Smider et al., 1994; Taccioli et al., 1994a). In vitro reconstitution experiments of *E. coli*-produced Ku subunits or baculovirus-expressed Ku subunits have shown that heterodimerization is needed for DEB (Ono et al., 1994; Tuteja et al., 1994). Also, in vitro translated Ku subunits have no activity in DEB unless co-translated (Griffith et al., 1992). Therefore, both genetic and biochemical data argue strongly that the two Ku subunits function in complex with one another. The phenotypes defined for the yeast Ku homologs are similarly impacted by deletion mutation of either gene (Milne et al., 1996).

Ku-DNA association may have functional implications in addition to the stimulation of DNA-PK activity, if Ku-mediated roles in DNA joining events can be demonstrated. One model would be that the Ku complexes directly stimulate joining of DNA breaks. For the analysis of DNA joining events, recent progress with the roles of the yeast Ku genes has been revealing. In yeast, Ku is required for DNA end joining of linearized plasmid DNA and of chromosomal DSBs (Milne et al., 1996). The efficiency of both of these DNA end joining processes was reduced >10 fold in *ku80Δ, hdf1Δ*, or *ku80Δ hdf1Δ* strains, implying that the two Ku subunits function together and are necessary for the same DNA joining events. These DNA joining defects also correlated with DNA damage sensitivity as *ku80Δ* and *hdf1Δ* strains were sensitive to methylmethane sulfonate (MMS) (Milne et al., 1996; Siede et al., 1996). Again, *ku80Δ hdf1Δ* strains are as MMS sensitive as single mutants, indicative of epistasis (Milne et al., 1996). Whether Ku-deficient mammalian cells are also defective in DNA end joining processes as in yeast has not yet been delineated. The composition of the DNA ends can vary and does not appear to be important for the Ku-dependence on the process of joining in vivo (Milne et al., 1996). These preliminary indications are supportive of a direct and positive role of Ku in DNA joining events.

In mammalian cells, although Ku-deficient mutants are highly radiation sensitive, the decrease in ability to repair DSBs is not so striking (Jeggo, 1990). These observations are paradoxical due to the extensive effects of Ku mutations on both of the V(D)J recombination product formation steps. In an effort to further elucidate the mechanisms of homology-independent DSB repair, a method was devised by Jasin and Dujon and co-workers for introducing specific DSBs independently of V(D)J recombination (Choulika et al., 1995; Rouet et al., 1994a, 1994b). The yeast endonuclease I-SceI has an 18-bp recognition sequence so that infrequently cuts DNA, and may not have any recognition sites in mammalian chromosomes (Rouet et al., 1994b). I-SceI-stimulated DSBs in normal cells can be repair by homology-dependent or independent pathways where the independent pathway resembles the coding joining step of V(D)J recombination (Rouet et al., 1994b). If a homologous DNA sequence is not present in tandem on the integrated plasmid substrate containing an I-SceI site, then most of the breaks that are formed are repaired by illegitimate recombination in the template. When I-SceI sites are introduced into the Ku-deficient cell line, $xrs6$, the repair of I-SceI-mediated breaks is dysfunctional (Liang et al., 1996). Ku-deficient cells have a striking decrease in recovered events indicating an inability to repair chromosome damage at a unique site per cell in a sufficient manner to allow restoration of the marker in which the I-SceI site is located. These observations are consistent with the extensive deletions noted for these same cells in V(D)J recombination product formation steps, and also suggests that Ku is required for the efficiency of the repair process. Since the disparity between cell survival and DSB repair measured in short range assays such as PFGE or neutral filter elution is high, it must be concluded that there are alternative Ku-independent strategies for healing DSBs, but that these mechanisms likely lead to chromosome deletions and/or rearrangement events that are not compatible with cell survival.

DNA-PK Functions in DSB Repair

Several observations indicate that the DNA-PK kinase activity is dependent on Ku for providing the localization to DNA repair sites, and stimulating the protein kinase function. Nevertheless, additional DNA-PK$_{cs}$ functions may occur that are Ku-independent, although none have currently been described. The DNA-PK activity was originally described as a DNA-dependent function. Yet, the phosphorylation function may operate in the absence of DNA because immunoprecipitation with anti-Ku or anti-DNA-PK$_{cs}$ antibodies can stimulate DNA-PK activity in vitro. Thus, formally there may be circumstances where the kinase is activatable in the absence of DNA breaks. DNA-PK$_{cs}$ does not negatively effect the stability of Ku, and likewise Ku is not needed for stable levels of DNA-PK$_{cs}$. This has been concluded most precisely by the analysis of Ku- and DNA-PK$_{cs}$ deficient mutants, where extracts of either types or reactivatable for DNA-PK phosphorylation activity by the introduction of the missing subunit (Finnie et al., 1995; Rathmell and Chu, 1994a). Furthermore, Ku and DNA-PK$_{cs}$ are able to associate in vitro once dissociated by high salt concentrations (Suwa et al., 1994). Measurements of DNA-PK components in dividing cells supports the notion that Ku and DNA-PK$_{cs}$ may only be associated a fraction of the time normally (S. Inoue and D. Weaver, unpublished). Likewise DNA-PK is generally inactive without a DNA association (Boubnov and Weaver, 1995; Finnie et al., 1995; Gottlieb et al., 1993).

Therefore, Ku and DNA-PK$_{cs}$ may form activated complexes at chromosome sites of biological significance (Figure 3). For V(D)J recombination, these conditions may be restricted to the putative coding junction intermediates, such as hairpins.

The recognition of DNA intermediates following RAG1/RAG2-mediated cleavages would accomplish two functions: localization to the specific DNA repair sites
where DSBs have occurred, and secondly, activation of DNA-PK. Because Ku is
essential for joining both products, perhaps Ku is first associated with VDJ rearrangement intermediates that are DNA ends or hairpins. Following Ku DNA
binding to these structures, DNA-PK$_{cs}$ may then associate with such a protein-
DNA structure.

If Ku and DNA-PK$_{cs}$ are associated on DNA prior to a need for the complex in
VDJ joining, then the complex would be expected to be "inactive". Considering the
possibility that Ku has a DNA helicase activity and is able to transit along DNA,
some conformational changes in the complex might occur when Ku binds to DNA
ends or hairpins. Whether biologically significant conformational changes of
DNA-PK accompany its associations with V(D)J joining is still unexplored.

Although significant emphasis has currently been placed on the protein phosphorylation activity of DNA-PK, there is as yet no evidence directly linking kinase
function with some aspect of V(D)J joining or DSB repair. DNA-PK may provide a
structural framework, or protein "bridge" for holding VDJ ends together. It is likely
that protein–protein interactions, in the form of a large multiprotein complex,
instead of DNA sequence-base annealing is responsible for the DNA joining steps
in the reaction. As already discussed, DNA homology is not required for V(D)J
recombination. Instead, the formation of particular protein contacts in the complex
may be the required steps for stimulating repair. The DNA-PK$_{cs}$ protein rather than
its kinase activity may be what is necessary in VDJ joining.

RSS joining appears to only require Ku and not DNA-PK$_{cs}$ because signal joining
is essentially normal in the *XRCC7* mutant backgrounds (Lieber et al., 1988). Since
RSS and coding junction formation steps can proceed independently (Sheehan and
Lieber, 1993) and accumulate as products with different kinetics and temperature
dependence (Ramsden and Gellert, 1995). Perhaps the protein requirements for
these two products do differ. For example, the RAG-dependent cleavages may be
coordinated with secondary DNA intermediate and product formation steps by the
activity of DNA-PK (Blunt et al., 1995). RAG1 and RAG2 each have potential
DNA-PK phosphorylation sites (SQ), where phosphorylation by DNA-PK could
regulate RAG activity.

In addition to potential RAG1/2 phosphorylation by DNA-PK, a number of
additional protein substrates may have activities that are influenced by DNA-PK
phosphorylation in the V(D)J recombination reaction. In vitro, DNA-PK phosphorylates many proteins at SQ or TQ sequences (Anderson et al., 1992; Lees-Miller et
al., 1992). Both Ku subunits are phosphorylated in DNA-PK complexes in a DNA-
dependent fashion. In pull-down experiments with DNA beads, Ku70 is phosphorylated approximately 5 times more than the Ku80 protein in the same complexes
(Boubnov and Weaver, 1995), arguing that Ku70 is more efficiently phosphorylated. Ku phosphorylation is dependent on DNA-PK$_{cs}$, as human and rodent
XRCC7 mutants have severely decreased Ku phosphorylation potential even
though Ku is quite stably expressed in these cells (Boubnov and Weaver, 1995; S. Jin
and D. Weaver, unpublished data). Perhaps the Ku phosphorylation that is stimulated by DNA end binding and DNA-PK influences the functions of Ku in V(D)J
recombination and DSB repair. These models await testing in the in vitro system for
V(D)J recombination.

XRCC4

Significant progress has been made towards the understanding of one of the genes impacting V(D)J recombination and IR repair. The XR-1 mutation originated by screening of Chinese hamster cells for radiation sensitivity (Giaccia et al., 1985), and was derived by much the same route as several of the Ku and DNA-PK$_{cs}$ mutants (reviewed in Weaver, 1995). With regard to V(D)J recombination mutant phenotypes, XR-1 cells resemble Ku-deficient cell lines in that both coding and signal junction formation are disrupted (Figure 3). In the standard transient transfection assays, neither coding or signal junction products are appreciably recovered (Taccioli et al., 1993). Also, for the rare events that are scored, nonspecific deletions not resembling V(D)J products are found.

The recent utilization of chromosomally integrated substrates to examine the XR-1 mutation has revealed that mutations in this gene do lead to subtly different outcomes. Li et al. used an assay whereby inversional rearrangement products could be analyzed following introduction of RAG1 and RAG2 into XR-1 (Li et al., 1995). The substrate, termed G12, was normally rearranged in controls, but in the XR-1 background, G12 was poorly rearranged. Furthermore, low frequency inversional recombination events could be selectively recovered and examined following a strategy pioneered by Lewis and coworkers (Lewis et al., 1984). XR-1 cells produced rearrangement events that were hybrid junctions at an elevated level relative to wildtype events and other V(D)J recombination-deficient mutants. Following DNA sequence analysis of recovered junctions, Li et al. found a novel outcome. The deleted junctions had signal joining that was imprecise, and coding joints that were almost normal. In addition to appropriate coding junctional deletions, they observed a high incidence of P nucleotides (7/7 events for which there was DNA sequencing). Furthermore, the junctions of RSS ends were not consistent with the use of terminal DNA homology. These observations are intriguing and imply that the XR-1 mutation disrupts a feature of V(D)J joining that has not been seen in other mutant backgrounds. As discussed, possibly the absence of XR-1 reveals an alternative joining pathway that does not require DNA homology.

Li et al. used the chromosomal rearrangement strategy as an effective device for cloning genes complementing the XR-1 V(D)J joining defect (Li et al., 1995). This strategy resembles the methods used to isolate the RAG1 gene by a functional assay (Schatz et al., 1989). XR-1 G12 cells were made RAG1-expression positive by transfection and were subsequently co-transfected with RAG2 and a human cDNA expression library. They found a single gene (XRCC4) that was able to restore V(D)J recombination product formation potential using this approach. Also, the XRCC4 gene transfected into XR-1 cells then complemented each of the mutant phenotypes: V(D)J recombination RSS and coding product formation in transient transfection assays, and restoration of IR sensitivity and DSB repair. The functional complementation was matched with gene localization. XRCC4 was localized to human chromosome 5q11.2-13.3, a region previously identified as the site of the XR-1 mutation (Giaccia et al., 1990; Otevrel and Stamato, 1995). Importantly, the XR-1 mutation was shown to be a deletion, indicating that the mutant phenotypes ascribed resulted from the absence of the protein.

The human and mouse XRCC4 genes were cloned, and DNA sequence analysis does not reveal any similarity to other genes in eukaryotic or prokaryotic databases (Li et al., 1995). XRCC4 encodes a putative 334 amino acid protein with an expected size of 38 kDa. Human and mouse XRCC4 genes are approximately 75% identical. A possible lead into XRCC4 function is that this protein contains several phosphorylation sites for DNA-PK, although there are also sites for cytoplasmic tyrosine and ser,thr kinases.

Several ideas have been put forward to speculate about XRCC4 molecular functions (Li et al., 1995). XRCC4 protein might be functional in a complex with the DNA-PK components, either by regulating the accessibility to DNA joining sites or modifying the activities of these other proteins. Because there is no evidence for DNA end binding defects in XR-1 extracts (Getts et al., 1994), DNA joining may be normal without XRCC4 (Stamato and Hu, 1987). XRCC4 could regulate and/or be a component of a nuclease. Alternatively, XRCC4 might stimulate the DNA ligase needed for V(D)J joining, that has not yet been identified. The XR-1 mutant was shown to be radiosensitive in G1 and early S phases of the cell cycle (Giaccia et al., 1985; Stamato et al., 1983), implying that XRCC4 protein may ordinarily function at these times. Although the identification of the XRCC4 gene has not defined its function for V(D)J recombination, cloning of XRCC4 has propelled the field forward. The next phase of analysis of XRCC4 will likely involve an association of this interesting protein with a biochemical activity, and the determination of its functions in in vitro VDJ joining.

The Future: Putting DNA Ends Together

Having identified four of the gene products necessary for VDJ joining and IR repair, are there others that are essential? Undoubtedly the answer to this question will be yes. The route to delve further into the joining mechanisms is now open to biochemical investigations. It is likely that the next research phase will include the description of each of the protein activities and how they are utilized in V(D)J recombination. An important remaining problem is to understand the molecular basis of the rearrangement phase of the reaction. In other words, what controls the ability of the reaction to create novel junctions rather than the reformation of breaks in DNA without rearrangement? An additional challenge ahead is to decipher how coding ends and RSS ends are differentially formed. Several indications have been made that the enzymology of these two joining steps are separable. Furthermore, there is evidence that the rate of joining of RSS and coding junctions can be significantly different (Ramsden et al., 1995). Coding end hairpins are processed much more rapidly than RSS ends to products in reactions that can be coordinated by a temperature shift to activate recombination initiation. Thus, following cleavages, a reordering of the enzymology of the reaction may ensue so that the proteins required for joining now substitute for the RAG1/RAG2 proteins required for initiation. Furthermore, although RAG1 and RAG2 are necessary for cleavages, these proteins may also orchestrate the later rearrangement and joining steps. Undoubtedly, a series of intricate protein:protein associations and possibly protein modifications will be the means by which this redistribution occurs.

REFERENCES

Alt, F.W., and D. Baltimore. 1982. Joining of immunoglobulin heavy chain gene segments: Implications from a chromosome with evidence of three D-J_H fusions. *Proc. Natl. Acad. Sci. USA*, 79, 4118–4122.

Anderson, C.W. 1993. DNA damage and the DNA-activated protein kinase. *TIBS*, 18, 433–437.

Anderson, C.W., and S.P. Lees-Miller. 1992. The nuclear serine/threonine protein kinase DNA-PK. *Crit. Rev. Euk. Gene Exprsn.*, 2, 283–314.

Banga, S., K. Hall, A. Sandhu, D. Weaver, and R. Athwal. 1994. Complementation of V(D)J recombination defect and X-ray sensitivity of *scid* mouse cells by human chromosome 8. *Mutat. Res.*, 315, 239–247.

Beall, E.L., A. Admon, and D.C. Rio. 1994. A Drosophila protein homologous to the human p70 Ku autoimmune antigen interacts with the P transposable element inverted repeats. *Proc. Nat. Acad. Sci. USA*, 91, 12681–12685.

Blier, P.R., A.J. Griffith, J. Craft, and J.A. Hardin. 1993. Binding of Ku protein to DNA: measurement of affinity for ends and demonstration of binding to nicks. *J. Biol. Chem.*, 268, 7594–7601.

Blunt, T., N.J. Finnie, G.E. Taccioli, G.C.M. Smith, J. Demengeot, T.M. Gottlieb, R. Mizuta, A.J. Varghese, F.W. Alt, P.A. Jeggo, and S.P. Jackson. 1995. Defective DNA-dependent protein kinase activity is linked to V(D)J recombination and DNA repair defects associated with the murine scid mutation. *Cell*, 80, 813–823.

Boubnov, N.V., and Weaver, D.T. 1995. Scid cells are deficient in Ku and RPA phosphorylation by the DNA-dependent protein kinase. *Molec. Cell. Biol.* 15, 5700–5706.

Boubnov, N.V., Z.P. Wills, and D.T. Weaver. 1993. V(D)J recombination coding junction formation without DNA homology: processing of coding termini. *Mol. Cell. Biol.*, 13, 6957–6968.

Boubnov, N.V., K.T. Hall, Z. Wills, S.E. Lee, D.M. He, D.M. Benjamin, C.R. Pulaski, H. Band, W. Reeves, E.A. Hendrickson, and D.T. Weaver. 1995. Complementation of the ionizing radiation sensitivity, DNA end binding, and V(D)J recombination defects of double-strand break repair mutants by the p86 Ku autoantigen. *Proc. Nat. Acad. Sci. USA*, 92, 890–894.

Cai, Q.Q., A. Plet, J. Imbert, M. Lafagepochitaloff, C. Cerdan, and J.M. Blanchard. 1994. Chromosomal location and expression of the genes coding for Ku p70 and p80 in human cell lines and normal tissues. *Cytogen. and Cell Genet.*, 65, 221–227.

Carter, T., and C.W. Anderson. 1991. The DNA-activated protein kinase. *Prog. Mol. Subcell. Biol.* 12, 37–47.

Choulika, A., A. Perrin, B. Dujon, and J.-F. Nicolas. 1995. Induction of homologous recombination in mammalian chromosomes by using the I-SceI system of Saccharomyces cerevisiae. *Molec. and Cell. Biol.*, 15, 1963–1973.

Cortes, P., Z.S. Ze, and D. Baltimore. 1994. RAG-1 interacts with the repeatd amino acid motife of the human homologue of the yeast protein SRP1. *Proc. Nat. Acad. Sci. USA*, 91, 7633–7637.

Cuomo, C., and M.A. Oettinger. 1994. Analysis of regions of RAG-2 important for V(D)J recombination. *Nuc. Acids Res.*, 22, 1810–1814.

Cuomo, C.A., S.A. Kirch, J. Gyuris, R. Brent, and M.A. Oettinger. 1994. Rch1, a protein that specifically interacts with the RAG-1 recombination activating protein. *Proc. Nat. Acad. Sci. USA*, 91, 6156–6160.

deVries, E., W. van Driel, W.G. Bergsma, A.C. Arnberg, and P.C. van der Vliet. 1989. HeLa nuclear protein recognizing DNA termini and translocating on DNA forming a regular DNA-multimeric protein complex. *J. Mol. Biol.*, **208**, 65–78.

Eastman, Q.M., T.M.J. Leu, and D.G. Schatz. 1996. Initiation of V(D)J recombination in vitro: the 12/23 rule. *Nature*, **380**, 85–88.

Errami, A., V. Smider, W.K. Rathmell, D.M. He, E.A. Hendrickson, M.Z. Zdzienicka, and G. Chu. 1996. Ku86 defines the genetic defect and restores X-ray resistance and V(D)J recombination to complementation group 5 hamster cell mutants. *Molec. Cell. Biol.*, **16**, 1519–1526.

Falzon, M., J.W. Fewell, and E.L. Kuff. 1993. EBP-80, a transcription factor closely resembling the human autoantigen Ku, recognizes single- to double-strand transitions in DNA. *J. Biol. Chem.*, **268**, 10546–10552.

Feldmann, H., and E.L. Winnacker. 1993. A putative homologue of the human autoantigen Ku from Saccharomyces cerevisiae. *J. Biol. Chem.* **268**, 12895–12900.

Finnie, N.J., T.M. Gottlieb, T. Blunt, P.A. Jeggo, and S.P. Jackson. 1995. DNA-dependent protein kinase activity is absent in xrs-6 cells: Implications for site-specific recombination and DNA double-strand break repair. *Proc. Nat. Acad. Sci. USA*, **92**, 320–324.

Gatti, R., E. Boder, H.V. Vinters, R.S. Sparkes, A. Norman, and K. Lange. 1994. Ataxia telangiectasia: An interdisciplinary approach to pathogenesis. *Medicine*, **70**, 99–117.

Gellert, M. 1992a. Molecular analysis of V(D)J recombination. *Annu. Rev. Genet.*, **22**, 425–446.

Gellert, M. 1992b. V(D)J recombination gets a break. *TIG*, **8**, 408–412.

Getts, R.C., and T.D. Stamato. 1994. Absence of a Ku-like DNA end binding activity in the *xrs* Double-strand DNA repair-deficient mutant. *J. Biol. Chem.*, **269**, 15981–15984.

Giaccia, A., R. Weinstein, J. Hu, and T.D. Stamato. 1985. Cell cycle-dependent repair of double-strand DNA breaks in a gamma-ray-sensitive Chinese hamster cell. *Somat. Cell Mol. Genet.*, **11**, 485–491.

Giaccia, A.J., N. Denko, R. MacLaren, D. Mirman, C. Waldren, I. Hart, and T.D. Stamato. 1990. Human chromosome 5 complements the DNA double-strand break-repair deficiency and gamma-ray sensitivity of the XR-1 hamster variant. *Am. J. Hum. Genet.*, **47**, 459–469.

Gilfillan, S., A. Dierich, M. Lemeur, C. Benoist, and D. Mathis. 1993. Mice lacking TdT: mature animals with an immature lymphocyte repertoire. *Science*, **261**, 1175–1178.

Gottlieb, T.M., and S.P. Jackson. 1993. The DNA-dependent protein kinase: requirement for DNA ends and association with Ku antigen. *Cell*, **72**, 131–142.

Greenwell, P.W., S.L. Kronmal, S.E. Porter, J. Gassenhuber, B. Obermaier, and T.D. Petes. 1995. TEL1, a gene involved in controlling teleomere length in *S. cerevisiae*, is homologous to the human ataxia telangiectasia gene. *Cell*, **82**, 823–829.

Griffith, A.J., P.R. Blier, T. Mimori, and J.A. Hardin. 1992. Ku polypeptides synthesized in vitro assemble into complexes which recognize ends of double-stranded DNA. *J. Biol. Chem.*, **267**, 331–338.

Hari, K.L., A. Santerre, J.J. Sekelsky, K.S. McKim, J.B. Boyd, and R.S. Hawley. 1995. The mei-41 gene of D. melanogaster is a structural and functional homolog of the human ataxia telangiectasia gene. *Cell*, **82**, 815–822.

Hartley, K.O., D. Gell, G.C.M. Smith, H. Zhang, N. Dvecha, M.A. Connelly, A. Admon, S.P. Lees-Miller, C.W. Anderson, and S.P. Jackson. 1995. DNA-dependent protein kinase catalytic subunit: a relative of phosphatidylinositol 3-kinase and the ataxia telangiectasia gene product. *Cell*, **82**, 849–856.

Hsieh, C.L., C. Arlett, and M.R. Lieber. 1993. V(D)J recombination in ataxia telangiectasia, Bloom's syndrome, and a DNA ligase I-associated immunodeficiency disorder. *J. Biol. Chem.*, **268**, 20105–20109.

Jackson, S.P. 1996. The recognition of DNA damage. *Curr. Op. Genet. Devel.*, **6**, 19–25.

Jacoby, D.B., and P.C. Wensink. 1994. Yolk protein factor-1 is a Drosophila homolog of Ku, the DNA-binding subunit of a DNA-dependent protein kinase from humans. *J. Biol. Chem.*, **269**, 11484–11491.

Jeggo, P. 1990. Studies on mammalian mutants defective in rejoining double-strand breaks in DNA. *Mutat. Res.*, **239**, 1–16.

Jeggo, P.A., and L.M. Kemp. 1983. X-ray-sensitive mutants of Chinese hamster ovary cell line. Isolation and cross-sensitivity to other DNA-damaging agents. *Mutat. Res.*, **112**, 313–327.

Kastan, M.B., Q. Zhan, W.S. El-Deiry, F. Carrier, T. Jacks, W.V. Walsh, B.S. Plunkett, B. Vogelstein, and A.J. Fornace. 1992. A mammalian cell cycle checkpoint pathway utilizing p53 and *GADD45* Is defective in ataxia-telangiectasia. *Cell*, **71**, 587–597.

Keith, C.T., and S.L. Schreiber. 1995. PIK-related kinases: DNA repair, recombination, and cell cycle checkpoints. *Science*, **270**, 50–51.

Kirchgessner, C., L. Tosto, K. Biederman, M. Kovacs, D. Araujo, E. Stanbridge, and J. Brown. 1993. Complementation of the radiosensitive phenotype in severe combined immunodeficient mice by human chromosome 8. *Cancer Res.*, **53**, 6011–6016.

Kirchgessner, C.U., C.K. Patil, J.W. Evans, C.A. Cuomo, L.M. Fried, T. Carter, M.A. Oettinger, and J.M. Brown. 1995. DNA-dependent kinase (p350) as a candidate gene for the murine SCID defect. *Science*, **267**, 1178–1183.

Komatsu, K., T. Ohta, Y. Jinno, N. Niikawa, and Y. Okumura. 1993. Functional complementation in mouse–human radiation hybrids assigns the putative murine scid gene to the pericentric region of human chromosome 8. *Human Molec. Genet.*, **2**, 1031–1034.

Komori, T., A. Okada, V. Stewart, and F.W. Alt. 1993. Lack of N regions in antigen receptor variable region genes of TdT-deficient lymphocytes. *Science*, **261**, 1171–1175.

Kurimasa, A., Y. Nagata, M. Shimizu, M. Emi, Y. Nakamura, and M. Oshimura. 1993. A human gene that restores the DNA-repair defect in scid mice is located on 8p11.1-q11.1. *Human Genet.*, **93**, 21–26.

Lafaille, J.J., A. DeCloux, M. Bonneville, Y. Takagaki, and S. Tonegawa. 1989. Junctional sequences of T cell receptor γδ genes: implications for γδ T cell lineages and for a novel intermediate of V–(D)–J joining. *Cell*, **59**, 859–870.

Lee, S.E., C.R. Pulaski, D.M. He, D.M. Benjamin, M.J. Voss, J. Um, and E.A. Hendrickson. 1995. Isolation of mammalian cell mutants that are X-ray sensitive, impaired in DNA double-strand break repair and defective for V(D)J recombination. *Mutat. Res.*, **336**, 279–291.

Lees-Miller, S.P., Y. Chen, and C.W. Anderson. 1990. Human cells contain a DNA-activated protein kinase that phosphorylates simian virus 40 T antigen, mouse p53, and the human Ku autoantigen. *Molec. and Cell. Biol.*, **10**, 6472–6481.

Lees-Miller, S.P., K. Sakaguchi, S.J. Ullrich, E. Appella, and C.W. Anderson. 1992. Human DNA-activated protein kinase phosphorylates serines 15 and 37 in the amino-terminal transactivation domain of human p53. *Molec. and Cell. Biol.*, **12**, 5041–5049.

Lees-Miller, S.P., R. Godbout, D.W. Chan, M. Weinfeld, R.S. Day, G.M. Barron, and J. Al-lalunis-Turner. 1995. Absence of p350 subunit of DNA-activated protein kinase from a radiosensitive human cell line. *Science*, **267**, 1183–1185.

Leu, T.J., and D.G. Schatz. 1995. Rag-1 and rag-2 are components of a high-molecular-weight complex, and association of rag-2 with this complex is rag-1 dependent. *Molec. and Cell. Biol.*, **15**, 5657–5670.

Lewis, S., A. Gifford, and D. Baltimore. 1984. Joining of Vk to Jk gene segments in a retroviral vector introduced into lymphoid cells. *Nature*, **308**, 425–428.

Lewis, S.M. 1994. The mechanism of V(D)J joining: Lessons from molecular, immunological, and comparative analyses. *Adv. Immunol.*, **56**, 27–150.

Li, Z., T. Otevrel, Y. Gao, H.-L. Cheng, B. Seed, T.D. Stamato, G.E. Taccioli, and F.W. Alt. 1995. The XRCC4 gene encodes a novel protein involved in DNA double-strand break repair and V(D)J recombination. *Cell*, **83**, 1079–1089.

Liang, F., P. Romanienko, D. Weaver, P. Jeggo, and M. Jasin. 1996. Chromosomal double-strand break repair in Ku80 deficient cells. In press.

Lieber, M.R., J.E. Hesse, S. Lewis, G.C. Bosma, N. Rosenberg, K. Mizuuchi, M.J. Bosma, and M. Gellert. 1988. The defect in murine severe combined immune deficiency: joining of signal sequences but not coding segments in V(D)J recombination. *Cell*, **55**, 7–16.

Lin, W.-C., and S. Desiderio. 1993. Regulation of V(D)J recombination activator protein RAG-2 by phosphorylation. *Science*, **260**, 953–959.

Lin, W.-C., and S. Desiderio. 1994. Cell cycle regulation of V(D)J recombination activating protein RAG-2. *Proc. Nat. Acad. Sci. USA*, **91**, 2733–2737.

Lu, X., and D.P. Lane. 1993. Differential induction of transcriptionally active p53 following UV or ionizing radiation: defects in chromsome instability syndromes? *Cell*, **75**, 765–778.

Lustig, A.J., and T.D. Petes. 1986. Identification of yeast mutants with altered telomere structure. *Proc. Nat. Acad. Sci. USA*, **83**, 1398–1402.

McBlane, J.F., D.C. van Gent, D.A. Ramsden, C. Romeo, C.A. Cuomo, M. Gellert, and M.A. Oettinger. 1995. Cleavage at a V(D)J recombination signal requires only RAG1 and RAG2 proteins and occurs in two steps. *Cell*, **83**, 387–395.

McCormack, W.T., L.W. Tjoelker, L.M. Carlson, B. Petryniak, C.F. Barth, E.H. Humphries, and C.B. Thompson. 1989. Chicken Ig$_L$ Gene Rearrangement Involves Deletion of a Circular Episome and Addition of Single Nonrandom Nucleotides to Both Coding Segments. *Cell*, **56**, 785–791.

Meier, J.T., and S.M. Lewis. 1993. P nucleotides in V(D)J recombination: A fine-structure analysis. *Mol. Cell Biol.*, **13**, 1078–1092.

Milne, G.T., S.F. Jin, K. Shannon, and D.T. Weaver. 1996. Mutations in two Ku homologues define a DNA end-joining repair pathway in Saccharomyces cerevisiae. *Mol. Cell Biol.*, **16**, 4189–4198.

Mimori, T., and J.A. Hardin. 1986. Mechanism of interaction between Ku protein and DNA. *J. Biol. Chem.*, **261**, 10375–10379.

Mimori, T., M. Akizuki, H. Yamagata, S. Inada, S. Yoshida, and M. Homma. 1981. *J. Clin. Invest.*, **68**, 611–620.

Mimori, T., J.A. Hardin, and J.A. Steitz. 1986. Characterization of the DNA-binding protein antigen Ku recognized by autoantibodies from patients with rheumatic disorders. *J. Biol. Chem.*, **261**, 2264–2278.

Mombaerts, P., J. Iacomini, R.S. Johnson, K. Herrup, and S. Tonegawa. 1992. RAG-1-deficient mice have no mature B and T lymphocytes. *Cell*, **68**, 869–877.

Morrow, D.M., D.A. Tagle, Y. Shiloh, F.S. Collins, and P. Hieter. 1995. TEL1, an *S. cerevisiae* homolog of the human gene mutated in ataxia telangiectasia, is functionally related to the yeast checkpoint gene MEC1. *Cell*, **82**, 831–840.

Oettinger, M.A. 1992. Activation of V(D)J recombination by RAG1 and RAG2. *TIGS*, **8**, 413–416.

Oettinger, M.A., D.G. Schatz, C. Gorka, and D. Baltimore. 1990. RAG-1 and RAG-2, adjacent genes that synergistically activate V(D)J recombination. *Science*, **248**, 1517–1523.

Ono, M., P.W. Tucker, and J.D. Capra. 1994. Production and characterization of recombinant human Ku antigen. *Nuc. Acids Res.*, **22**, 3918–3924.

Otevrel, T., and T.D. Stamato. 1995. Regional localization of the XRCC4 human radiation repair gene. *Genomics*, **27**, 211–214.

Paillard, S., and F. Strauss. 1991. Analysis of the mechanism of interaction of simian Ku protein with DNA. *Nuc. Acids Res.*, **19**, 5619–5624.

Painter, R.B., and B.R. Young. 1980. Radiosensitivity in ataxia-telangiectasia: A new explanation. *Proc. Natl. Acad. Sci. USA*, **77**, 7315–7317.

Peterson, S.R., A. Kurimasa, M. Oshimura, W.S. Dynan, E.M. Bradbury, and D.J. Chen. 1995. Loss of the 350kD catalytic subunit of the DNA-dependent protein kinase in DNA double-strand break repair mutant mammalian cells. *Proc. Nat. Acad. Sci. USA*, **92**, 3171–3174.

Porter, S.E., P.W. Greenwell, K.B. Ritchie, and T.D. Petes. 1996. The DNA-binding protein Hdf1p (a putative Ku homolog) is required for maintaining normal teleomere length in Saccharomyces cerevisiae. *Nuc. Acids Res.*, **24**, 582–585.

Ramsden, D.A., and M. Gellert. 1995. Formation and resolution of double-strand break intermediates in V(D)J rearrangement. *Genes and Devel.*, **9**, 2409–2420.

Rathmell, W.K., and G. Chu. 1994a. A DNA end-binding factor involved in double-strand break repair and V(D)J recombination. *Mol. Cell Biol.*, **14**, 4741–4748.

Rathmell, W.K., and G. Chu. 1994b. Involvement of the Ku autoantigen in the cellular response to DNA double-strand breaks. *Proc. Nat. Acad. Sci. USA*, **91**, 7623–7627.

Reeves, W. 1985. Usse of monoclonal antibodies for the characterization of novel DNA-binding proteins recognized by human autoimmune sera. *J. Exp. Med.*, **161**, 18–39.

Roth, D.B., J.P. Menetski, P.B. Nakajima, M.J. Bosma, and M. Gellert. 1992a. V(D)J recombination: broken DNA molecules with covalently sealed (hairpin) coding ends in scid mouse thymocytes. *Cell*, **70**, 983–991.

Roth, D.B., P.B. Nakajima, J.P. Menetski, M.J. Bosma, and M. Gellert. 1992b. V(D)J recombination in mouse thymocytes: double-strand breaks near T cell receptor δ rearrangement signals. *Cell*, **69**, 41–53.

Roth, D.B., C. Zhu, and M. Gellert. 1993. Characterization of broken DNA molecules associated with V(D)J recombination. *Proc. Natl. Acad. Sci. USA*, **90**, 10788–10792.

Rouet, P., F. Smith, and M. Jasin. 1994a. Expression of a site-specific endonuclease stimulates homologous recombination in mammalian cells. *Proc. Nat. Acad. Sci. USA*, **91**, 6064–6068.

Rouet, P., F. Smith, and M. Jasin. 1994b. Introduction of double-strand breaks into the genome of mouse cells by expression of a rare-cutting endonuclease. *Molec. and Cell. Biol.*, **14**, 8096–8106.

Sadofsky, M., J.E. Hesse, J.F. McBlane, and M. Gellert. 1993. Expression and V(D)J recombination activity of mutated RAG-1 proteins. *Nuc. Acids Res.*, **21**, 5644–5650.

Sadofsky, M., J.E. Hesse, and M. Gellert. 1994. Definition of a core region of RAG-2 that is functional in V(D)J recombination. *Nuc. Acids Res.*, **22**, 1805–1809.

Sadofsky, M., J.E. Hesse, D.C. van Gent, and M. Gellert. 1995. RAG-1 mutations that affect the target specificity of V(D)J recombination: a possible direct role of RAG-1 in site recognition. *Genes Dev.*, **9**, 2193–2199.

Satoh, M., J. Wang, and W.H. Reeves. 1995. Role of free p70 (Ku) subunit in posttranslational stabilization of newly synthesized p80 during DNA-dependent protein kinase assembly. *Eur. J. Cell Biol.*, **66**, 127–135.

Savitsky, K., A. Bar-Shira, S. Gilad, G. Rotman, Y. Ziv, L. Vanagaite, D.A. Tagle, S. Smith, T. Uziel, S. Sfez, M. Ashkenazi, I. Pecker, M. Frydman, R. Harnik, S.R. Patanjali, A. Simmons, G.A. Clines, A. Sartiel, R.A. Gatti, L. Chessa, O. Sanal, M.F. Lavin, N.G.J. Jaspers, A.M.R. Taylor, C.F. Arlett, T. Miki, S.M. Weissman, M. Lovett, F.S. Collins, and Y. Shiloh. 1995. A single ataxia telangiectasia gene with a product similar to PI-3 kinase. *Science*, **268**, 1749–1753.

Schatz, D., M.A. Oettinger, and D. Baltimore. 1989. The V(D)J recombination activating gene RAG-1. *Cell*, **59**, 1035–1048.

Schatz, D., M. Oettinger, and M. Schlissel. 1992. V(D)J recombination: molecular biology and regulation. *Ann. Rev. Immunol.*, **10**, 359–383.

Schlissel, M., A. Constantinescu, T. Morrow, M. Baxter, and A. Peng. 1993. Double-strand signal sequence breaks in V(D)J recombination are blunt, 5′-phosphorylated, RAG-dependent, and cell cycle regulated. *Genes and Dev.*, **7**, 2520–2532.

Sheehan, K.M., and M.R. Lieber. 1993. V(D)J recombination: signal and coding joint resolution are uncoupled and depend on parallel synapsis of the sites. *Mol. Cell. Biol.* **13**, 1363–1370.

Shimma, Y., and I. Uno. 1990. Isolation and characterization of neomycin-sensitive mutants in Saccharomyces cerevisiae. *J. Gen. Microbiol.*, **136**, 1753–1761.

Shinkai, Y., G. Rathbun, K. Lam, E. Oltz, V. Stewart, M. Mendelsohn, J. Charon, M. Datta, F. Young, A. Stall, and F. Alt. 1992. RAG-2 deficient mice lack mature lymphocytes due to an inability to initiate V(D)J recombination. *Cell*, **68**, 855–867.

Siede, W., A.A. Friedl, I. Dianova, F. Eckardt-Schupp, and E.C. Friedberg. 1996. The Saccharomyces cerevisiae Ku autoantigen homologue affects radiosensitivity only in the absence of homologous recombination. *Genetics*, **142**, 91–102.

Silver, D., E. Spanopoulou, R. Mulligan, and D. Baltimore. 1993. Dispensable sequence motifs in the RAG-1 and RAG-2 genes for plasmid V(D)J recombination. *Proc. Nat. Acad. Sci., USA.*, **90**, 6100–6104.

Sipley, J.D., J.C. Menninger, K.O. Hartley, D.C. Ward, S.P. Jackson, and C.W. Anderson. 1995. The gene for the catalytic subunit of the human DNA-activated protein kinase maps to the site of the XRCC7 gene on chromosome 8. *Proc. Nat. Acad. Sci. USA*, **92**, 7515–7519.

Smider, V., W.K. Rathmell, M.R. Lieber, and G. Chu. 1994. Restoration of X-ray resistance and V(D)J recombination in mutant cells by Ku cDNA. *Science*, **266**, 288–291.

Stamato, T.D., and J. Hu. 1987. Normal DNA ligase activity in a gamma-ray-sensitive Chinese hamster mutant. *Mutat. Res.* **183**, 61–67.

Stamato, T.D., R. Weinstein, A. Giaccia, and L. Mackenzie. 1983. Isolation of cell cycle-dependent gamma-ray-sensitive Chinese hamster ovary cell. *Somat. Cell Genet.*, **9**, 165–173.

Suwa, A., M. Hirakata, Y. Takeda, S.A. Jesch, T. Mimori, and J.A. Hardin. 1994. DNA-dependent protein kinase (Ku protein-p350 complex) assembles on double-stranded DNA. *Proc. Nat. Acad. Sci. USA*, **91**, 6904–6908.

Taccioli, G.E., G. Rathbun, E. Oltz, T. Stamato, P.A. Jeggo, and F.W. Alt. 1993. Impairment of V(D)J recombination in double-strand break repair mutants. *Science*, **260**, 207–210.

Taccioli, G., T.M. Gottlieb, T. Blunt, A. Priestly, J. Demengeot, R. Mizuta, A.R. Lehmann, F.W. Alt, S.P. Jackson, and P.A. Jeggo. 1994a. Ku80: product of the XRCC5 gene and its role in DNA repair and V(D)J recombination. *Science*, **265**, 1442–1445.

Taccioli, G.E., H.-L. Cheng, A.J. Varghese, G. Whitmore, and Alt F.W. 1994b. A DNA Repair Defect in Chinese Hamster Ovary Cells Affects V(D)J Recombination Similarly to the Murine *Scid* Mutation. *J. Biol. Chem.*, **269**, 7439–7442.

Tonegawa, S. 1983. Somatic generation of antibody diversity. *Nature*, **302**, 575–581.

Tuteja, N., R. Tuteja, A. Ochem, P. Taneja, N.W. Huang, A. Simoncsits, S. Susic, K. Rahman, L. Marusic, J. Chen, J. Zhang, S. Wang, S. Pongor, and A. Falaschi. 1994. Human DNA helicase II: a novel DNA unwinding enzyme identified as the Ku autoantigen. *EMBO J.,* **13**, 4991–5001.

van Gent, D.C., J.F. McBlane, D.A. Ramsden, M.J. Sadofsky, J.E. Hesse, and M. Gellert. 1995. Initiation of V(D)J recombination in a cell-free system. *Cell*, **81**, 925–934.

van Gent, D.C., K. Mizuuchi, and M. Gellert. 1996. Similarities between initiation of V(D)J recombination and retroviral integration. *Science*, **271**, 1592–1594.

Walker, A.I., T. Hunt, R.J. Jackson, and C.W. Anderson. 1985. Double-stranded DNA induces the phosphorylation of several proteins including the 90,000 Mr heat-shock protein in animal cell extracts. *EMBO J.*, **4**, 139–145.

Wang, J., M. Satoh, A. Pierani, J. Schmitt, C.-H. Chou, H.G. Stunnenberg, R.G. Roeder, and W.H. Reeves. 1994. Assembly and DNA binding of recombinant Ku (p70/p80) autoantigen defined by a novel monoclonal antibody specific for p70/p80 heterodimers. *J. Cell Science*, **107**, 3223–3233.

Weaver, D. 1995. V(D)J recombination and double-strand break repair. *Adv. Immunol.*, **58**, 29–85.

Weaver, D., N. Boubnov, Z. Wills, K. Hall, and J. Staunton. 1995. V(D)J recombination: Double-strand break repair gene products in the joining mechanism. *Ann. N.Y. Acad. Sci.*, **764**, 99–111.

Weaver, D.T. 1995. What to do at an end: DNA double-strand break repair. *TIGS*, **11**, 388–392.

Yoshida, M., Y.I. Shimma, I. Uno, and A. Toh-e. 1994. Cloning and sequencing of the NES24 Gene of Saccharomyces cerevisiae. *Yeast*, **10**, 371–376.

Zakian, V.A. 1995. ATM-related genes: what do they tell us about functions of the human gene. *Cell*, **82**, 685–687.

Zdzienicka, M.Z., and J.W.I.M. Simons. 1987. Mutagen-sensitive cell lines are obtained with a high frequency in V79 Chinese hamster cells. *Mutat. Res.*, **178**, 235–244.

Zhu, C., and D.B. Roth. 1995. Characterization of coding ends in thymocytes of scid mice: implications for the mechanism of V(D)J recombination. *Immunity*, **2**, 101–112.

Chapter
TWO

The Ku Autoantigen

WESTLEY H. REEVES, JINGSONG WANG, AJAY K. AJMANI, LOVORKA STOJANOV and MINORU SATOH

Division of Rheumatology and Immunology, UNC Lineberger Comprehensive Cancer Center, University of North Carolina at Chapel Hill, Chapel Hill, NC 27599-7280, USA

I. INTRODUCTION

Autoantibodies found in the sera of patients with systemic autoimmune diseases are useful clinical markers and also have been instrumental in unraveling the biology of their target antigens. For example, autoantibodies to small nuclear ribonucleoproteins (snRNPs) occurring in sera of patients with systemic lupus erythematosus (SLE) were crucial reagents in determining the role of the U1 and other snRNPs in RNA processing [1]. A subset of autoantibodies reactive with the Sm B′/B and D proteins shared by U1, U2, U4-6, and U5 snRNPs is a marker for SLE, having virtually 100% specificity for the disease [2]. Autoantibodies to the Ku antigen are a more recent example of the value of autoimmune sera in understanding both autoimmunity and the molecular biology of target antigens.

The Ku antigen is a heterodimer consisting of M_r ~70 and 80–86 kDa proteins that is the DNA binding component of a DNA-dependent protein kinase (DNA-PK). The catalytic subunit of DNA-PK is a protein of ~460 kDa (DNA-PK$_{cs}$, Figure 1). Autoantibodies to Ku antigen were identified initially in 1981 as a novel precipitin line in double immunodiffusion formed by sera from Japanese patients with an unusual autoimmune syndrome characterized by features of scleroderma and

Send correspondence to Westley H. Reeves, MD, Division of Rheumatology and Immunology, University of North Carolina at Chapel Hill, 3330 Thurston Building, CB# 7280, Chapel Hill, NC 27599-7280; Phone (919) 966-4191, Fax (919) 966-1739.

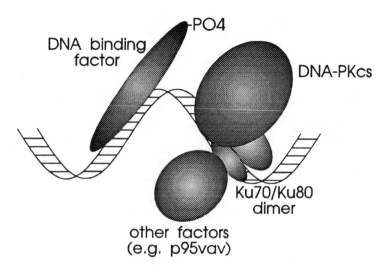

Figure 1. Diagram of the structure of DNA-PK bound to chromatin. Both subunits of the p70/p80 Ku heterodimer are illustrated interacting with DNA-PK$_{cs}$ on a strand of dsDNA, although it is not yet clear which Ku subunit(s) actually contact DNA-PK$_{cs}$. Engagement of DNA by Ku may facilitate subsequent interactions of Ku with DNA-PK$_{cs}$ [88]. Once DNA-PK assembles on chromatin, it can phosphorylate DNA-bound substrates on serine or threonine. Other factors, such as p95^{vav} or sequence-specific DNA binding proteins, also may interact with the complex.

polymyositis overlap syndrome [3]. The designation Ku was derived from the initial letters of the first patient's name. The 70 and 80–86 kDa Ku polypeptides (designated p70 or Ku70 and p80 or Ku80, respectively) and the association of these proteins with DNA were reported in 1985 [4,5]. A DNA-dependent serine-threonine kinase activity in mammalian cells first identified in 1990 [6,7] was later shown to be associated with Ku [8,9]. The identification of a Ku-associated kinase activity coupled with the molecular cloning of the Ku70 and Ku80 genes has led to rapid progress in understanding the role of Ku antigen in repairing double stranded DNA breaks and in V(D)J recombination. Recent advances in this rapidly changing field will be reviewed here, emphasizing their implications for the pathogenesis of autoimmunity, B and T cell development, and immunodeficiency.

I.1. Other Factors That Are Similar or Identical to Ku Antigen

Numerous factors with properties similar or identical to the Ku antigen have been reported (Table 1). Primate-specific, proliferation-sensitive nuclear proteins of 64–82 kDa identified by isoelectric focusing are reactive with anti-Ku monoclonal antibodies and appear identical to Ku [10,11]. Several factors thought to be involved in transcriptional activation also are probably identical to Ku antigen, including nuclear factor IV (NFIV) [12], PSE1 [13], TREF [14,15], EBP80 [16–18], E1BF [19,20], YPF1 [21], Ku-2 [22], CTC box binding factor (CTCBF) [23], constitutive heat shock element binding factor (CHBF) [24,25], and proteins that bind to the interferon-inducible transcriptional enhancer following interferon stimulation [26]. Ku antigen is also identical to the DNA dependent ATPase [27,28] and DNA

Table 1. Partial List of Factors Related to Ku Antigen

Factor	Reference	Size (kDa)	Similarity to Ku*	Proposed function
NFIV	[12,73]	72, 84	DNA, prot, imm	binds adenovirus DNA
PSE1	[13]	73, 83	prot, imm	binds U1 snRNA promoter
TREF	[14,15]	62, 82	prot, imm	binds transferrin receptor promoter
EBP-80	[17,18]	75, 80	DNA, prot, imm	binds regulatory sequence of retroviral LTR
E1BF	[19]	72, 85	imm	RNA Pol I transcription
Ku-2	[22]	83, 72	prot, imm	B cell Ku homologue
YPF1	[21,243]	69 (β), 85 (α)	DNA, imm	Drosophila Ku homologue
HDF	[68]	70, 85	DNA	yeast cell cycle regulation
unnamed	[26]	73, 84	prot	IFN-inducible enhancer
DNA helicase II	[29]	72, 87	DNA	DNA helicase
DNA-ATPase	[29]	68, 83	prot, imm	DNA dependent ATPase
CHBF	[24,25]	70, 86	imm	binds heat shock element
CTCBF	[23]	75, 85	prot, imm	binds collagen promoter

*DNA = DNA sequence homology; prot = amino acid sequence homology; imm = immunological crossreactivity.

helicase II [29]. Finally, there has been some confusion in the literature regarding the relationship of the Ku and Ki autoantigens [30,31]. Although these specificities are frequently present in the same serum, the Ki antigen is a 29.5 kDa protein that is identical to the SL antigen, but immunologically and biochemically unrelated to Ku [32,33].

II. BIOCHEMICAL CHARACTERISTICS OF THE ANTIGENS

II.1. Ku Antigen

The Ku autoantigen originally was described as an acidic nuclear protein forming a precipitin line distinct from Sm, RNP, Ro (SS-A) and La (SS-B), which was sensitive to trypsin, mild heating, and pH >10 or <5. It was found later that the Ku antigen consists of a dimer, or possibly a tetramer, of noncovalently linked ~70 kDa and ~80 kDa protein subunits migrating at ~10 S on sucrose density gradients [4,5]. However, a broader peak of DNA-associated Ku antigen was also detectable at 10–20 S. Although gel filtration studies of Ku in crude extracts initially suggested an M_r of ~300 kDa [3], analysis of purified Ku complex in nondenaturing gels indicated a molecular mass of approximately 173 ± 21 kDa [22], in close agreement with the size of approximately 160 kDa estimated by electron microscopy [12]. The Ku dimer has an ellipsoidal shape, approximately 16 nm long and 8 nm wide [12]. Taken together, the physical properties of Ku are most consistent with a 1:1 p70/p80 heterodimer. The initial estimates of an M_r of 300 kDa may reflect binding of the Ku complex to other components, such as DNA, histones, and/or DNA-PK$_{cs}$ [34,35]. A free form of p70 also has been detected in human cells [36] (see also §4.3),

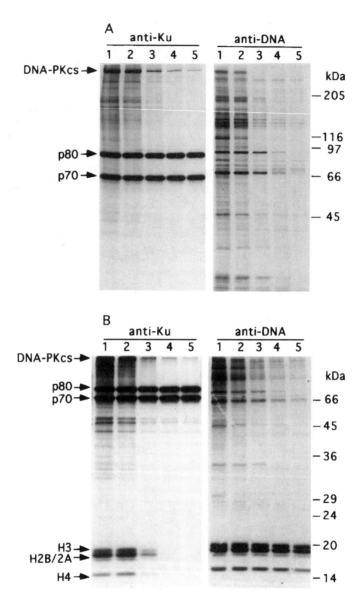

Figure 2. Ku is dissociated from DNA-PK$_{cs}$ under conditions causing its dissociation from DNA. Human K562 (erythroleukemia cells) were labeled with [^{35}S] methionine and cysteine and cell extract was immunoprecipitated using mAbs specific for Ku (162) or DNA (3H9) as described [36]. The immunoprecipitates were washed with buffers containing the following concentrations of NaCl: 0.1 M (lane 1), 0.2 M (lane 2), 0.3 M (lane 3), 0.4 M (lane 4), 0.5 M (lane 5), and analyzed on 8% (top) and 12.5% (bottom) SDS-polyacrylamide gels. Note that anti-Ku and anti-DNA antibodies both immunoprecipitate histones (H3, H2A/H2B, H4), p70 and p80 Ku, and DNA-PK$_{cs}$ after low salt washing. At higher salt concentrations, however, anti-Ku antibodies immunoprecipitate only p70 and p80, and the anti-DNA antibodies immunoprecipitate histones and/or HMG proteins that remain bound to fragmented DNA in the sonicated cell extract. Positions of molecular weight markers are shown on the right.

and free p70 may be the predominant form of Ku antigen in certain insect cells [37,38].

There is evidence that Ku heterodimers assemble into larger multimeric complexes after binding to DNA [12]. At high concentrations in vitro, Ku antigen binds to the ends of double stranded (ds) DNA followed by a non-energy dependent translocation to internal positions along the DNA strand. Translocation away from the termini allows binding of more Ku, which also can translocate along the DNA, resulting in a multimeric Ku-DNA complex. Binding of sequence-specific factors to sites adjacent to the termini enhances binding of Ku strongly, and blocks its further translocation [12]. The possibility that certain sequence-specific DNA binding factors could also interact directly with Ku has been raised [15].

II.2. DNA-PK Catalytic Subunit (DNA-PK$_{cs}$)

A eukaryotic DNA dependent serine-threonine kinase activity designated DNA-dependent protein kinase (DNA-PK) was shown to be associated with a large (~300–350 kDa) protein [6,7]. More recently, the size of this protein has been shown to be ~460 kDa [39]. Phosphorylation mediated by the purified kinase is activated by linear dsDNA molecules in a sequence-independent manner; closed circular plasmids, single stranded (ss) DNA, and DNA–RNA heteroduplexes are poor activators [6,7,9].

Although the initial studies suggested that the kinase consists of a single subunit, it was later found to be associated with the Ku autoantigen [8,9]. Interestingly, although the Ku antigen had been studied intensively, and cDNAs encoding its subunits cloned, several years before the identification of the kinase subunit (now termed DNA-PK catalytic subunit or DNA-PK$_{cs}$), the association of Ku with this component was not recognized due to the low affinity of the interaction. Indeed, the Ku antigen is dissociated from DNA-PK$_{cs}$ under conditions leading to its dissociation from DNA (Figure 2). Thus, even relatively mild washing of antigenic complexes immunoprecipitated by anti-Ku antibodies causes nearly complete loss of DNA-PK$_{cs}$. In the first reports of the association between Ku and DNA-PK$_{cs}$, immunoprecipitates were washed with 0.1 M NaCl, conditions under which a series of DNA-associated proteins, including histones, remain associated with anti-Ku immunoprecipitates (Figure 2). Despite the lack of clear evidence in immunoprecipitation studies for the formation of a specific complex, there is strong functional evidence that the interaction of Ku with DNA-PK$_{cs}$ is not a consequence of their colocalization on the same strand of DNA: 1) DNA-dependent protein kinase activity requires DNA ends; 2) DNA-PK$_{cs}$ cannot be UV crosslinked to DNA in the absence of Ku but can be in the presence of Ku; 3) DNA-PK$_{cs}$ must be associated with Ku for optimal enzymatic activity; and 4) antisera to Ku inhibit DNA-PK activity [9].

The in vitro substrates for DNA-PK are primarily DNA binding proteins, including a number of transcription factors [40,41], the RNA polymerase II carboxyl-terminal domain [8], replication factor A (RPA) [42–44], and the Ku antigen itself [6,45] (Table 2). However, several non-DNA binding proteins also can be phosphorylated by DNA-PK in vitro [45], although it is unclear whether they represent physiological substrates. It has been shown that the transcription factor Sp1 must colocalize on the same strand of DNA as DNA-PK in order to be phosphorylated optimally

Table 2. Partial List of in vitro DNA-PK Substrates

Protein	DNA binding protein	Target sequence*
p53 tumor suppressor protein	yes	SQ/TQ
Sp-1 transcription factor	yes	SQ/TQ
c-Jun transcription factor	yes	SQ/TQ
c-Fos transcription factor	yes	non-SQ/TQ
Oct-1 transcription factor	yes	n.a.
c-Myc transcription factor	yes	n.a.
TFIID transcription factor	yes	n.a.
Ku (p70 and p80)	yes	n.a.
Replication protein A	yes	n.a.
SV40 large T antigen	yes	SQ/TQ
RNA polymerase II (large subunit)	yes	non-SQ/TQ
Heat shock protein 90 (hsp-90)	no	SQ/TQ
Casein	no	n.a.
Phosvitin	no	n.a.

*Target site recognized by DNA-PK classified as either serine-glutamine/threonine-glutamine (SQ/TQ) type, or non-SQ/TQ type, see references [41,45]. n.a. = not available.

[9]; this is likely to be true for other substrates, as well. Although the substrates of DNA-PK in vivo remain poorly defined, it has been shown recently that radiation-induced hyperphosphorylation of RPA is deficient in vivo in severe combined immunodeficiency (SCID) cells compared with wild type controls, or SCID cells carrying human chromosome 8 [44].

DNA-PK phosphorylates only serine and threonine residues [6,7]. The preferred substrates have been investigated further using synthetic peptides derived from the c-Jun protein [41] and the p53 tumor suppressor protein [46]. The minimal kinase recognition motif appears to consist of either a serine-glutamine (SQ) or threonine-glutamine (TQ) sequence, sometimes flanked by acidic residues [41]. However, some SQ/TQ sequences are not phosphorylated, and other proteins that do not contain SQ or TQ sequences also can be phosphorylated efficiently by DNA-PK, including the carboxyl-terminal domain of the large subunit of RNA polymerase II and c-Fos [45].

II.3. Immunological Reagents

Biochemical studies of the Ku/DNA-PK antigens and determination of their subcellular distribution have been facilitated by the availability of a wide variety of murine monoclonal antibodies (mAbs), some of which are listed in Table 3. These include mAbs specific for p70, p80, the p70/p80 heterodimer, and DNA-PK$_{cs}$ [4,5,7,10,13,47–53]. All anti-p80 mAbs described so far are reactive with primate

Table 3. Partial List of Murine Monoclonal Antibodies Specific
for Components of DNA-PK

mAb	Isotype	Specificity	Reference	Notes*
111	IgG1	p80 (aa 610–705)	[4,50]	recognizes primate Ku only; IP, IF, IB
S10B1	IgG1	p80 (aa 8–221)	[13,50]	recognizes primate Ku only; IP, IF, IB
N9C1	IgG1	p80 (aa 1–374)	[13,36,50]	recognizes only free p80; IP, IF, IB
N3H10	IgG2b	p70 (aa 506–541)	[13,50]	human p70: IF, IB, IB; murine p70: IB only
S5C11	IgG1	p70[†]	[13,50]	IF, IB, IP
162	IgG2a	p70/p80 dimer	[4,51]	recognizes human or rodent heterodimer; IP, IF
18-2	IgG[†]	DNA-PK$_{cs}$	[7,52]	IF, IP, IB
25-4	IgG[†]	DNA-PK$_{cs}$	[52]	IF, IP, IB
42-27	IgG[†]	DNA-PK$_{cs}$	[53]	IF, IP, IB

*Species specificity, if known and applications; IF = immunofluorescence; IP = immunoprecipitation; IB = immunoblotting. [†]Incomplete information.

(human or simian) Ku, but not with rodent or insect homologues, whereas other mAbs, such as 162 (anti-p70/p80 dimer) and N3H10 (anti-p70) exhibit at least partial crossreactivity. The large number of anti-Ku mAbs may reflect the strong antigenicity of human Ku in mice. In contrast to the many anti-Ku mAbs, only three mAbs specific for DNA-PK$_{cs}$ are available ([7,52,53]; see Table 3).

II.4. Subcellular Distribution of Ku and DNA-PK$_{cs}$

Ku antigen was originally reported to have a speckled nucleoplasmic distribution by indirect immunofluorescence staining of human liver section cells using polyclonal autoimmune sera [3]. However, in later studies utilizing mAbs, intense nucleolar staining of human tissue culture cells was seen (Figure 3) [4,5]. The explanation for this discrepancy remains unclear, and could lie in the cell substrate used for immunofluorescence or else differences in the epitopes recognized by autoimmune sera and murine mAbs. There have been reports that the Ku antigen is a cell surface antigen [54–56], but so far there is not definitive evidence that Ku is an intrinsic membrane protein. In addition, although there is little evidence at present for a cytoplasmic form of Ku antigen, that possibility has not been excluded completely.

In mitosis, Ku is associated with the condensing chromosomes in early prophase cells (Figure 4). However, by late prophase, it appears in some studies to be distributed within the cytoplasm ([57]; see Figure 4). Ku remains in a cytoplasmic

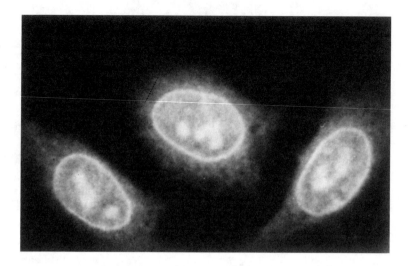

Figure 3. Intracellular distribution of Ku in interphase cells. Interphase HeLa cells were stained with anti-Ku mAb 162 followed by FITC-conjugated goat anti-mouse IgG antibodies. Cells were photographed using an MRC-600 Confocal Laser Scanning System equipped with filters for FITC (anti-Ku). Note the irregular nuclear and intense nucleolar staining by anti-Ku mAbs, and the bright staining at the nuclear periphery.

distribution until late telophase. Double staining with antibodies to lamin B (a nuclear envelope protein) and Ku also suggests that Ku antigen is largely cytoplasmic during most of mitosis, and that its transport into the nucleus after cell division is delayed until after the nuclear envelope reforms (Figure 5). However, other studies suggest that Ku remains associated with the chromosomes at least through metaphase [49].

Immunofluorescence studies of DNA-PK$_{cs}$ reveal that its intracellular distribution is similar to that of Ku [7]. In mitosis, DNA-PK$_{cs}$ is distributed primarily in the cytoplasm, consistent with the distribution of Ku (Figure 6).

II.5. Tissue and Species Distribution of Ku and DNA-PK$_{cs}$

For reasons that are unexplained, primate cells contain 40- to 60-fold more Ku antigen than rodent cells, whereas the level of Ku in bovine cells is intermediate between primate and rodent cells (Figure 7) [10,30,50,58], despite comparable levels of Ku mRNA in mice and humans [58]. It also has been shown that DNA-PK activity is reduced greatly in rodent cells [45]. However, since enzymatic activity is Ku-dependent, it is not yet certain whether this reflects the absence of Ku or of DNA-PK$_{cs}$. The functional significance of low levels of Ku antigen in non-primate cells is not known. Interestingly, human cells contain ~400,000 Ku molecules per cell [59], far higher than the 16–40 double strand breaks induced by 1 Gy of ionizing irradiation. Thus, it has been pointed out that the amount of Ku in a human cell appears to far exceed what is needed for DNA repair ([60]; see §5.1). The low levels of Ku in rodent cells might, therefore, be of little consequence for

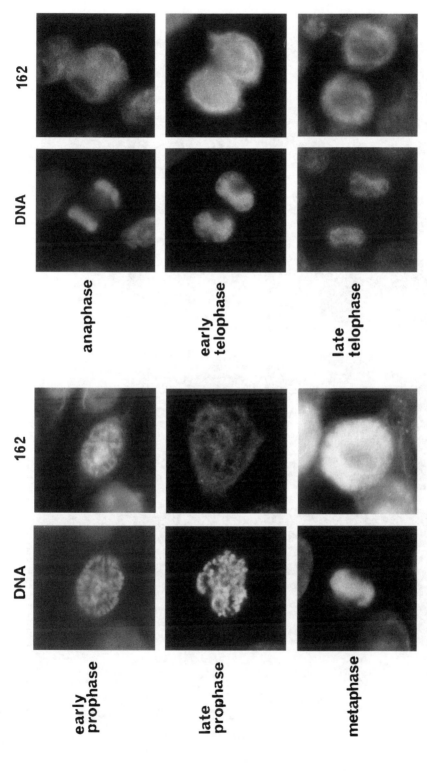

Figure 4. Double staining of mitotic cells for DNA and Ku. Mitotic HeLa cells in early prophase, late prophase, metaphase, anaphase, early telophase, and late telophase were stained with propidium iodide (PI) to demonstrate DNA (left), and with anti-Ku mAb 162 (right). Binding of 162 was detected using FITC-conjugated goat anti-mouse IgG antibodies. Single cells were photographed using an MRC-600 Confocal Laser Scanning System equipped with filters for FITC (anti-Ku) and rhodamine (used to detect PI staining). Note the co-localization of Ku and DNA staining in early prophase, but not later in mitosis.

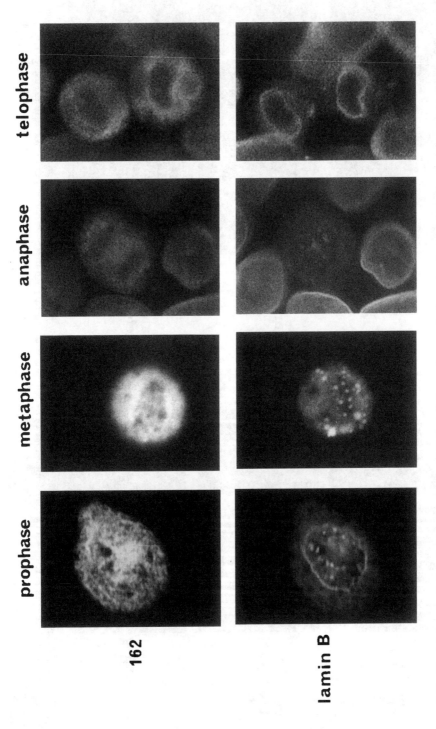

Figure 5. Double staining of mitotic cells for Ku and lamin B. HeLa cells in prophase, metaphase, anaphase, and telophase were stained with anti-Ku mAb 162 plus human autoimmune serum containing anti-lamin B antibodies. Binding of 162 was detected using rhodamine-conjugated goat anti-mouse IgG, and binding of human anti-lamin B antibodies with FITC-conjugated goat anti-human IgG antibodies. Single cells were viewed and photographed using an MRC-600 Confocal Laser Scanning System equipped with FITC and rhodamine filters.

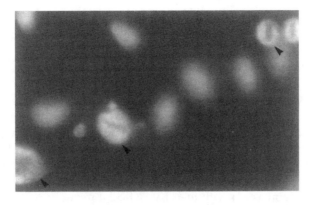

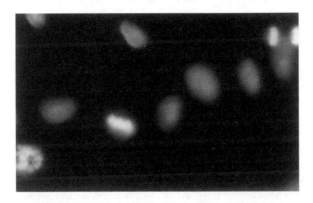

Figure 6. Intracellular distribution of DNA-PK$_{cs}$. HeLa cells were double stained with anti-DNA-PK$_{cs}$ mAb 25-4 plus propidium iodide (PI). Binding by mAb 25-4 was detected using FITC-conjugated goat anti-mouse IgG antibodies. Cells were viewed and photographed using a Leitz epifluorescence microscope equipped with FITC and rhodamine (for PI staining) filters. FITC staining (DNA-PK$_{cs}$) is shown above (mitotic cells are indicated by arrowheads); PI staining of DNA in the same cells is shown below.

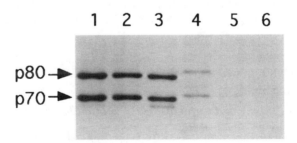

Figure 7. Ku antigen in various species. HeLa (human cervical carcinoma, lane 1), K562 (human erythroleukemia, lane 2), COS (green monkey kidney, lane 3), MDBK (bovine kidney, lane 4), SP2/0 (murine myeloma, lane 5) and L929 (murine fibroblast, lane 6) cell lines were labeled with [^{35}S] methionine and cysteine and cell extract (1.5×10^6 cell equivalents per lane) was immunoprecipitated using anti-Ku mAb 162 as described [36]. The immunoprecipitates were analyzed by SDS-PAGE. Note low levels of Ku antigen in murine and bovine cell lines, compared with human and simian cells.

DNA repair. However, the low level of DNA-PK in non-primate cells could cause other functional differences (see §5).

Ku and DNA-PK$_{cs}$ have been detected in all normal human cell types and tissues examined to date with the exception of mature neutrophils [61]. Immature neutrophils and the promyelocytic leukemia cell line HL-60 contain Ku as well as DNA-PK$_{cs}$ ([61]; A.K. Ajmani et al., unpublished data). Preliminary observations in our laboratory suggest that the components of DNA-PK are lost during the myelocyte stage of granulocyte differentiation. The loss of Ku and DNA-PK$_{cs}$ appears to be an active process, since the half-life of both subunits is several days [61]. This may be related to the fact that mature neutrophils are committed to undergo cell death by apoptosis (see §5.2). Interestingly, mature neutrophils are highly sensitive to ionizing radiation [62], consistent with their Ku-deficient phenotype.

II.6. Posttranslational Modification of Ku and DNA-PK$_{cs}$

The first evidence for posttranslational modification of the Ku70 and Ku80 subunits was the demonstration of multiple isoforms having slightly different pI values on 2D-gels [10,11,63]. Interestingly, the distribution of these isoforms differed between growth-arrested and proliferating cells [10,63]. Although phosphorylation of Ku could not be confirmed in the original studies, it was shown later that both p70 and p80 are phosphorylated on serine [35]. Phosphothreonine or phosphotyrosine residues have not been detected. The p80 subunit carries a site that potentially could be phosphorylated by nuclear kinase II [64]. Both p70 and p80 Ku are also targets for DNA-PK in vitro, and DNA-PK$_{cs}$ is autophosphorylated [6]. The consequences, if any, of phosphorylation of these proteins on DNA-PK function are unknown.

It also has been shown that p80 can undergo site-specific proteolytic cleavage if it is bound to DNA [65]. This releases an 18 kDa carboxyl-terminal polypeptide, converting Ku into a dimer (termed Ku') of p70 with a truncated (69 kDa) fragment derived from the amino-terminal portion of p80. The Ku' dimer is resistant to further proteolysis, and retains end-binding activity. The protease(s) responsible for this site are sensitive to leupeptin and chymostatin, and are inhibited by raising the pH from 7.0 to 8.0. Cleavage of the carboxyl-terminal domain of Ku80 could have important consequences for the function of DNA-PK, particularly in the inactivation and/or disassembly of the DNA-PK complex once it has phosphorylated its DNA-bound substrates.

III. MOLECULAR CLONING, CHROMOSOMAL LOCATION, AND EXPRESSION

III.1. Molecular Cloning and Chromosomal Location Ku70 Gene

Human Ku70 cDNAs were obtained by screening γt11 expression libraries with high titer human autoimmune sera [54,66,67]. A single mRNA of ~2.4 kb hybridizing with p70 cDNAs is identified by northern blot analysis in human cells and tissues [54,66]. The predicted amino acid sequence encoded by the open reading frame was verified by sequencing peptides generated by protease treatment of the intact p70 protein (the N-terminus of the protein is blocked) [66]. The cDNAs encode a 609 amino acid protein of predicted molecular mass 69,842 Da and pI 6.19 (Figure 8A). Homologues of human p70 in mouse [58], hamster (E. Hendrickson,

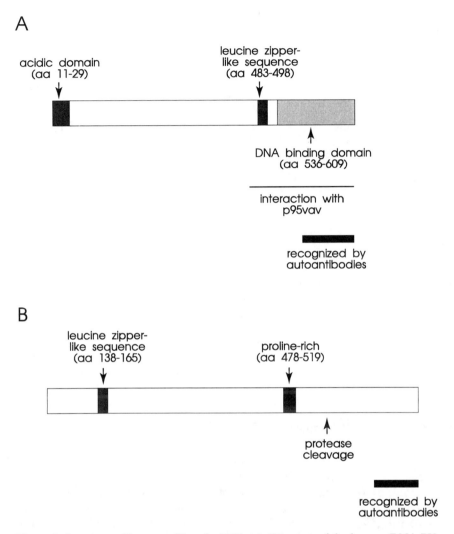

Figure 8. Structure of human p70 and p80 Ku. **A**: Diagram of the human DNA-PK$_{cs}$ protein, showing locations of prominent structural features. Amino acids 11–29, acidic domain; amino acids 483–498, leucine zipper-like sequence; amino acids 536–609, DNA binding domain; amino acids 460–609, interaction with p95^{vav}; amino acids 560–609, major epitope recognized by human autoantibodies on western blots. **B**: Diagram of the human p80 protein, showing locations of prominent structural features. Amino acids 138–165, leucine zipper-like sequence; amino acids 478–519, proline-rich region; amino acids 682–732, major epitope recognized by human autoantibodies on western blots. Approximate location is indicated of a site that is proteolytically cleaved when p80 is bound to DNA, releasing a ~18 kDa fragment.

personal communication), and *Drosophila* [21,38], as well as putative tick (*Rhipicephalus appendiculatus*, G.C. Paesen and P.A. Nuttall, unpublished data, GENBANK accession number 1063592), and yeast (*Saccharomyces cerevisiae*, [68]) homologues also have been identified (Table 4A). The human and murine sequences are 83% identical at the amino acid level, and the human and *Drosophila* sequences are

Table 4A. Ku70 Homologues in Other Species

Species	% identity with human	kDa (aa)	Reactivity with mAbs	Chromosome
Human	(100)	69.9 (609)	N3H10, S5C11	22q13
Mouse	82.9	(608)	N3H10*	n.a.
Drosophila	24	72.4 (631)	none	3, position 86E
Yeast	21.8[†]	(602)	none	–

*Reactive on immunoblots but not with native antigen. [†]Overlap of 298 amino acids (aa 226–578 of yeast protein and aa 213–556 of human p70). n.a. = not available.

Table 4B. Ku80 Homologues in Other Species

Species	% identity with human	kDa (aa)	Reactivity with mAbs	Chromosome
Human	(100)	(732)	111, S10B1, N9C1	2q34-36
Mouse	77.6	(732)	none	n.a.
Hamster	80.3	(732)	n.a.	n.a.
Drosophila	n.a.	85 (n.a.)	none	n.a.

n.a. = not available.

24% identical and 51% similar [21]. The candidate yeast p70 protein exhibits 21.8% identity with human Ku70 over a 298 amino region (aa 226–578), but considerably lower sequence similarity over the rest of the sequence (Table 4A). The Ku70 gene has been localized to human chromosome 22q13 using fluorescence in situ hybridization (Table 5) [69]. The *Drosophila* homologue appears to be located on the right arm of chromosome 3 ([38] and P. Wensink, personal communication).

The deduced amino acid sequence of Ku70 does not have significant homology with other proteins in the PIR database. However, several structural features of the antigen are apparent. All mammalian Ku70 proteins studied thus far have a strongly acidic domain located at the amino-terminus (Figure 8A). This region is also present in *Drosophila*. The acidic domain resembles, in some respects, acidic transcriptional activator domains found in certain transcription factors. These regions are thought to interact with other components of the transcriptional [70] or DNA replication [71] machinery. However, it is not known whether or not the acidic amino-terminal domain of p70 influences the level of transcriptional activation. Finally, a leucine zipper-like sequence is found between amino acids 483 and 498, although it is not known whether or not this region is involved in protein–protein interactions.

III.2. Molecular Cloning and Chromosomal Location of the Ku80 Gene

Human Ku80 cDNAs encoding a 732 amino acid protein were obtained by screening expression libraries with either murine mAbs or human autoimmune sera

Table 5. Chromosomal Locations of V(D)J Recombination Mutants

Protein	Chromosome[a]	Group[b]	DSB repair[c]	V(D)J[d]
Ku70	22q13	mutants not yet reported	expected to be deficient	expected to be abnormal
Ku80	2q33-35	XRCC5 (sxi, xrs)	deficient	coding and signal
DNA-PK$_{cs}$	8p11-q12	XRCC7 (scid)	deficient	coding only
38 kDa	5q11.2-13.3	XRCC4 (XR-1)	deficient	signal → coding
RAG1	11p13	[RAG1 knockout]	normal	coding and signal
RAG2	11p13	[RAG2 knockout]	normal	coding and signal

[a]Human chromosome location. [b]Complementation group. [c]Repair of double-stranded DNA breaks induced by ionizing radiation. [d]Defect in V(D)J recombination after transfection with RAG1/RAG2 plus either pJH200 (signal joining) or pJH290 (coding joining).

[64,72–74]. Sequence analysis of cDNAs obtained from human liver and spleen libraries has shown that the p80 protein is encoded by mRNAs of ~2.7 and 3.4 kb [64,72] that may be derived from a common gene containing alternative poly-adenylation sites [72]. The deduced amino acid sequence of human p80 indicates a molecular mass of 82,592 Da and pI 5.34 (Figure 8B). The predicted sequence was verified by N-terminal amino acid sequencing. Mouse [75], Chinese hamster (*Cricetulus griseus*, [60]), but not yeast or insect, homologues have been sequenced (Table 4B). The human and mouse sequences are 77.6% identical at the amino acid level. A *Drosophila* homologue of ~85 kDa has been reported, but cDNAs have not been cloned. The Ku80 gene is located on human chromosome 2q34-36 [69]. Analysis of the Ku80 sequence reveals a leucine zipper-like sequence at positions 138–165, and a proline-rich domain (amino acids 478–519). Like Ku70, the deduced amino acid sequence of Ku80 does not have significant homology with other proteins.

III.3. Molecular Cloning and Chromosomal Location of the DNA-PK$_{cs}$ Gene

The sequence of the human DNA-PK$_{cs}$ protein was reported within the past few months [39,76] after screening a γt10 library with oligonucleotides based on partial amino acid sequences. A single mRNA of >12 kb hybridizing with the cDNAs is identified by northern blot analysis. Although initial estimates suggested the size of the protein was ~350 kDa, the cDNAs isolated encode a 4,096 amino acid protein having a predicted molecular mass of 465,482 Da and pI 6.9 (Figure 9A). The DNA-PK$_{cs}$ gene has been localized to chromosome 8p11-q12 [77–79] (Table 5). In addition to an extensive domain showing sequence homology with the phospha-tidylinositol 3-kinase superfamily (see §4.5), DNA-PK$_{cs}$ contains multiple SQ motifs (potential autophosphorylation sites) as well as a long leucine zipper sequence, which may mediate interactions with Ku or other proteins (Figure 9).

A

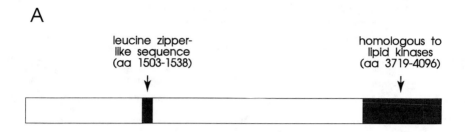

B

Protein	Identity with DNA-PKcs	similarity to DNA-PKcs
TOR2 (yeast)	34% (42/123)	51% (63/123)
TOR1 (yeast)	34% (42/123)	49% (61/123)
FRAP (human)	28% (42/149)	44% (67/149)
ATM (human)	36% (28/76)	57% (44/76)
PI3-kinase (human)	30% (17/56)	58% (33/56)

Figure 9. Structure of human DNA-PK$_{cs}$. **A**: Diagram of human DNA-PK$_{cs}$ protein, showing locations of prominent structural features. Amino acids 1503–1538, leucine zipper-like sequence; amino acids 3719–4096, domain exhibiting homology to lipid kinases. **B**: Comparisons of DNA-PK$_{cs}$ sequence with the sequences of selected members of the phosphatidylinositol 3-kinase (PI3-kinase) superfamily. Amino acids 3719–4096 of were compared with database sequences of yeast TOR-1 and TOR-2, human FKBP-rapamycin associated protein (FRAP), the ataxia telangiectasia protein (ATM), and human PI3-kinase using the BLASTP algorithm (National Center for Biotechnology Information). Percent identity and similarity, as well as the number of identical or similar residues over the total length of the overlap, are indicated.

IV. FUNCTIONAL DOMAINS OF DNA-PK

IV.1. DNA Binding

The association of Ku with DNA was first suggested by its release from nuclei by deoxyribonuclease I (DNase) treatment [4,5] and by the co-immunoprecipitation of DNA along with Ku antigen by mAbs [4,34]. Ku antigen also is associated with chromosomes in early prophase cells [57] (Figure 4). Specific binding of Ku to ends of double stranded (ds) DNA was reported in 1986 [59]. DNA–RNA heteroduplexes, supercoiled closed circular DNA, and yeast tRNA bind very poorly to Ku. Binding to linear dsDNA is independent of whether the ends are blunt, or 5'- or 3'-recessed. In DNase I footprinting assays, both 3' and 5' end-labeled double stranded DNA termini are protected, providing further evidence that Ku has end-binding activity. In addition to dsDNA ends, there is evidence that Ku interacts with closed circular single-stranded DNA [12], single-stranded nicks or gaps, single to double strand transitions, and closed stem-loop "dumbbell" structures [22, 80,81].

Although Ku will bind to any dsDNA end regardless of its sequence [82], there have been reports that certain sequences are bound preferentially. This could be explained by preferential binding to A-T-rich termini [12,73], or to specific sequences, such as promoter sequences [12–14,22]. However, the protection of DNA by Ku binding is influenced by the translocation of Ku along DNA fragments and by the prior binding of other factors [12,15]. Thus, interactions with site-specific DNA binding factors might enhance the apparent binding affinity, causing the binding of Ku to appear specific for particular sequences.

Southwestern blot analysis suggests that p70 can bind DNA, whereas p80 cannot [59,83,84]. The binding of DNA to p70 on nitrocellulose membranes requires a prolonged renaturation step, but not the formation of p70/p80 heterodimers [83, 84]. The domain mediating interactions of p70 with DNA has been mapped by southwestern blotting and DNA immunoprecipitation assays [84]. The minimal sequence required for binding to linear target DNA in vitro consists of amino acids 536–609. Deletion of amino acids 601–609 abrogates DNA binding as well as reactivity with human autoimmune sera containing autoantibodies to this region (see §8.3). In contrast to these data, however, studies using in vitro translated p70 and p80 subunits suggest that dimerization may be necessary for efficient DNA binding [85]. Nevertheless, the binding of recombinant (vaccinia virus) p70 to DNA exhibits comparable salt sensitivity to that of the p70/p80 heterodimer [86]. Moreover, the p70 protein binds preferentially to ends of dsDNA, one of the defining features of Ku DNA binding activity [86]. Thus, p70 appears to have a critical role in DNA binding. The contribution of p80 is an area of continuing research interest. It is possible that p80 increases the affinity of DNA binding, or alters the interaction in some other, thus far undefined, manner.

IV.2. Nuclear Localization

Expression of Ku antigen in rabbit kidney (RK13) cells using a recombinant vaccinia viruses suggests that p70 contains a nuclear localization sequence (NLS) [51]. The sequence KVTKRK (amino acids 539–544) resembles a "typical nuclear localization sequence," defined as four (K + R) residues in a hexapeptide stretch [87]. Using recombinant baculoviruses to express fragments of human p70 in Sf-9 insect cells, we have obtained evidence that a nuclear localization sequence is carried on amino acids 505–609 (J. Wang et al., unpublished data), consistent with the possibility that the sequence KVTKRK mediates nuclear import. Interestingly, dimerization of p70 fragments carrying the putative NLS with NLS-less p80 constructs led to nuclear import of p80 as well as p70, suggesting that one subunit of Ku can mediate nuclear localization of the other.

The free p80 protein also undergoes nuclear transport, suggesting that it too carries a nuclear localization signal. It has been suggested that the sequence TAKKLK (amino acids 563–568) could be the p80 NLS [64]. The DNA-PK$_{cs}$ sequence also has several potential "typical" nuclear localization sequences, but there is little information at present to indicate which portion of the protein mediates nuclear transport. However, since assembly with Ku antigen appears to occur on DNA [88], it is likely that DNA-PK$_{cs}$ contains one or more nuclear localization sequences, or else interacts transiently with another factor that facilitates its nuclear transport.

IV.3. p70/p80 Dimerization

The p70 and p80 Ku subunits consistently appear at approximately equal intensities in immunoprecipitates and comigrate in sucrose density gradients, strongly suggesting that they form a dimer [4,5]. In addition, an mAb that recognizes the p70/p80 dimer and prevents its dissociation has been described [51]. Although both p70 and p80 contain leucine zipper-like sequences [64,66], it remains uncertain whether or not these regions mediate dimerization. Studies to address this question have been hampered by the difficulty in assembling p70/p80 heterodimers in vitro, although some progress has been made in this respect recently [29]. Small quantities of intact p70/p80 heterodimer can also be assembled by in vitro translation of the two subunits [85]. However, assembly occurs most efficiently in the intracellular milieu. The assembly of Ku heterodimers has been investigated using viral expression systems [51,89]. Since non-primate cells contain exceedingly low levels of Ku antigen (see above), the recombinant human Ku antigen can be detected readily using anti-Ku mAbs when expressed in non-primate cells.

Ku (p70/p80) heterodimers form efficiently in RK13 cells coinfected with recombinant vaccinia viruses expressing each of the two subunits (p70-vacc and p80-vacc, respectively) [36,51]. The half-life of the heterodimer is >16 h in vaccinia-infected cells; in uninfected cells, the half-life is five days or more [36,61]. The free p70 subunit also is expressed efficiently in RK13 cells, with a half-life comparable to that of the p70/p80 dimer. In striking contrast, however, the half-life of free p80 is <1.5 h [36]. In contrast, the half-life of p80 in coinfected RK13 cells is comparable to that of p70, suggesting that p80 is rescued from intracellular degradation by dimerizing with p70. Figure 10 illustrates the stabilization of p80 by dimerization with p70 in RK13 cells. Although p70 can be expressed well in singly infected cells, p80 is expressed at high levels only if co-expressed with p70. Marked differences in the half-lives of the free Ku subunits are observed between different cell lines. In murine L-929 cells, both free p70 and free p80 have extremely short half-lives, and dimerization rescues both subunits from proteolytic degradation. This pattern also is exhibited by the Chinese hamster V79 derivative XR-V15B [60]. This p80 mutant cell line contains very low levels of p70, and the p70 levels can be restored by transfecting the cells with hamster p80. A third pattern is seen in Sf-9 insect cells infected with recombinant baculoviruses expressing the subunits of human Ku. In these cells, both p70 and p80 both can be expressed at high levels without dimerization ([89] and J. Wang et al., unpublished data). There is also evidence that human-rabbit [51] and human-hamster [90–92] dimers can form, although the human p80-hamster p70 dimer seems to have reduced activity in double strand break repair [60,90–92].

The phenomenon of subunit stabilization as a consequence of dimerization also is seen in pulse-chase studies of uninfected human K562 (erythroleukemia) cells [36]. The effects of DNA-PK$_{cs}$ binding on the p70, p80, and DNA-PK$_{cs}$ subunit half-lives are not known. Posttranslational stabilization of individual subunits of DNA-PK conferred by assembly into complexes complicates the analysis of cell

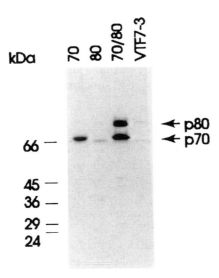

Figure 10. Post-translational stabilization of p80 as a consequence of dimerization with p70. RK13 cells were transfected with plasmids pBKS-p70 and/or pBKS-p80 in which human p70 and p80, respectively, were cloned behind the T7 promoter of the vector pBKS (+). After transfection, cells were infected with recombinant vaccinia virus VTF7-3 directing the synthesis of T7 RNA polymerase [242]. Cells were labeled with [^{35}S] methionine and cysteine, and extracts were analyzed 20 h after infection by immunoprecipitation with anti-Ku mAbs N3H10 (anti-p70), 111 (anti-p80), or 162 (anti-p70/p80 dimer). Immunoprecipitation of control transfected cells after VTF-7 infection using mAb 162 is shown on the right. Positions of molecular weight markers in kDa are indicated on the left. Note that p80 protein is expressed at high levels only in cells co-transfected with both p70 and p80 plasmids, whereas p70 protein is expressed at high levels either after transfecting p70 plasmid alone, or after cotransfecting the p70 and p80 plasmids.

lines with DNA-PK mutations. For example, knocking out p70 expression in the K562 cell line would be predicted to decrease the cellular level of p80 considerably. This may make it difficult to establish which subunit of DNA-PK is abnormal in a mutant cell line without actually sequencing the mutation. For example, p70 expression is deficient xrs-5 cells, even though these cells are thought to carry a mutation in the p80 gene [90,93].

The posttranslational stabilization of Ku subunits by dimerization may have consequences for regulating cellular levels of DNA-PK. Pulse-chase studies indicate that K562 cells contain a pool of unassembled p70 subunits that is available to dimerize with newly synthesized p80 [36]. The availability of unassembled p70 subunits may ensure that newly synthesized p80 assembles into dimers before it can be degraded. It is of interest that certain insect cells, including salivary gland cells from *Trichosia pubescens* [37] and *Drosophila* Kc [38], but not Kc0 [21,94] cells appear to contain predominantly, or exclusively, unassembled p70 subunits. The explanation for the absence of p80 in Kc cells is uncertain, however, since the p80 positive Kc0 cell line is a Kc derivative adapted for growth in serum-free medium (P. Wensink, personal communication). So far, although a pool of free p70 can be detected in some cell lines, human or other mammalian cells that express exclusively unassembled p70 have not been described. Identification of p70(+)/p80(–) mammalian cells would be of interest in relationship to the insect cell lines reported previously. Since free p70 has DNA end-binding activity, the expression of p70 in the absence of p80 could have important functional consequences.

IV.4. Interaction of Ku with p95^{vav}

Although Ku appears to function primarily in the nucleus, it may bind to certain cytoplasmic factors, with possible implications for cellular signaling. An interaction of p70 Ku with p95^{vav}, a protooncogene product expressed in hematopoietic cells, has been reported recently [95]. Using the yeast two-hybrid system, it was shown that p70 Ku interacts with amino acids 813–837 of Vav, part of the carboxyl-terminal Src homology 3 (SH3) domain. The interaction does not involve binding of the SH3 domain to a proline-rich domain of Ku, as would be expected. Instead, p95^{vav} binds to amino acids 463–609 of p70, a region containing the DNA binding domain as well as a leucine zipper-like motif. The leucine zipper (amino acids 483–498) is not sufficient for the interaction with p95^{vav}. p95^{vav} is a cytoplasmic protein expressed only in cells of the hematopoietic lineage [96]. It contains a series of structural motifs found in intracellular signaling molecules, and is tyrosine phosphorylated upon activation of hematopoietic cells through their surface receptors, such as the B cell IgM receptor complex [97] or the T cell receptor–CD4 complex [96]. However, the precise role of Vav in cellular signaling is unknown. Interestingly, in addition to containing phosphotyrosine residues, p95^{vav} is phosphorylated on serine and threonine [96] and contains three SQ and one TQ sequences.

   Although Vav has been reported to be a cytoplasmic protein [98], it contains two possible nuclear localization sequences, although these normally are inactive. It is possible that posttranslational modification could expose these sequences, allowing Vav to enter the nucleus and bind to Ku. Alternatively, the association of p95^{vav} with p70 could facilitate its nuclear transport.

IV.5. Homology Of DNA-PK$_{cs}$ with Members of the Phosphatidylinositol (PI) 3-Kinase Family

Analysis of the predicted amino acid sequence of DNA-PK$_{cs}$ revealed that the carboxyl-terminal ~380 amino acids exhibit sequence homology with the catalytic domains of members of the phosphatidylinositol (PI) 3-kinase superfamily [39,76] (Figure 9B). These proteins fall into two subgroups. The first includes the 110 kDa subunit (p110) of mammalian PI3 kinase and several other proteins. DNA-PK$_{cs}$ falls into the second subgroup, which includes the yeast FKBP12 rapamycin binding proteins Tor1p, Tor2p, and their human homologue FRAP, the yeast rad3 protein, and the ataxia telangiectasia gene product (ATM). Despite significant sequence homology with PI3 kinases, DNA-PK$_{cs}$ does not appear to phosphorylate lipids [39]. The proteins in subgroup 2 are involved in cell cycle control, DNA repair, and DNA damage responses, and lipid phosphorylation does not appear to be a feature of any of the proteins of this subgroup. Like DNA-PK$_{cs}$, the other proteins in this subgroup may be protein kinases instead of lipid kinases. The lipid kinase p110 is associated with a regulatory component that links it to activated growth factor receptors. Similarly, the Ku subunit links DNA-PK$_{cs}$ to DNA. Since ATM and rad3, like DNA-PK$_{cs}$, are involved in DNA repair, it is possible that Ku-like factors targeting the other members of subgroup 2 to DNA will be found [99,100].

IV.6. Interaction of Ku with DNA-PK$_{cs}$

In view of the sequence homology of the carboxyl-terminal portion of DNA-PK$_{cs}$ with the catalytic domains of lipid kinases, it is likely that this region carries the protein kinase activity. This may imply that the large amino-terminal portion of the protein is involved in interactions with Ku antigen or other proteins. Thus far, little is known concerning the domains of Ku mediating its interaction with DNA-PK$_{cs}$. Since DNA-PK$_{cs}$ appears to assemble with Ku on DNA [88], it is possible that Ku antigen undergoes a conformational change upon binding DNA that allows DNA-PK$_{cs}$ to bind. That possibility would be consistent with preliminary evidence from our laboratory suggesting that both p70 and p80 may contribute to the interaction with DNA-PK$_{cs}$ (J. Wang et al., unpublished data).

V. FUNCTIONS OF DNA-PK

V.1. DNA Repair and V(D)J Recombination

There has been considerable interest recently in the role of DNA-PK in repairing double stranded DNA breaks. This has been reviewed recently [101,102], and will be discussed here only in general terms. Hamster and mouse cell mutants with increased sensitivity to ionizing radiation have been studied extensively to identify genes involved in DNA repair [103,104]. Hamster cell lines have been especially useful for generating double strand break (DSB) repair mutants because they are functionally haploid, making it easier to obtain mutants. DSB repair mutants fall into nine or more complementation groups. Three groups, designated XRCC4, XRCC5, and XRCC7 (Table 6) exhibit similar phenotypes, characterized by the inability to repair X-ray induced DSBs as well as defective V(D)J recombination in transfection assays [101,103,104]. They retain the ability to repair single-stranded breaks induced by UV irradiation or other agents. Efforts to identify the defective gene in the XRCC5 complementation group by transferring single human chromosomes using the microcell-mediated chromosome transfer technique led to the realization that this mutation is located on human chromosome 2q25 [105,106]. Interestingly, this region was close to the location of the p80 gene identified previously [69]. This led to investigation of whether the end binding activity of Ku might be involved in DSB repair. Indeed, it was found that cells in the XRCC-5 group were defective in DNA end-binding activity, and that the X-ray sensitivity of the XRCC5 cell lines xrs-6, XR-V15B, and sxi-3 could be corrected partially by stably transfecting the human p80 gene, but not by transfecting the human p70 gene [90–92]. All XRCC5 mutants exhibit decreased stable transfection efficiencies suggesting that Ku antigen may be involved in nonhomologous recombination [107]. Interestingly, this property is not shared by XRCC7 (scid) mutants ([101,108]; see Table 7).

Table 6. Double Strand Break Repair Mutants

Group	Cell line	Derivative of	Species
XRCC5	xrs-1, xrs-2, xrs-3, xrs-4, xrs-5, xrs-6	CHO-K1	Chinese hamster
	sxi-1, sxi-2, sxi-3, sxi-4	V79-4	Chinese hamster
	XR-V15B*	V79	Chinese hamster
	XR-V9B*	V79B	Chinese hamster
XRCC7	scid	BALB/c scid mouse	Mouse
	V-3	AA8 (CHO-K1 derivative)	Chinese hamster
XRCC4	XR-1	CHO-K1	Chinese hamster

*Mutations have been characterized: XR-V15B has a 138 bp deletion (46 amino acids, from codon 372-417 of p80); XR-V9B has a 252 bp deletion (84 amino acids, from codon 267-350 of p80); neither of these mutations shifts the reading frame [60].

Table 7. Comparison of *XRCC5* (Ku80) and *XRCC7* (DNA-PK$_{cs}$) Mutations

Characteristic	XRCC5	XRCC7
V(D)J recombination: coding joints	defective	defective
V(D)J recombination: signal joints	defective	normal
X-irradiation; γ-irradiation	sensitive	sensitive
Stable transfection (non-homologous recombination)	decreased efficiency	normal
Topoisomerase II inhibitors (etoposide)	sensitive	normal
UV irradiation	normal	normal
Alkylating agents (MMS)	normal	normal

Since V(D)J recombination is defective in cells with defective DSB repair [109–112], the effect of transfecting Ku80 on the V(D)J recombination defect in *XRCC-5* mutant cells was investigated. The V(D)J recombination mechanism has been reviewed recently [101,113], and will summarized only briefly. In the process of V(D)J recombination, three separate gene segments encoding the variable (V), diversity (D) and joining (J) regions are juxtaposed to form a contiguous exon. The V, D, and J segments are each flanked by recombination signal sequences (RSS) [114]. V(D)J recombination involves cleavage of the DNA at two recombination signal sequences (RSS) by the lymphocyte-specific recombination activating proteins RAG-1 and RAG-2 (reviewed in [115]). The RSS sequences consist of a highly conserved palindromic heptamer sequence and a less conserved nonamer sequence, separated by 12 or 23 base pair spacers. One of each type of spacer is required (reviewed in [101]). This process results in the generation of DSBs that are subsequently repaired by non-lymphocyte specific components of the DSB repair machinery.

After the cleavage step, noncoding sequences are circularized, and the coding ends are modified further by the addition of non-templated nucleotides by the lymphocyte-specific enzyme terminal deoxytransferase (TdT). It has been proposed that a hairpin-ended DNA serves as an intermediate prior to joining the two coding ends, thus explaining the presence of additional "palindromic" or P residues at certain coding ends (reviewed in [101,116]). The imprecise joining of coding ends is an additional source of variable region diversity. Until recently, the non-lymphocyte-specific proteins that repair DSBs generated by V(D)J recombination have been poorly characterized.

RAG-1 and RAG-2 are the lymphocyte-specific protein components required for introducing site-specific DNA breaks during V(D)J recombination [117–119]. Expression of RAG-1 and RAG-2 in a non-lymphoid cell is sufficient to enable V(D)J recombination to take place if plasmids carrying recombination substrates are cotransfected [112,117,120]. Mutant cell lines from the XRCC5 group exhibit defective formation of signal (RSS) joints as well as coding joints when transfected with RAG-1, RAG-2, and the recombination template plasmids pJH200 (RSS joints) or pJH290 (coding joints) [90–92,112]. These defects can be corrected by stably transfecting the cells with the p80 gene, suggesting that a mutation in p80 Ku is responsible for both the V(D)J recombination defect and their X-ray sensitivity [90–92]. This was proved recently in the case of the XR-V15B and XR-V9B mutants (Table 6), both of which contain deletions in the p80 coding sequence [60].

It has been known for some time that severe combined immunodeficiency (SCID) defect in mice is associated with the lack of V(D)J recombination (reviewed in [121]), as well as a generalized defect in DSB repair [109–111]. However, in contrast to the V(D)J recombination defect in XRCC5 cells, the scid mutation causes abnormal joining of coding segments, but not signal sequences ([122]; see Table 5). Minicell transfer experiments have shown that human chromosome 8 can complement the scid defect [123]. In addition, SCID cell lines (hamster V3, murine SCVA2, the human glioma cell line M059J, and fibroblast lines from equine SCID) as well as primary murine SCID fibroblasts are deficient in DNA-PK$_{cs}$ protein expression [53,78,124,125]. Moreover, DNA-PK activity is deficient in SCID cells [78,125]. However, DNA-PK$_{cs}$ mRNA is present in equine SCID cells [125]. These data suggest that the SCID mutation affects the DNA-PK$_{cs}$ gene itself, or that it is a mutation in a gene influencing the expression of DNA-PK$_{cs}$ protein. The former possibility is supported by the localization of the DNA-PK$_{cs}$ gene to chromosome 8q11 by in situ hybridization [79]. This is the same chromosomal location as XRCC7. Thus, although it is not yet formally proved, the bulk of available information strongly suggests that the scid defect is caused by mutation of the DNA-PK$_{cs}$ gene.

V.2. Apoptosis

In view of the role of DNA-PK in DSB repair, it was of interest to examine its effects on the DSBs introduced during apoptosis. Apoptosis is a process of programmed cell death in which cells are eliminated in a controlled fashion [126,127]. It is characterized by cell shrinkage, chromatin condensation, and DNA fragmentation, although there are reports that apoptosis can occur without DNA fragmentation in certain cell lines [128]. A variety of signals lead to induction of, or protection from, apoptosis. These signals may be external, e.g., withdrawal of viability factors, growth factors or glucocorticoid hormones, signaling through cell surface receptors, such as APO-1 (fas), or exposure to cytotoxic anticancer agents or ionizing radiation [129,130]. Alternatively, the signals may be internal, as in the case of deregulated cellular oncogene expression.

One of the features common to many forms of apoptosis is the generation of DSBs by protease-activated nucleases [131]. DNA-PK would be expected to oppose this process by facilitating the repair of these breaks. Consistent with that possibility, human neutrophils, a cell type that is irreversibly committed to undergo programmed cell death, are devoid of Ku antigen [61] (Figure 11). Interestingly, neutrophils are also sensitive to ionizing radiation [62]. In contrast, both Ku and DNA-PK$_{cs}$ are present at relatively high levels in the human promyelocytic leukemia cell line HL-60. However, both antigens are absent by FACS analysis of HL-60 cells undergoing spontaneous apoptosis [61]. The same is true of T cells undergoing activation-induced apoptosis. Since the half-lives of Ku and DNA-PK$_{cs}$ are considerably longer than the 48 h between mitogen stimulation and analysis of the apoptotic cells for antigen expression, these data suggest that the components of DNA-PK undergo active degradation, presumably by proteases activated during apoptosis. In support of that interpretation, it has been shown recently that DNA-PK$_{cs}$ is cleaved by an interleukin 1 converting enzyme (ICE)-like protease within 3 h of an apoptosis-inducing stimulus, resulting in the appearance of a stable 150 kDa degradation product [132]. No detectable cleavage of Ku is seen at this early timepoint, however. The protease mediating this cleavage is sensitive to iodoacetamide and tosyl-L-lysine chloromethyl ketone (TLCK), but not to leupeptin, antipain, pepstatin A, chymostatin, phenylmethylsulfonyl fluoride (PMSF), E-64, acetyl-leucyl-leucyl-normethional, or the ICE-specific inhibitor N-(N-Ac-tyr-val-ala)-3-amino-4-oxobutanoic acid [132], suggesting that the protease is not ICE itself. However, the pattern of inhibitor sensitivity was identical to that displayed by poly-(ADP-ribose) polymerase, which is cleaved by the ICE homologue CPP32 [133]. The same enzyme also may be involved in cleavage of DNA-PK$_{cs}$ in apoptotic cells.

V.3. DNA-Dependent ATPase and Helicase Activity

Besides serving as the DNA end binding activity of DNA-PK, there is some evidence that Ku itself may have enzymatic activity. For instance, it has been reported recently that Ku antigen has a single stranded DNA-dependent ATPase activity [28]. A cellular DNA-dependent ATPase activity upregulated by DNA-PK mediated phosphorylation appears to be similar or identical to Ku on the basis of the molecular weights of its subunits, sequence analysis of tryptic peptides, and immunological crossreactivity with anti-Ku antibodies. Moreover, photoaffinity labeling studies suggest that both p70 and p80 contain ATP binding sites [28,29]. The ATPase activity of this complex is not associated with helicase activity [27].

In contrast, Ku was reported by another group to have helicase activity as well as single-stranded DNA dependent ATPase activity [29]. The preferred substrate for the helicase activity appears to be a fork-like structure containing a single to double

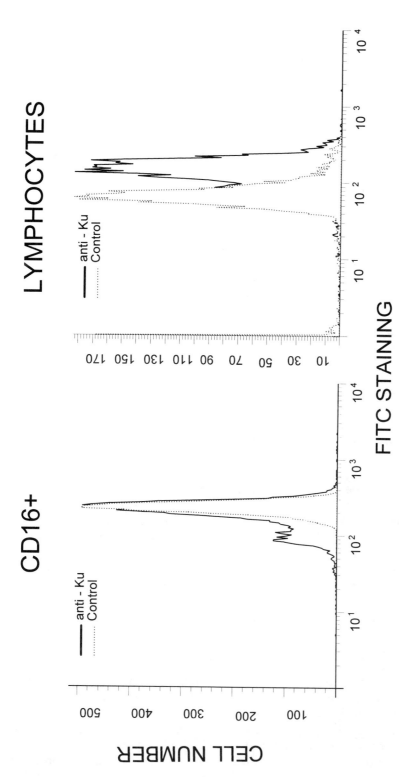

Figure 11. Absence of Ku in human neutrophils. Human peripheral blood neutrophils and lymphocytes were isolated and surface stained with anti-CD16 mAb followed by intracellular staining with anti-Ku mAb 162 or isotype control (PAb 101, anti-SV40 large T antigen) [61]. Intracellular staining was analyzed by FACS after gating on the neutrophil (CD16+ cells, left) or lymphocyte (right) populations. Staining of neutrophils (left) by 162 is no different than the negative control. In contrast, 162 staining of lymphocytes is considerably more intense than the control staining (right).

strand transition. Although this activity required single stranded DNA, Ku binds poorly to single stranded DNA substrates [59]. However, single to double strand transitions are bound efficiently [80]. The genes encoding the 72 and 87 kDa subunits of this factor were cloned, and have sequences identical to those of p70 and p80 Ku. Recombinant subunits expressed in bacteria could be assembled into dimers displaying partial DNA binding and helicase activity, but it was not shown that the biochemically purified factor or recombinant heterodimer had ATPase activity. Moreover, the possibility that Ku copurifies with helicases present mammalian cells and in prokaryotic cells cannot be excluded entirely. The problem of copurification of other antigens with Ku also has arisen in examining the role of Ku in transcription (see §5.5).

In addition, single stranded DNA binding proteins, including the T4 gene 32 product, *E. coli* single stranded DNA binding protein (SSB), and replication factor A (RPA) appear to cause ATP-independent DNA strand separation [134,135]. It may be relevant, therefore, that DNA-PK$_{cs}$ phosphorylates the 34 kDa subunit of RPA, raising the possibility that DNA-PK is associated, at least transiently, with RPA [42–44]. Moreover, the 70 kDa subunit of RPA could comigrate with p70 Ku on SDS gels. For the above reasons, the designation of Ku antigen as a helicase should probably be viewed as tentative until confirmed by further studies.

V.4. Possible Role of Ku in Chromosomal Translocations

Chromosomal translocations involving certain oncogenes play an important role in the pathogenesis of lymphomas, leukemias, and other neoplastic diseases [136]. The distribution of chromosomal translocations in a particular disease, such as t(14;18) translocations in follicular B cell lymphomas or t(9;22) in chronic myeloid leukemia, is not random. For example, in follicular lymphomas, in which the *BCL2* gene is fused to the immunoglobulin heavy chain locus, 70% of the translocations occur within a 100 bp segment of the untranslated portion of *BCL2* exon 3 [137,138]. This short segment has been termed the major breakpoint region. In view of the importance of specific DSBs and the possible involvement of the V(D)J recombinase system in some B and T cell tumors [139], DNA-PK and/or Ku antigen could play a role in the pathogenesis of chromosomal translocations. Consistent with that possibility, it has been shown recently that a portion of the BCL2 major breakpoint region carries a helicase binding site, and that Ku antigen is at least one component of the helicase binding complex [138]. The interaction of Ku with this region appears to be cell cycle regulated, suggesting that Ku or associated factors might play a direct role in generating chromosomal translocations, instead of merely recognizing fortuitously generated DSBs.

V.5. Transcription

Ku has been proposed to serve a role in transcription because of its association of with DNase I hypersensitive sites and certain transcriptionally active nuclear domains such as the nucleolus [35], its association with transcriptionally active chromosome puffs in insects [37], and the structure of the p70 subunit [66]. Many studies suggest that binding of Ku to specific DNA sequences can enhance or repress transcription [12–15,18–20,22,24,25,94,140–143]. However, it is difficult to be certain whether the transcriptional effects of Ku are mediated through binding to a particular sequence or class of sequences or by interactions with other sequence-specific DNA binding factors, or if it is a general property related to the "nonspecific" end binding activity of Ku to DNA.

One possibility is that Ku antigen exhibits both specific and nonspecific DNA binding activity under different conditions. This may be the case for yolk protein factor I (YPF1), a transcription factor that is likely to be a *Drosophila* homologue of Ku. YPF1 activity is required for normal steady state levels of yolk protein 1 (yp1) mRNA in vivo, and is detected at high levels in late stages of *Drosophila* oogenesis and embryogenesis, but is present only at low levels in larvae or adult males ([94,140]; P. Wensink, personal communication). The β subunit (69 kDa) displays 24% identity with the human p70 sequence (Table 4A) [21]. Antibodies raised against the 85 kDa α subunits are immunologically crossreactive with human (HeLa cell) Ku, but human autoantibodies do not recognize the *Drosophila* protein [21]. The sequence of the α subunit is not yet known. YPF1, a heterodimer of the two subunits, exhibits binding to a 31 bp sequence within the coding region of the yp1 gene as well as "nonspecific" end binding. In the presence of 0.1 M NaCl, YPF1 has nonspecific, extremely high affinity, end binding activity, whereas at 0.4 M NaCl, the sequence specific DNA binding activity is seen after the factor moves to an internal site on the DNA strand (P. Wensink, personal communication). Interestingly, the DNA binding properties of the α/β dimer may be quite different from those of the free β subunit, which appears to exhibit sequence specific binding to inverted repeats of the P transposable element [38].

Another explanation for apparent sequence specific binding is that Ku could interact with other sequence-specific DNA binding proteins, as in the case of TREF, a Ku-like factor that binds the transferrin promoter [14,15]. TREF interacts specifically with the transcriptional control element (TRA) of the transferrin promoter [14]. The purified factor contains two subunits (TREF-1 and TREF-2) that are probably identical to p70 and p80 Ku. However, highly purified fractions containing these proteins no longer exhibit sequence-specific binding to TRA, while displaying nonspecific DNA binding characteristic of Ku [15]. The sequence specific binding activity of less highly purified fractions appears to be carried by an additional factor termed TRAC that co-purifies with Ku. Interestingly, the sequence recognized by TRAC is similar to other promoter sequences with which Ku associates, including the proximal sequence element of the U1 snRNA gene [13], the 31 bp sequence element recognized by YPF1 [140,144], the E3 enhancer of the T cell receptor β chain [141], and the cAMP responsive element CRE [15]. One interpretation of these data is that the apparent sequence specificity of Ku binding to DNA seen in several systems is a consequence of its association with sequence-specific factors. This could reflect either a direct, functional association with Ku or an in vitro artifact of the techniques used to purify sequence specific DNA-binding factors.

The behavior of DNA-PK in nucleoli is perhaps the best evidence so far implicating Ku and/or DNA-PK in transcriptional regulation. The fact that DNA-PK phosphorylates several transcription factors in vitro, including Sp1, c-Jun, c-Fos, and others, as well as RNA polymerase II (Table 2), provides indirect evidence that Ku is involved in transcriptional regulation. The intense nucleolar immunofluorescence in tissue culture cells stained by anti-Ku mAbs [4,5,49] contrasts with the lack of nucleolar immunofluorescence in liver sections stained with human autoimmune serum. Nucleolar localization of Ku antigen also has been shown in quiescent (G0) human peripheral blood lymphocytes [145]. However, 48–72 h after mitogen stimulation, nucleolar staining is nearly absent, despite increased levels of p70 and p80 mRNAs. It is unclear why the B cells, which would should not be activated by PHA, also apparently exhibited little nucleolar staining. The absence of Ku in nucleoli after PHA activation was interpreted as indicating that nucleolar localization was limited to early G1. However, an alternative explanation is that nucleolar expression of Ku is lost as a consequence of growing the cells in culture. Another possibility is that Ku associates with nucleoli only in quiescent cells, and that it either is absent in the nucleoli of cycling cells, or else extracted during fixation of cells that have entered the cell cycle, as seen in the case of proliferating cell nuclear antigen [146].

Studies with human autoimmune sera suggest that Ku antigen is associated with certain transcriptionally active regions of the genome of the sandfly *Trichosia pubescens* [37]. Interestingly, Ku was present in transcriptionally active chromosome puffs characterized by RNA polymerase II transcription. In contrast, the chromosome puff containing the nucleolar organizer region was devoid of Ku, despite having high transcriptional activity, as indicated by intense incorporation of RNA precursors and the presence of large amounts of DNA/RNA hybrids.

The negative association of Ku antigen with the level of ribosomal gene transcription was confirmed using in vitro RNA polymerase I transcription systems [147–149]. As is true of transcription by RNA polymerases II and III, RNA polymerase I transcription involves assembly on the ribosomal promoter of a multiprotein complex consisting of RNA polymerase I as well as a series of additional factors [150,151]. In mice, the factor TIF-IB (equivalent to SL1 in humans and Rib1 in *Xenopus*), which is itself a multisubunit complex containing the TATA binding protein, recognizes the ribosomal promoter. This complex binds to an abundant DNA-binding protein called upstream binding factor (UBF). UBF is identical to NOR-90, an autoantigen recognized by sera from certain patients with scleroderma [152,153]. UBF stimulates RNA polymerase I transcription by facilitating the formation of transcription complexes and by competing with a repressor factor for the binding of TIF-IB (SL1, Rib1). The repressor factor is a dimer of 75 and 90 kDa proteins, both of which can be crosslinked to DNA by UV light [151]. This activity can be removed by immunodepleting with human anti-Ku antibodies, suggesting that the repressor is identical or closely related to Ku. The repression is ATP-independent, and it is thought that Ku mediates repression at the ribosomal DNA promoter by a "promoter occlusion" mechanism [148,151].

It was found subsequently that DNA-PK represses RNA polymerase I transcription approximately ten times more efficiently than Ku alone [148]. Moreover, transcriptional repression by DNA-PK required ATP hydrolysis, since unlike repression by Ku alone, it was inhibited by the nonhydrolyzable ATP and GTP analogues AMP-PNP and GMP-PNP, and by the protein kinase inhibitor 6-dimethylaminopurine (DMAP). Moreover, it could be inhibited by human anti-Ku antibodies. Interestingly, RNA polymerase II transcription is not repressed, strongly suggesting that DNA-PK acts on a factor specific for promoter-directed RNA polymerase I transcription [149]. The repression of RNA polymerase I transcription appears to have little effect on factor-independent transcriptional initiation or elongation [148]. Finally, phosphorylation of TIF-IB (or a cofractionating protein) by DNA-PK decreases RNA polymerase I transcription in vitro [148,149]. It also has been suggested that DNA-PK and protein phosphatase I may affect the level of phosphorylation of TIF-IB (SL1) antagonistically [149].

The recently described localization of the overexpressed RAG-1 and RAG-2 proteins to the nucleoli and the nuclear periphery [154] is reminiscent of the distribution of Ku in HeLa cells (Figure 3). This raises the possibility that the nuclear and/or nucleolar localization of the RAG proteins is due to protein–protein interactions with components of DNA-PK, or that Ku, RAG-1, and RAG-2 interact with the same nucleic acid targets. Binding to DNA breaks introduced during V(D)J recombination could explain the colocalization of the RAG proteins with Ku at the nuclear periphery, since there is evidence that immunoglobulin genes are anchored on insoluble components of the nucleus, such as the nuclear matrix or nuclear lamina [155]. Anchorage of DNA to the nuclear periphery or matrix appears to be important for both DNA replication [156] and transcriptional activation [155,157], and also could facilitate V(D)J recombination. It is not yet clear, however, why the RAG-1 and RAG-2 proteins, which assemble at recombination sequences found in the immunoglobulin and T cell receptor genes [119], become associated with ribosomal DNA.

VI. MECHANISMS OF AUTOANTIBODY PRODUCTION IN SLE

The Ku antigen was identified originally during the course of investigating the mechanisms of autoantibody production in SLE, and the genes for p70 and p80 were cloned using SLE sera. As has been the case for many of the autoantigens recognized by autoantibodies in SLE patients, the antigen recognized by anti-Ku autoantibodies has proved to be interesting biologically. Conversely, the extensive information now available regarding the function of Ku and its interactions with other factors is likely to have an important impact on future studies of the mechanisms of autoimmunity to chromatin in general, and to double stranded DNA in particular. Studies of the biology of Ku antigen function may facilitate understanding of how immune responses to macromolecular particles arise in SLE. Most, if not all, of the major lupus autoantigens consist of multicomponent particles, frequently consisting of both proteins and nucleic acid [2]. Before discussing what is known about how autoimmunity to Ku develops, the general features of autoantibody production in SLE will be reviewed, emphasizing current understanding of how multicomponent antigens, such as Ku, are seen by the immune system.

VI.1. Characteristics of Autoantibody Production in SLE

Antinuclear antibodies are central to the pathogenesis of SLE, but the mechanisms of autoantibody production remain incompletely understood. Several characteristics of lupus autoantibodies are consistent with the view that they are produced in response to antigen in a T cell dependent manner. First, these antibodies are produced at extremely high titers, and may represent up to 15% of the total immunoglobulin in certain patients [158]. For instance, the titers of anti-Ku sera used for cloning the Ku cDNAs ranged from 10^{-6} to 10^{-7} [66,74]. Second, only a small subset of the thousands of nuclear proteins is selected for an autoimmune response, and certain types of autoantibodies are highly specific markers for disease subsets [2]. For example, anti-Sm, anti-double stranded (ds) DNA, and anti-ribosomal P antibodies are virtually pathognomonic of SLE [2,159]. In contrast, autoantibodies to tRNA synthetases are associated almost exclusively with polymyositis or dermatomyositis, and are rare in SLE unless there is coexisting myositis [160]. Third, the antigens recognized by autoantibodies in these diseases are generally constituents of macromolecular complexes. "Linked sets" of autoantibodies to the individual components of a complex tend to be produced tandemly, and the autoantibodies frequently recognize multiple structurally and spatially distinct epitopes of that complex, suggesting that they are generated in response to antigen [58,161,162]. This view also is supported by the existence of numerous somatic mutations in the immunoglobulin V regions of murine autoantibody genes [163]. Thus, most evidence suggests that both B and T cells participate in autoantibody production in lupus. In healthy individuals, however, both B and T cell tolerance prevents this from occurring. There are three main mechanisms for avoiding autoimmunity. Autoreactive cells may be deleted (clonal elimination) or rendered anergic (clonal anergy). Alternatively, some self antigens are sequestered or prevented in other ways from encountering the immune system, resulting in a state of immunological ignorance.

VI.2. B Cell Tolerance

Studies with immunoglobulin and/or antigen transgenic mice have shown that all three of the above mechanisms, clonal elimination, clonal anergy, and ignorance, apply to B cells. In the case of multivalent antigens or membrane bound proteins, such as MHC class I molecules, immature B cells expressing transgenes encoding the rearranged genes for both chains of an autoantibody specific for the antigen never develop, and die by a two stage process terminating in apoptosis (reviewed in [164]). In contrast, B cells expressing a transgenic autoantibody specific for a soluble self antigen expressed in the bone marrow can mature, but do not secrete immunoglobulin — i.e., they become anergic. More recent studies suggest that B cell tolerance is multifactorial, and that the use of broad terms such as "deletion" or "anergy" may be insufficient to describe the multiple checkpoint mechanisms involved [164].

B cells recognizing certain soluble autoantigens expressed outside the bone marrow or sequestered away from the immune system can escape clonal elimination and anergy, and may escape to the periphery [164,165]. However, they generally do not proliferate or mature to autoantibody secreting cells because they require T cell help for activation. B cell non-responsiveness to many self antigens that are present at low levels (probably including nuclear antigens) appears to be controlled primarily by a lack of appropriate T cell help.

VI.3. T Cell Tolerance

The major mechanism for removing autoreactive T cells with high affinity antigen receptors involves clonal deletion in the thymus [166]. However, T cells expressing receptors specific for antigens not expressed in the thymus or T cells expressing low avidity/affinity receptors cannot be eliminated in this manner. Immunological tolerance to antigens not expressed in the thymus is maintained by peripheral inactivation of T cells [167,168]. Ligation of the T cell antigen receptor is insufficient, by itself, to activate naive T cells to proliferate or differentiate. Clonal expansion of T cells requires a second, costimulatory, signal that is delivered by antigen presenting cells [167]. In the absence of a costimulatory signal, T cell receptor occupancy by antigen can result in unresponsiveness (clonal anergy) or cell death by apoptosis.

Some self proteins are encountered by the immune system at levels too low to trigger either T cell activation or tolerance. This may reflect either low abundance or sequestration in immunologically privileged sites (reviewed in [169]). T cells able to recognize these antigens will not be activated nor will they be deleted or rendered anergic. They remain ignorant.

VI.4. Effect of Antigen Processing on the Expressed T Cell Repertoire

The expressed repertoire of T cells responsive to an exogenous antigen is focused onto a limited number of major T cell inducing determinants rather than being broadly directed against all portions of the antigen [170,171]. T cell repertoire is controlled, in part, by MHC-linked genes through a determinant selection mechanism in which immunodominant peptides bind to MHC molecules that can present the peptide, but not to MHC molecules that are unable to present the peptide [170,172]. Another factor influencing T cell repertoire is the existence of hindering structures on naturally processed fragments that differentially affect presentation by different MHC molecules [170,173]. Hindering structures that affect presentation by MHC molecules can include structural constraints imposed by the tertiary structure of a protein [174] as well as intermolecular contacts between the subunits of an oligomeric antigen [175,176]. For example, recognition of the human chorionic gonadotropin (hCG) α/β dimer by α-specific T cell hybridomas is dramatically reduced compared to free hCG-α or heat dissociated dimers, suggesting that the quaternary structure of hCG affects presentation of antigenic determinants of the monomers by interfering with proteolytic degradation into peptides capable of binding MHC molecules.

T cells responsive to minor antigenic determinants can evade tolerance by remaining ignorant due to the relatively low amounts of peptides suitable for MHC binding after in vivo processing of the intact antigen [177]. Autoreactive T cells can be activated under special circumstances, such as immunization with artificially processed self peptides. Although T cell responses to minor determinants are not stimulated under normal circumstances, they could be induced by crossreactive microbial antigens [178] or by altering the structure of a self antigen [179,180]. Once a response to a minor determinant is initiated, it can be perpetuated by self antigen because the conditions required to recall memory T cell responses are less stringent than those required to activate naive T cells [177,181].

VII. INDUCTION OF AUTOANTIBODIES IN EXPERIMENTAL SYSTEMS

VII.1. Molecular Mimicry

Immunological crossreactivity of a microbial antigen with a self antigen could lead to the production of a population of anti-microbial antibodies crossreacting with autoantigens. This has been termed "molecular mimicry" [182]. For instance, immunologically significant crossreactions have been reported between herpes simplex virus and intermediate filaments [183] and between a retroviral p30^{gag} protein and the U1 small nuclear ribonucleoprotein (snRNP) 70K protein [184]. Autoantibody production might begin as a monospecific response to an epitope shared by a microbial antigen and a self antigen, and receptor-mediated uptake of autoantigen by autoreactive B cells could broaden the autoantibody response by generating autoreactive T cells [184], a possibility supported by experimentally induced autoimmunity to cytochrome c [185]. Immunization of mice with foreign cytochrome c induces a population of antibodies cross-reactive with self cytochrome c. Adoptive transfer of B cells from mice primed with foreign cytochrome c to naive mice causes T cells of the recipient mice to respond to murine cytochrome c, suggesting that the autoreactive B cells can prime autoreactive T cells. Thus, although molecular mimicry may be limited initially to a single crossreactive epitope, B cells serving as APCs can cause diversification of the immune response. This could explain the diversity of autoantibodies specific for different epitopes of self antigens typical of SLE.

VII.2. Role of Intermolecular-Intrastructural Help

Another factor that may potentiate the spreading of autoimmunity is the activation of multiple B cell clones specific for components of a multicomponent antigen by T cells reactive with a single component. This has been termed "intermolecular-intrastructural help" [186]. There is considerable evidence that intermolecular-intrastructural help is involved in humoral immune responses to viral particles [187–190]. For example, T cells specific for the influenza nucleoprotein can help B cells specific for the hemagglutinin [187–189]. This also appears to be true for multicomponent self antigens, such as the U1 snRNP [191]. In the special case of a complex consisting of both foreign and self antigens, T cells specific for nonself components might drive the production of autoantibodies to the self components. For example, transgenic mice expressing the membrane-associated glycoprotein of vesicular stomatitis virus (VSV-G) do not produce autoantibodies to this "self" antigen when immunized with VSV-G in adjuvant or recombinant vaccinia virus expressing VSV-G, whereas autoantibodies are induced readily by infection with wild type VSV [192]. B cells specific for the transgenic self protein VSV-G may process intact VSV particles, resulting in presentation of nonself VSV peptides to T_h cells and autoantibody production.

Two recent reports are consistent with this mode of intermolecular-intrastructural spreading of autoimmunity [193,194]. Anti-Ro (SS-A) and anti-La (SS-B) antibodies frequently coexist in the sera of SLE patients, and the two antigens are at least transiently associated with one another in cells [2,195]. Immunization of mice with recombinant murine La protein resulted in the production of anti-La autoantibodies, suggesting that immunological ignorance may govern nonresponsiveness to La [194]. Interestingly, immunization with La also led to the production of anti-Ro antibodies. Conversely, immunization with Ro led to the production of anti-La as well as anti-Ro antibodies. Similar observations were made in the Sm/RNP system after immunizing with peptides derived from the Sm-B protein [193]. The simplest explanation for these observations is that T cells specific for the immunizing antigen are capable of stimulating B cells carrying receptors for different components of the Ro-La complex or U1 snRNP.

VII.3. *Altered Antigen Processing in Autoimmunity*

Since T cell tolerance to minor determinants self antigens may be incomplete [177,196], anything that increases the exposure of the immune system to minor antigenic determinants potentially could trigger autoimmunity. The possibility that complexes of self and nonself antigens can alter the normal pattern of antigen processing is raised by the pattern of processing of the oligomeric antigen, hCG [176]. The binding of a number of well-characterized viral oncoproteins, including SV40 large T antigen (SVT) [197,198], the 58 kDa E1B protein of adenovirus types 2 and 5 [199], and the E6 proteins of human papillomavirus [200], to the p53 tumor suppressor protein offers an opportunity to investigate whether the binding of foreign antigens to self proteins can promote autoimmunity. Mice immunized with purified complexes of murine p53 with SVT develop autoantibodies to p53 at titers up to 1:25,000, whereas mice immunized with either protein separately do not [179]. Once autoimmunity is established by immunizing with p53/SVT complexes, the anti-p53, but not the SVT, response can be boosted by immunizing the mice with murine p53. Thus, once autoimmunity to p53 is established, it can be maintained by self antigen. More recently it has been shown that p53-specific, class II restricted, CD4+ T cells become activated after immunizing mice with p53/SVT complexes (X. Dong et al., submitted for publication). Moreover, priming the mice with SVT did not enhance the production of autoantibodies when the mice were challenged subsequently with p53/SVT complexes, strongly suggesting that T cells specific for SVT did not provide intermolecular-intrastructural help to B cells specific for self p53. The simplest explanation of these results is that the binding of SVT alters the pattern of processing of p53 by antigen presenting cells, resulting in the presentation of cryptic self epitopes to which T cell tolerance in incomplete. Similar mechanisms could participate in the induction of autoantibody production in lupus or other autoimmune diseases.

VIII. AUTOIMMUNITY TO Ku AND DNA-PK$_{cs}$

New information on the roles of molecular mimicry, intermolecular-intrastructural help, and altered antigen processing in generating immune responses to multicomponent complexes may be relevant to the immunopathogenesis of anti-Ku antibodies. Obviously, understanding how these autoantibodies develop will require detailed information regarding the interactions of Ku antigen with other structures. As indicated above, that information is increasingly available.

VIII.1. *Ku as a Model of Autoimmunity to Chromatin Particles*

The autoimmune response to Ku in SLE is of interest because of the association of Ku antigen with DNA and in view of the pivotal role proteins may play in supplying T cell epitopes for anti-DNA antibody production [162,201]. Autoantibodies to double stranded (ds) DNA are produced nearly exclusively by patients with systemic lupus erythematosus (SLE), and are a useful diagnostic marker for the disease [2]. There is evidence that anti-dsDNA antibodies are involved directly in the pathogenesis of the kidney disease characteristic of SLE [202,203]. Anti-dsDNA antibody levels frequently increase when the disease is more active, and decrease during periods reduced activity [202]. Also, anti-dsDNA antibodies are enriched selectively in the renal glomeruli of patients with lupus nephritis [203]. Idiotypic markers of pathogenic anti-dsDNA antibodies have been identified [204–206], and finally, certain monoclonal anti-dsDNA antibodies are pathogenic when injected into mice [207] or expressed as transgenes [208,209].

Anti-DNA antibodies are produced by two subsets of B cells. Anti-DNA antibodies produced by the B1 (CD5+) subset are generally more specific for single-stranded (ss) DNA, and are predominantly IgM with low affinity and crossreactivity with other antigens [210,211]. Their role in the pathogenesis of lupus nephritis is uncertain [212]. In contrast, anti-DNA antibodies produced by the conventional B cell subset are typically IgG, have higher affinity for antigen, and are less crossreactive than those produced by the B1 subset. Pathogenic anti-dsDNA antibodies in both humans and lupus-prone mice frequently are of T cell dependent isotypes such as IgG2a and IgG2b in mice, and IgG1 in humans [213,214]. This is of interest because there is little evidence that T cells can recognize nucleic acids. For that reason, the possibility has been considered that proteins associated with DNA might be important in the pathogenesis of anti-DNA antibodies by providing epitopes recognized by the T cells helping anti-dsDNA antibody production [201]. Murine T cells that recognize epitopes of histones or HMG proteins can provide help for anti-DNA antibody production [201,215]. However, an immune response to histones is not always accompanied by the production of pathogenic anti-DNA antibodies. For instance, procainamide and certain other drugs induce a lupus-like syndrome associated with the production of anti-histone antibodies, but patients with drug-induced lupus rarely develop anti-dsDNA antibodies or kidney disease [216,217]. Similarly, patients with mixed connective tissue disease (MCTD) make autoantibodies to the 70K, A, and C proteins of U1 snRNP particles, whereas lupus patients make antibodies to the same proteins plus additional epitopes located on the physically associated B'/B, D, E/F, and G proteins [191,218]. It is not known why autoimmunity does not spread from the 70K, A, and C proteins to the other components of U1 snRNPs in MCTD.

VIII.2. General Features of Autoimmunity to Ku Antigen

Our laboratory encountered the Ku antigen while trying to identify DNA binding protein autoantigens that could provide T cell epitopes for anti-DNA antibodies [4]. Autoantibodies to Ku can be detected in a variety of autoimmune conditions. They were originally reported as a precipitin line distinct from other known lines in double immunodiffusion found in sera of 6 of 11 Japanese patients with polymyositis-scleroderma overlap syndrome (55% of patients in this rare subset), compared with 3 of 319 patients (1%) with other connective tissue diseases [3]. The high frequency of autoantibodies in the Japanese polymyositis-scleroderma overlap subset has been confirmed in subsequent studies [219–221]. However, by immunoprecipitation and ELISA, non-precipitating autoantibodies to Ku are relatively common in Japanese patients with SLE or scleroderma [221]. In American and European patients, anti-Ku antibodies are associated with SLE, scleroderma, and MCTD, but also have been detected in polymyositis, Sjögren's syndrome, rheumatoid arthritis, Grave's disease and primary pulmonary hypertension [4,54, 222,223]. Estimates of the prevalence of anti-Ku antibodies in American SLE patients vary widely [4,30,221,222]. This is likely to reflect at least partly marked differences in the prevalence of these antibodies in different racial groups ([224] and L. Stojanov et al., unpublished data). The titers of anti-Ku antibodies may be extremely high, and levels can increase during periods of increased disease activity in some patients [4,162].

Information regarding the HLA associations of anti-Ku antibodies is limited. However, there is some evidence for an association with the class II allele Dqw1 [222]. DQw1 was present in 17 of 19 (89%) anti-Ku positive patients, compared with 58% and 61% in white and black controls, respectively (relative risk 5.8). However, the number of patients was small, and HLA-DQw1 is a common allele in healthy individuals that is found at increased frequency in white SLE patients in general. Additional studies involving larger numbers of patients will be necessary to further define the influence of race and HLA alleles on the production of autoantibodies to Ku.

VIII.3. Specificities of Anti-Ku Antibodies

The association of anti-Ku antibodies with SLE as well as other diseases not characterized by anti-dsDNA antibody production suggests that poorly understood differences in the immune response could determine whether or not autoimmunity spreads from a DNA-binding protein to DNA. Although there is information on the fine specificities of anti-Ku antibodies, little is known about whether or not they exhibit disease-specific patterns.

The majority of human anti-Ku positive sera have little reactivity with p70 or p80 on immunoblots, but react strongly with the native antigen, suggesting that the major autoepitopes are conformational [74,162]. However, some sera do contain autoantibodies that recognize p70 or p80 after denaturation [30,50,162]. These autoepitopes have been mapped using fragments of p70 and p80 expressed as fusion proteins in bacteria [47,58,74,225,226]. At least four B cell epitopes of p70 have been reported. A major conformational autoepitope recognized by human autoimmune sera lies on amino acids 560–609 of p70 [58,74,226]. Interestingly, this region is located within the DNA binding domain (Figure 8A). Deletion of amino acids 560–571 or 601–609 eliminates antigenicity, and mutations in the vicinity of amino acids 585–595 reduce antigenicity substantially [58,227]. Deleting amino acids 601–609 also abrogates DNA binding activity, suggesting that DNA binding and autoantibody binding may both depend on the same structure. In another study, amino acids 315–609 appeared to be required for antigenicity of p70, and there was no reactivity of ten human autoimmune sera with fusion proteins carrying amino acids 551–609 or 514–609 [225]. The explanation for this apparent discrepancy is unclear, but could be related to the use of TrpE fusion proteins in some studies [58,74,226] and β-galactosidase fusion proteins in others [225]. Alternatively, it could reflect differences in the patient populations examined. Several minor epitopes of p70 also have been defined (amino acids 1–115, 506–535, and 115–467, respectively) [74,225]. Unfortunately, little is known at present about epitopes of native p70 that are recognized.

Like p70, p80 contains one or more major autoepitope(s) near its C-terminus [47,74,226] (Figure 8B). Minor autoepitopes have been localized to amino acids 1–374 and 558–681, respectively [74,226]. Functional domains of p80 remain poorly characterized, and it is unclear whether or not the major antigenic domain at the C-terminus of the molecule is a functional site. It is of interest that many human autoimmune sera with Ku activity have been reported to inhibit the interaction of Ku with DNA-PK$_{cs}$ [9], suggesting that they may contain autoantibodies to the interaction sites of either Ku or DNA-PK$_{cs}$. In view of the rarity of anti-DNA-PK$_{cs}$ antibodies (see below), the antibodies are more likely to recognize the interaction site of Ku. However, it is not known whether this site is located on p80, p70, or both proteins. Preferential reactivity of lupus sera with active or functional sites has been reported previously [228], but the explanation for this phenomenon is not known. It could reflect the fact that active/functional sites are generally located on the surface of a molecule, making them more accessible to B cell surface immuno-globulin, or biochemical features typical of both active sites and autoepitopes.

VIII.4. Autoantibodies to p70, p80, and DNA-PK$_{cs}$ Are Produced Tandemly

In certain patients, the levels of anti-p70 and anti-p80 antibodies rise and fall tandemly, consistent with an immune response directed against the Ku particle as a unit [162]. Studies of the recognition of recombinant, native p70 and p80 suggest that although autoantibodies to both subunits occur together in many sera, some sera contain extremely high titers of antibodies to p70 or p80 alone (J. Wang et al., manuscript in preparation).

Autoantibodies that recognize DNA-PK$_{cs}$ have been reported recently in association with anti-Ku antibodies (M. Satoh et al., *Clin. Exp. Immunol.* 105, 460, 1996). One type of autoantibody stabilizes the molecular interaction of DNA-PK$_{cs}$ with Ku, while another type recognizes biochemically purified DNA-PK$_{cs}$. Both types were strongly associated with anti-Ku antibodies. Notably, there is a hierarchy of autoantibodies recognizing different components of DNA-PK: autoantibodies recognizing biochemically purified DNA-PK$_{cs}$ were always associated with "stabilizing" antibodies, which were, in turn, always associated with anti-Ku antibodies. It is of interest that autoimmunity to DNA-PK$_{cs}$ is tightly linked to an anti-Ku response, despite the weak association between the two components. Since Ku is associated weakly with many other antigens, including DNA, histones, and p95^{vav}, autoimmunity to these antigens also may be linked to the production of anti-Ku antibodies. These data suggest that autoimmunity to Ku spreads to DNA-PK$_{cs}$, and raise the possibility that "stabilizing" autoantibodies could play a role in this process. Stabilizing antibodies could, for example, increase the concentration of intact DNA-PK available for uptake by antigen presenting cells. Stabilizing antibodies specific for components of the U1 snRNP have also been reported (M. Satoh et al., submitted for publication).

The physical linkage of many proteins to the same DNA fragment suggests that autoimmunity to any of these proteins could potentially spread to any of the other associated antigens as a consequence of intermolecular-intrastructural help. More-over, it is possible that under certain conditions, an immune response to a foreign DNA-binding protein, such as SV40 large T antigen, might spread to self antigens bound on the same fragment of DNA. The rules for this process are not yet understood. For instance, it is not known why anti-p80 antibodies sometimes occur at high titers in the complete absence of anti-p70. In the p53/SVT model, intermolecular-intrastructural help may facilitate the spreading of autoimmunity inefficiently (§7.3). Thus, other factors, such as altered antigen processing, could play a significant role in spreading.

Autoantibodies themselves could be a mechanism driving the spreading of autoimmunity. The binding of an antibody to an antigen might mimic the effect of the binding of SVT to p53 [179]. Thus, the interaction of antibodies with antigen could alter how the antigen is processed by antigen presenting cells, exposing cryptic epitopes. It has been shown previously that antibodies can either enhance or inhibit the processing of certain peptides [229–231]. In addition, there is evidence for the preferential coupling of T and B cell epitopes [232], and several recent studies suggest that epitopes recognized by T cells specific for lupus autoantigens are frequently located in close proximity to major B cell epitopes [193,232,233]. The fine specificity of autoantibodies produced against an antigen could play a key role in intramolecular diversification of the T cell response as well as intermolecular spreading [234,235]. Stabilizing antibodies that arise during an immune response to one protein could potentially alter antigen processing of an interacting antigen, either by physically covering it, or by impeding the dissociation of the complex. We are currently investigating whether this could explain the hierarchy of antibodies to different components of DNA-PK seen in lupus.

VIII.5. Potential Role of Molecular Mimicry in Spreading of Autoimmunity

In addition to associations between autoantibodies directed at different components of the same particle, there are associations between autoantibodies to apparently unrelated antigens. One example of this is the association of autoantibodies to Ku with autoantibodies to RNA polymerase II [236,237] and the Su antigen [238]. These associations are not readily explained by either intermolecular-intrastructural help or by the altered antigen processing model. It may be of interest, however, to note that the carboxyl-terminal domain (CTD) of RNA polymerase II is phosphorylated by DNA-PK [8] as well as other kinases [239]. Ku antigen, itself, as well as a series of other proteins, including replication protein A (RPA), another antigen recognized by human autoimmune sera [240,241], are also phosphorylated, primarily on SQ/TQ sequences, by DNA-PK (Table 2). It is conceivable that the structures recognized by DNA-PK also can be recognized by a subset of autoantibodies. An autoantibody recognizing a Ku sequence that is phosphorylated by DNA-PK might potentially crossreact with a phosphorylated DNA-PK site of another protein. In fact, certain human autoantibodies are highly specific for the phosphorylated form of the large subunit of RNA polymerase II [236,237], possibly explaining the association between anti-Ku and anti-RNA polymerase II antibodies. The striking association of autoantibodies specific for the phosphorylated form or RNA polymerase II and topoisomerase I (also a phosphoprotein) could be explained in this way, as well. Besides crossreacting with epitopes found on other phosphoproteins, autoantibodies to crossreactive phosphorylated epitopes could mediate spreading of autoimmunity to new epitopes of a crossreactive antigen by altering antigen processing (see above).

IX. CONCLUSION

The Ku antigen was discovered because it is the target of autoantibodies in patients with SLE and other systemic autoimmune disorders. It is one of a group of chromatin-associated autoantigens that may be important in generating pathogenic anti-DNA antibodies implicated in the development of lupus nephritis. Autoantibodies to Ku have been instrumental in the biochemical characterization of this antigen. The past several years have witnessed dramatic progress in understanding the biological role of Ku. Progress in this area is likely to lead to a more complete understanding of how autoimmunity to Ku and other components of chromatin develops. Autoimmunity might initiate as a consequence of altered antigen processing restricted to one or more chromatin components. Once autoimmunity to a single protein is induced, other mechanisms could spread autoimmunity to other components, including intermolecular-intrastructural help, molecular mimicry, and/or antibody-mediated spreading in which the binding of autoantibodies to an antigen alters processing of that antigen, resulting in the recruitment of additional populations of autoreactive T cells specific for cryptic epitopes.

ACKNOWLEDGMENTS

We thank Drs. Eric Hendrickson (Brown University), Pieter C. Wensink (Brandeis University), and Aziz Sancar (University of North Carolina) for helpful discussions. We also are grateful to Dr. B. Batten (BioRad) for assisting with the confocal microscopy, and Drs. T. Carter (St. John's University) and M. Knuth (Promega) for providing monoclonal antibodies N3H10 and 25-4, respectively. The vTF7-3 vector vaccinia virus was obtained from Drs. T. Fuerst and B. Moss through the AIDS Research and Reference Reagent Program, Division of AIDS, NIAID, NIH. This work was supported by grants R01-AR40391, P50-AR42573, P60-AR30701, T32-AR7416, and RR00046 from the United States Public Health Service. Dr. Wang is the recipient of a postdoctoral fellowship from the Arthritis Foundation.

NOTES

1. Lerner, M.R., and J.A. Steitz. 1979. Antibodies to small nuclear RNAs complexed with proteins are produced by patients with systemic lupus erythematosus. *Proc. Natl. Acad. Sci. USA* **76**, 5495–5499.
2. Tan, E.M. 1982. Autoantibodies to nuclear antigens (ANA): their biology and medicine. *Adv. Immunol.* **33**, 167–240.
3. Mimori, T., M.H. Akizuki, H. Yamagata, S. Inada, S. Yoshida, and M. Homma. 1981. Characterization of a high molecular weight acidic nuclear protein recognized by autoantibodies from patients with polymyositis-scleroderma overlap. *J. Clin. Invest.* **68**, 611–620.
4. Reeves, W.H. 1985. Use of monoclonal antibodies for the characterization of novel DNA-binding proteins recognized by human autoimmune sera. *J. Exp. Med.* **161**, 18–39.
5. Yaneva, M., R. Ochs, D.K. McRorie, S. Zweig, and H. Busch. 1985. Purification of an 86–70 kDa nuclear DNA-associated protein complex. *Biochim. Biophys. Acta* **841**, 22–29.

6. Lees-Miller, S.P., Y.R. Chen, and C.W. Anderson. 1990. Human cells contain a DNA-activated protein kinase that phosphorylates simian virus 40 T antigen, mouse p53, and the human Ku autoantigen. *Mol. Cell. Biol.* **10**, 6472–6481.

7. Carter, T., I. Vancurova, I. Sun, W. Lou, and S. DeLeon. 1990. A DNA-activated protein kinase from HeLa cell nuclei. *Mol. Cell. Biol.* **10**, 6460–6471.

8. Dvir, A., S.R. Peterson, M.W. Knuth, H. Lu, and W.S. Dynan. 1992. Ku autoantigen is the regulatory component of a template-associated protein kinase that phosphory-lates RNA polymerase II. *Proc. Natl. Acad. Sci. USA* **89**, 11920–11924.

9. Gottlieb, T.M., and S.P. Jackson. 1993. The DNA-dependent protein kinase: require-ment for DNA ends and association with Ku antigen. *Cell* **72**, 131–142.

10. Celis, J.E., P. Madsen, S. Nielsen, G.P. Ratz, J.B. Lauridsen, and A. Celis. 1987. Levels of synthesis of primate-specific nuclear proteins differ between growth-arrested and proliferating cells. *Exp. Cell Res.* **168**, 389–401.

11. Stuiver, M.H., J.E. Celis, and P.C. van der Vliet. 1991. Identification of nuclear factor IV/Ku autoantigen in a human 2D-gel protein database. *FEBS* **282**, 189–192.

12. de Vries, E., W. van Driel, W.G. Bergsma, A.C. Arnberg, and P.C. van der Vliet. 1989. HeLa nuclear protein recognizing DNA termini and translocating on DNA forming a regular DNA-multimeric protein complex. *J. Mol. Biol.* **208**, 65–78.

13. Knuth, M.W., S.I. Gunderson, N.E. Thompson, L.A. Strasheim, and R.R. Burgess. 1990. Purification and characterization of PSE1, a transcription activating protein related to Ku and TREF that binds the proximal sequence element of the human U1 promoter. *J. Biol. Chem.* **265**, 17911–17920.

14. Roberts, M.R., W.K. Miskimins, and W.K. Ruddle. 1989. Nuclear proteins TREF1 and TREF2 bind to the transcriptional control element of the transferrin receptor gene and appear to be associated as a heterodimer. *Cell Regulation* **1**, 151–164.

15. Roberts, M.R., Y. Hań, A. Fienberg, L. Hunihan, and F.H. Ruddle. 1994. A DNA-bind-ing activity, TRAC, specific for the TRA element of the transferrin receptor gene copurifies with the Ku autoantigen. *Proc. Natl. Acad. Sci. USA* **91**, 6354–6358.

16. Falzon, M., and E.L. Kuff. 1990. A variant binding sequence for transcription factor EBP-80 confers increased promoter activity on a retroviral long terminal repeat. *J. Biol. Chem.* **265**, 13084–13090.

17. Falzon, M., and E.L. Kuff. 1991. Binding of the transcription factor EBP-80 mediates the methylation response of an intracisternal A-particle long terminal repeat pro-moter. *Mol. Cell. Biol.* **11**, 117–125.

18. Falzon, M., J.W. Fewell, and E.L. Kuff. 1993. EPB-80, a transcription factor closely resembling the human autoantigen Ku, recognizes single- to double-strand transi-tions in DNA. *J. Biol. Chem.* **268**, 10546–10552.

19. Hoff, C.M., and S.T. Jacob. 1993. Characterization of the factor E1BF from a rat hepatoma that modulates ribosomal RNA gene transcription and its relationship to the human Ku autoantigen. *Biochem. Biophys. Res. Commun.* **190**, 747–753.

20. Hoff, C.M., A.K. Ghosh, B.S. Prabhakar, and S.T. Jacob. 1994. Enhancer 1 binding factor, a Ku-related protein, is a positive regulator of RNA polymerase I transcription initiation. *Proc. Natl. Acad. Sci. USA* **91**, 762–766.

21. Jacoby, D.B., and P.C. Wensink. 1994. Yolk protein factor 1 is a Drosophila homolog of Ku, the DNA-binding subunit of a DNA-dependent protein kinase from humans. *J. Biol. Chem.* **269**, 11484–11491.

22. May, G., C. Sutton, and H. Gould. 1991. Purification and characterization of Ku-2, an octamer-binding protein related to the autoantigen Ku. *J. Biol. Chem.* **266**, 3052–3059.

23. Genersch, E., C. Eckerskorn, F. Lottspeich, C. Herzog, K. Kuhn, and E. Poschl. 1995. Purification of the sequence-specific transcription factor CTCBF, involved in the con-

trol of human collagen IV genes: subunits with homology to Ku antigen. *EMBO J.* **14**, 791–800.

24. Li, G.C., S. Yang, D. Kim, A. Nussenzweig, H. Ouyang, J. Wei, P. Burgman, and L. Li. 1995. Suppression of heat-induced hsp70 expression by the 70-kDa subunit of the human Ku autoantigen. *Proc. Natl. Acad. Sci. USA* **92**, 4512–4516.

25. Kim, D., H. Ouyang, S. Yang, A. Nussenzweig, P. Burgman, and G.C. Li. 1995. A constitutive heat shock element-binding factor is immunologically identical to the Ku autoantigen. *J. Biol. Chem.* **270**, 15277–15284.

26. Wedrychowski, A., W. Henzel, L. Huston, N. Pasidis, D. Ellerson, M. McRae, D. Seong, O.M.Z. Howard, and A. Deisseroth. 1992. Identification of proteins binding to interferon-inducible transcriptional enhancers in hematopoietic cells. *J. Biol. Chem.* **267**, 4533–4540.

27. Vishwanatha, J.K., and E.F. Baril. 1990. Single-stranded-DNA-dependent ATPase from HeLa cells that stimulates DNA polymerase alpha-primase activity: purification and characterization of the ATPase. *Biochemistry* **29**, 8753–8759.

28. Cao, Q.P., S. Pitt, J. Leszyk, and E.F. Baril. 1994. DNA-dependent ATPase from HeLa cells is related to human Ku autoantigen. *Biochemistry* **33**, 8548–8557.

29. Tuteja, N., R. Tuteja, A. Ochem, A. Simoncsits, S. Susic, K. Rahman, L. Marusic, J. Chen, J. Zhang, S. Wang, S. Pongor, and A. Falaschi. 1994. Human DNA helicase II: a novel DNA unwinding enzyme identified as the Ku autoantigen. *EMBO J.* **13**, 4991–5001.

30. Francoeur, A.M., C.L. Peebles, P.T. Gompper, and E.M. Tan. 1986. Identification of the Ki (Ku, p70/p80) autoantigens and analysis of anti–Ki autoantibody reactivity. *J. Immunol.* **136**, 1648–1653.

31. Fritzler, M.J. 1992. Antibodies to nonhistone antigens in systemic lupus erythematosus. In Systemic Lupus Erythematosus. R. G. Lahita, editor. Churchill Livingstone, New York. 273–291.

32. Bernstein, R.M., S.H. Morgan, C.C. Bunn, R.C. Gainey, G.R.V Hughes, and M.B. Mathews. 1986. The SL autoantibody-antigen system: clinical and biochemical studies. *Ann. Rheum. Dis.* **45**, 353–358.

33. Nikaido, T., K. Shimada, M. Shibata, M. Hata, M. Sakamotos, Y Takasaki, and C. Sato. 1990. Cloning and nucleotide sequence of a cDNA for Ki antigen, a highly conserved nuclear protein detected with sera from patients with systemic lupus erythematosus. *Clin. Exp. Immunol.* **79**, 209–214.

34. Mimori, T., J.A. Hardin, and J.A. Steitz. 1986. Characterization of the DNA-binding protein antigen Ku recognized by autoantibodies from patients with rheumatic disorders. *J. Biol. Chem.* **261**, 2274–2278.

35. Yaneva, M., and H. Busch. 1986. A 10 S particle released from deoxyribonuclease-sensitive regions of HeLa cell nuclei contains the 86-kilodalton–70-kilodalton protein complex. *Biochemistry* **25**, 5057–5063.

36. Satoh, M., J. Wang, and W.H. Reeves. 1995. Role of free p70 (Ku) subunit in post-translational stabilization of newly synthesized p80 during DNA-dependent protein kinase assembly. *Eur. J. Cell Biol.* **66**, 127–135.

37. Amabis, J.M., D.C. Amabis, J. Kaburaki, and B.D. Stollar. 1990. The presence of an antigen reactive with a human autoantibody in Trichosia pubescens (Diptera: Sciaridae) and its association with certain transcriptionally active regions of the genome. *Chromosoma* **99**, 102–110.

38. Beall, E.L., A. Admon, and D.C. Rio. 1994. A Drosophila protein homologous to the human p70 Ku autoimmune antigen interacts with the P transposable element inverted repeats. *Proc. Natl. Acad. Sci. USA* **91**, 12681–12685.

39. Hartley, K.O., D. Gell, G.C.M. Smith, H. Zhang, N. Divecha, M. Connelly, A. Admon, S.P. Lees-Miller, C.W. Anderson, and S. Jackson. 1995. DNA-dependent protein kinase catalytic subunit: a relative of Phospatidylinositol 3-kinase and the ataxia telangiectasia gene product. *Cell* **82**, 849–856.

40. Jackson, S.P., J.J. MacDonald, S. Lees-Miller, and R. Tjian. 1990. GC box binding induces phosphorylation of Sp1 by a DNA-dependent protein kinase. *Cell* **63**, 155–165.

41. Bannister, A.J., T.M. Gottlieb, T. Kouzarides, and S.P. Jackson. 1993. c-Jun is phosphorylated by the DNA-dependent protein kinase in vitro: definition of the minimal kinase recognition motif. *Nucleic Acids Res.* **21**, 1289–1295.

42. Brush, G.S., C.W. Anderson, and T.J. Kelly. 1994. The DNA-activated protein kinase is required for the phosphorylation of replication protein A during simian virus 40 DNA replication. *Proc. Natl. Acad. Sci. USA* **91**, 12520–12524.

43. Pan, Z.Q., A.A. Amin, E. Gibbs, H. Niu, and J. Hurwitz. 1994. Phosphorylation of the p34 subunit of human single-stranded-DNA-binding protein in cyclin A-activated G1 extracts is catalyzed by cdk-cyclin A complex and DNA-dependent protein kinase. *Proc. Natl. Acad. Sci. USA* **91**, 8343–8347.

44. Boubnov, N.V., and D.T. Weaver. 1995. scid cells are deficient in Ku and replication protein A phosphorylation by the DNA-dependent protein kinase. *Mol. Cell. Biol.* **15**, 5700–5706.

45. Anderson, C.W., and S.P. Lees-Miller. 1992. The nuclear serine/threonine protein kinase DNA-PK. *CRC Crit. Rev. Eukaryotic Gene Exp.* **2**, 283–314.

46. Lees-Miller, S., K. Sakaguchi, S.J. Ullrich, E. Appella, and C.W. Anderson. 1992. Human DNA-activated protein kinase phosphorylates serines 15 and 37 in the amino-terminal transactivation domain of human p53. *Mol. Cell. Biol.* **12**, 5041–5049.

47. Wen, J., and M. Yaneva. 1990. Mapping of epitopes on the 86 kDa subunit of the Ku autoantigen. *Mol. Immunol.* **27**, 973–980.

48. Li, L.L., and N.H. Yeh. 1992. Cell cycle-dependent migration of the DNA-binding protein Ku80 into nucleoli. *Exp. Cell Res.* **199**, 262–268.

49. Higashiura, M., Y. Shimizu, M. Tanimoto, T. Morita, and T. Yagura. 1992. Immunolocalization of Ku-proteins (p80/p70): localization of p70 to nucleoli and periphery of bith interphase nuclei and metaphase chromosomes. *Exp. Cell Res.* **201**, 444–451.

50. Wang, J., C.H. Chou, J. Blankson, M. Satoh, M.W. Knuth, R.A. Eisenberg, D.S. Pisetsky, and W.H. Reeves. 1993. Murine monoclonal antibodies specific for conserved and non-conserved antigenic determinants of the human and murine Ku autoantigens. *Mol. Biol. Rep.* **18**, 15–28.

51. Wang, J., M. Satoh, A. Pierani, J. Schmitt, C.H. Chou, H.G. Stunnenberg, R.G. Roeder, and W.H. Reeves. 1994. Assembly and DNA binding of recombinant Ku (p70/p80) autoantigen defined by a novel monoclonal antibody specific for p70/p80 heterodimers. *J. Cell Sci.* **107**, 3223–3233.

52. Konno-Sato, S., J.M. Wu, and T.H. Carter. 1993. Phosphorylation of a 72-kDa nucleoprotein (NP-72) in HL-60 cells is mediated by the double-stranded DNA-dependent protein kinase (DNA-PK). *Biochem. Mol. Biol. Int.* **31**, 113–124.

53. Kirchgessner, C.U., C.K. Patil, J.W. Evans, C.A. Cuomo, L.M. Fried, T. Carter, M.A. Oettinger, and J.M. Brown. 1995. DNA-dependent kinase (p350) as a candidate gene for the murine SCID defect. *Science* (Wash. DC) **267**, 1178–1183.

54. Chan, J.Y.C., M.I. Lerman, B.S. Prabhakar, O. Isozaki, P. Santisteban, R.C. Kuppers, E.L. Oates, A.L. Notkins, and L.D. Kohn. 1989. Cloning and characterization of a cDNA that encodes a 70-kDa novel human thyroid autoantigen. *J. Biol. Chem.* **264**, 3651–3654.

55. Prabhakar, B.S., G.P. Allaway, J. Srinivasappa, and A.L. Notkins. 1990. Cell surface expression of the 70-kD component of Ku, a DNA-binding nuclear autoantigen. *J. Clin. Invest.* **86**, 1301–1305.

56. Ginis, I., S.J. Mentzer, X. Li, and D.V. Faller. 1995. Characterization of a hypoxia-responsive adhesion molecule for leukocytes on human endothelial cells. *J. Immunol.* **155**, 802–810.

57. Reeves, W.H. 1987. Antinuclear antibodies as probes to explore the structural organization of the genome. *J. Rheumatol.* **14** (Suppl 13), 97–105.

58. Porges, A., T. Ng, and W.H. Reeves. 1990. Antigenic determinants of the Ku (p70/p80) autoantigen are poorly conserved between species. *J. Immunol.* **145**, 4222–4228.

59. Mimori, T., and J.A. Hardin. 1986. Mechanism of interaction between Ku protein and DNA. *J. Biol. Chem.* **261**, 10375–10379.

60. Errami, A., V. Smider, W.K. Rathmell, D.M. He, E.A. Hendrickson, M.Z. Zdzienicka, and G. Chu. 1996. Ku86 defines the genetic defect and restores X-ray resistance and V(D)J recombination to complementation group 5 hamster cell mutants. *Mol. Cell. Biol. In press.*

61. Ajmani, A.K., M. Satoh, E. Reap, P.L. Cohen, and W.H. Reeves. 1995. Absence of autoantigen Ku in mature human neutrophils and human promyelocytic leukemia line (HL-60) cells and lymphocytes undergoing apoptosis. *J. Exp. Med.* **181**, 2049–2058.

62. Terai, C., D.B. Wasson, C.J. Carrera, and D.A. Carson. 1991. Dependence of cell survival on DNA repair in human mononuclear phagocytes. *J. Immunol.* **147**, 4302–4306.

63. Bravo, R., and J.E. Celis. 1982. Human proteins sensitive to neoplastic transformation in cultured epithelial and fibroblast cells. *Clin. Chem.* **28**, 949–954.

64. Yaneva, M., J. Wen, A. Ayala, and R. Cook. 1989. cDNA-derived amino acid sequence of the 86-kDa subunit of the Ku antigen. *J. Biol. Chem.* **264**, 13407–13411.

65. Paillard, S., and F. Strauss. 1993. Site-specific proteolytic cleavage of Ku protein bound to DNA. *Proteins: Structure, function, and genetics* **15**, 330–337.

66. Reeves, W.H., and Z.M. Sthoeger. 1989. Molecular cloning of cDNA encoding the p70 (Ku) lupus autoantigen. *J. Biol. Chem.* **264**, 5047–5052.

67. Griffith, A.J., J. Craft, J. Evans, T. Mimori, and J.A. Hardin. 1992. Nucleotide sequence and genomic structure analyses of the p70 subunit of the human Ku autoantigen: evidence for a family of genes encoding Ku (p70)-related polypeptides. *Mol. Biol. Rep.* **16**, 91–97.

68. Feldmann, H., and E.L. Winnacker. 1993. A putative homologue of the human autoantigen Ku from Saccharomyces cerevisiae. *J. Biol. Chem.* **268**, 12895–12900.

69. Cai, Q.Q., A. Plet, J. Imbert, M. Lafage-Pochitaloff, C. Cerdan, and J.M. Blanchard. 1994. Chromosomal location and expression of the genes coding for Ku p70 and p80 in human cell lines and normal tissues. *Cytogenet. Cell Genet.* **65**, 221–227.

70. Triezenberg, S.J., R.C. Kingsbury, and S.L. McKnight. 1988. Functional dissection of VP16, the trans-activator of herpes simplex virus immediate early gene expression. *Genes Dev.* **2**, 718–729.

71. Li, R., and M.R. Botchan. 1993. The acidic transcriptional activation domains of VP16 and p53 bind the cellular replication protein A and stimulate in vitro BPV-1 DNA replication. *Cell* **73**, 1207–1221.

72. Mimori, T., Y. Ohosone, N. Hama, A. Suwa, M. Akizuki, M. Homma, A.J. Griffith, and J.A. Hardin. 1990. Isolation and characterization of cDNA encoding the 80-kDa subunit protein of the human autoantigen Ku (p70/p80) recognized by autoanti-

bodies from patients with scleroderma-polymyositis overlap syndrome. *Proc. Natl. Acad. Sci. USA* **87**, 1777–1781.

73. Stuiver, M.H., F.E.J. Coenjaerts, and P.C. van der Vliet. 1990. The autoantigen Ku is indistinguishable from NF IV, a protein forming multimeric protein-DNA complexes. *J. Exp. Med.* **172**, 1049–1054.

74. Reeves, W.H., A. Pierani, C.H. Chou, T. Ng, C. Nicastri, R.G. Roeder, and Z.M. Sthoeger. 1991. Epitopes of the p70 and p80 (Ku) lupus autoantigens. *J. Immunol.* **146**, 2678–2686.

75. Falzon, M., and E.L. Kuff. 1992. The nucleotide sequence of a mouse cDNA encoding the 80 kDa subunit of the Ku (p70/p80) autoantigen. *Nucleic Acids Res.* **20**, 3784.

76. Poltoratsky, V.P., X. Shi, J.D. York, M.R. Lieber, and T.H. Carter. 1995. Human DNA-activated protein kinase (DNA-PK) is homologous to phosphatidylinositol kinases. *J. Immunol.* **155**, 4529–4533.

77. Kurimasa, A., Y. Nagata, M. Shimizu, M. Emi, Y. Nakamura, and M. Oshimura. 1994. A human gene that restores the DNA-repair defect in SCID mice is located on 8p11.1→q11.1. *Hum. Genet.* **93**, 21–26.

78. Peterson, S.R., A. Kurimasa, M. Oshimura, W.S. Dynan, E.M. Bradbury, and D.J. Chen. 1995. Loss of the catalytic subunit of the DNA-dependent protein kinase in DNA double-strand-break-repair mutant mammalian cells. *Proc. Natl. Acad. Sci. USA* **92**, 3171–3174.

79. Sipley, J.D., J.C. Menninger, K.O. Hartley, D.C. Ward, S.P. Jackson, and C.W. Anderson. 1995. Gene for the catalytic subunit of the human DNA-activated protein kinase maps to the site of the *XRCC7* gene on chromosome. *Proc. Natl. Acad. Sci. USA* **92**, 7515–7519.

80. Morozov, V.E., M. Falzon, C.W. Anderson, and E.L. Kuff. 1994. DNA-dependent protein kinase is activated by nicks and larger single-stranded gaps. *J. Biol. Chem.* **269**, 16684–16688.

81. Blier, P.R., A.J. Griffith, J. Craft, and J.A. Hardin. 1993. Binding of Ku protein to DNA. Measurement of affinity for ends and demonstration of binding to nicks. *J. Biol. Chem.* **268**, 7594–7601.

82. Zhang, W.W., and M. Yaneva. 1992. On the mechanisms of Ku protein binding to DNA. *Biochem. Biophys. Res. Commun.* **186**, 574–579.

83. Allaway, G.P., A.A. Vivino, L.D. Kohn, A.L. Notkins, and B.S. Prabhakar. 1989. Characterization of the 70 kDa component of Ku autoantigen expressed in insect cell nuclei using a baculovirus vector. *Biochem. Biophys. Res. Commun.* **168**, 747–755.

84. Chou, C.H., J. Wang, M.W. Knuth, and W.H. Reeves. 1992. Role of a major autoepitope in forming the DNA binding site of the p70 (Ku) antigen. *J. Exp. Med.* **175**, 1677–1684.

85. Griffith, A.J., P.R. Blier, T. Mimori, and J.A. Hardin. 1992. Ku polypeptides synthesized in vitro assemble into complexes which recognize ends of double-stranded DNA. *J. Biol. Chem.* **267**, 331–338.

86. Wang, J., M. Satoh, C.H. Chou, and W.H. Reeves. 1994. Similar DNA binding properties of free p70 (Ku) subunit and p70/p80 heterodimer. *FEBS Lett.* **351**, 219–224.

87. Boulikas, T. 1994. Putative nuclear localization signals (NLS) in protein transcription factors. *J. Cell. Biochem.* **55**, 32–58.

88. Suwa, A., M. Hirakata, Y. Takeda, S. A. Jesch, T. Mimori, and J.A. Hardin. 1994. DNA-dependent protein kinase (Ku protein-p350 complex) assembles on double-stranded DNA. *Proc. Natl. Acad. Sci. USA* **91**, 6904–6908.

89. Ono, M., P.W. Tucker, and J.D. Capra. 1994. Production and characterization of recombinant human Ku antigen. *Nucleic Acids Res.* **22**, 3918–3924.

90. Smider, V., W.K. Rathmell, M.R. Lieber, and G. Chu. 1994. Restoration of X-ray resistance and V(D)J recombination in mutant cells by Ku cDNA. *Science* (Wash. DC) **266**, 288–291.

91. Taccioli, G.E., T.M. Gottlieb, T. Blunt, A. Priestley, J. Demengeot, R. Mizuta, A.R. Lehmann, F.W. Alt, S.P. Jackson, and P.A. Jeggo. 1994. Ku80: Product of the XRCC5 gene and its role in DNA repair and V(D)J recombination. *Science* (Wash. DC) **265**, 1442–1445.

92. Boubnov, N.V., K.T. Hall, Z. Wills, S.E. Lee, D.M. He, D.M. Benjamin, C.R. Pulaski, H. Band, W.H. Reeves, E.A. Hendrickson, and D.T. Weaver. 1995. Complementation of the ionizing radiation sensitivity, DNA end binding, and V(D)J recombination defects of double-strand break repair mutants by the p86 Ku autoantigen. *Proc. Natl. Acad. Sci. USA* **92**, 890–894.

93. Rathmell, W.K., and G. Chu. 1994. Involvement of the Ku autoantigen in the cellular response to DNA double-strand breaks. *Proc. Natl. Acad. Sci. USA* **91**, 7623–7627.

94. Mitsis, P.G., and P.C. Wensink. 1989. Purification and properties of yolk protein factor I, a sequence-specific DNA-binding protein from Drosophila melanogaster. *J. Biol. Chem.* **264**, 5195–5202.

95. Romero, F., C. Dargemont, F. Pozo, W.H. Reeves, J. Camonis, S. Gisselbrecht, and S. Fischer. 1996. p95vav associates with the nuclear protein Ku-70. *Mol. Cell. Biol.* **16**, 37–44.

96. Bustelo, X.R., J.A. Ledbetter, and M. Barbacid. 1992. Product of vav proto-oncogene defines a new class of tyrosine protein kinase substrates. *Nature* (Lond.) **356**, 68–71.

97. Bustelo, X.R., and M. Barbacid. 1992. Tyrosine phosphorylation of the vav proto-oncogene product in activated B cells. *Science* (Wash. DC) **256**, 1196–1199.

98. Hu, P., B. Margolis, and J. Schlessinger. 1993. Vav: a potential link between tyrosine kinases and Ras-like GTPases in hematopoietic signaling. *BioEssays* **15**, 179–183.

99. Hubbard, M.J., and P. Cohen. 1993. On target with a new mechanism for the regulation of protein phosphorylation. *Trends Biochem. Sci.* **18**, 172–177.

100. Zakian, V.A. 1995. ATM-related genes: what do they tell us about functions of the human gene? *Cell* **82**, 685–687.

101. Weaver, D.T. 1995. V(D)J recombination and double-strand break repair. *Adv. Immunol.* **58**, 29–85.

102. Jeggo, P.A., G.E. Taccioli, and S.P. Jackson. 1995. Menage a trois: double strand break repair, V(D)J recombination and DNA-PK. *BioEssays* **17**, 949–957.

103. Zdzienicka, M.Z. 1995. Mammalian mutants defective in the response to ionizing radiation-induced DNA damage. *Mutat. Res.* **336**, 203–213.

104. Collins, A.R. 1993. Mutant rodent cell lines sensitive to ultraviolet light, ionizing radiation and cross-linking agents: a comprehensive survey of genetic and biochemical characteristics. *Mutat. Res.* **293**, 99–118.

105. Jeggo, P.A., M. Hafezparast, A.F. Thompson, B.C. Broughton, G.P. Kaur, M.Z. Zdzienicka, and R.S. Athwal. 1992. Localization of a DNA repair gene (XRCC5) involved in double-strand-break rejoining to human chromosome 2. *Proc. Natl. Acad. Sci. USA* **89**, 6423–6427.

106. Hafezparast, M., G.P. Kaur, M. Zdzienicka, R.S. Athwal, A.R. Lehmann, and P.A. Jeggo. 1993. Subchromosomal localization of a gene (XRCC5) involved in double strand break repair to the region 2q34-36. *Somatic Cell Mol. Genet.* **19**, 413–421.

107. Jeggo, P.A., and J. Smith-Ravin. 1989. Decreased stable transfection frequencies of six X-ray-sensitive CHO strains, all members of the xrs complementation group. *Mutat. Res.* **218**, 75–86.

108. Staunton, J., and D. Weaver. 1994. Hairpin-ended DNA integrates efficiently in scid fibroblasts. *Mol. Cell. Biol.* **14**, 3876–3883.

109. Fulop, G.M., and R.A. Phillips. 1990. The scid mutation in mice causes a general defect in DNA repair. *Nature* (Lond.) **347**, 479–482.

110. Biedermann, K.A., J. Sun, A.J. Giaccia, L.M. Tosto, and J.M. Brown. 1991. scid mutation in mice confers hypersensitivity to ionizing radiation and a deficiency in DNA double-strand break repair. *Proc. Natl. Acad. Sci. USA* **88**, 1394–1397.

111. Hendrickson, E.A., X.Q. Qin, E.A. Bump, D.G. Schatz, M. Oettinger, and D.T. Weaver. 1991. A link between double-strand break-related repair and V(D)J recombination: the scid mutation. *Proc. Natl. Acad. Sci. USA* **88**, 4061–4065.

112. Taccioli, G.E., G. Rathbun, E. Oltz, T. Stamato, P.A. Jeggo, and F.W. Alt. 1993. Impairment of V(D)J recombination in double-strand break repair mutants. *Science* (Wash. DC) **260**, 207–210.

113. Gellert, M. 1992. Molecular analysis of V(D)J recombination. *Annu. Rev. Genet.* **22**, 425–446.

114. Tonegawa, S. 1983. Somatic generation of antibody diversity. *Nature* (Lond.) **302**, 575–581.

115. Thompson, C.B. 1996. New insights into V(D)J recombination and its role in the evolution of the immune system. *Immunity* **3**, 531–539.

116. Gellert, M. 1992. V(D)J recombination gets a break. *Trends Genet.* **8**, 408–446.

117. Schatz, D.G., M.A. Oettinger, and D. Baltimore. 1989. The V(D)J recombination activating gene, RAG-1. *Cell* **59**, 1035–1048.

118. Oettinger, M.A., D.G. Schatz, C. Gorka, and D. Baltimore. 1990. RAG-1 and RAG-2, adjacent genes that synergistically activate V(D)J recombination. *Science* (Wash. DC) **248**, 1517–1523.

119. McBlane, J.F., D.C. van Gent, D.A. Ramsden, C. Romeo, C.A. Cuomo, M. Gellert, and M.A. Oettinger. 1995. Cleavage at V(D)J recombination signal requires only RAG1 and RAG2 proteins and occurs in two steps. *Cell* **83**, 387–395.

120. Hesse, J.E., M.R. Lieber, M. Gellert, and K. Mizuuchi. 1987. Extrachromosomal DNA substrates in pre-B cells undergo inversion or deletion at immunoglobulin V–(D)–J joining signals. *Cell* **49**, 775–783.

121. Bosma, M., and A. Carroll. 1991. The scid mouse mutant: definition, characterization, and potential uses. *Annu. Rev. Immunol.* **9**, 323–350.

122. Lieber, M.R., J.E. Hesse, S. Lewis, G.C. Bosma, N. Rosenberg, K. Mizuuchi, M.J. Bosma, and M. Gellert. 1988. The defect in murine severe combined immune deficiency: joining of signal sequences but not coding segments in V(D)J recombination. *Cell* **55**, 7–16.

123. Kirchgessner, C.U., L.M. Tosto, K.A. Biedermann, M. Kovacs, D. Araujo, E.J. Stanbridge, and J.M. Brown. 1993. Complementation of the radiosensitive phenotype in severe combined immunodeficient mice by human chromosome 8. *Cancer Res.* **53**, 6011–6016.

124. Lees-Miller, S.P., R. Godbout, D.W. Chan, M. Weinfeld, R.S. Day, G.M. Barron, and J. Allalunis Turner. 1995. Absence of p350 subunit of DNA-activated protein kinase from a radiosensitive human cell line. *Science* (Wash. DC) **267**, 1183–1185.

125. Wiler, R., R. Leber, B.B. Moore, L.F. VanDyk, L.E. Perryman, and K. Meek. 1995. Equine severe combined immunodeficiency: a defect in V(D)J recombination and DNA-dependent protein kinase activity. *Proc. Natl. Acad. Sci. USA* **92**, 11485–11489.

126. Schwartz, L.M., and B.A. Osborne. 1993. Programmed cell death, apoptosis and killer genes. *Immunol. Today* **14**, 582–590.

127. Cohen, J.J. 1993. Apoptosis. *Immunol. Today* **14**, 126–130.

128. Cohen, G.M., X.M. Sun, R.T. Snowden, D. Dinsdale, and D.N. Skilleter. 1992. Key morphological features of apoptosis may occur in the absence of internucleosomal DNA fragmentation. *Biochem. J.* **286**, 331–334.

129. Ashwell, J.D., N.A. Berger, J.A. Cidlowski, D.P. Lane, and S.J. Korsmeyer. 1994. Coming to terms with death: apoptosis in cancer and immune development. *Immunol. Today* **15**, 147–151.

130. Strasser, A., A.W. Harris, T. Jacks, and S. Cory. 1994. DNA damage can induce apoptosis in proliferating lymphoid cells via p53-independent mechanisms inhibitable by Bcl-2. *Cell* **79**, 329–339.

131. Cohen, J.J., R.C. Duke, V.A. Fadok, and K.S. Sellins. 1992. Apoptosis and programmed cell death in immunity. *Annu. Rev. Immunol.* **10**, 267–293.

132. Casciola-Rosen, L.A., G.J. Anhalt, and A. Rosen. 1995. DNA-dependent protein kinase is one of a subset of autoantigens specifically cleaved early during apoptosis. *J. Exp. Med.* **182**, 1625–1634.

133. Nicholson, D.W., A. Ali, N.A. Thornberry, J.P. Vaillancourt, C.K. Ding, M. Gallant, Y. Gareau, P.R. Griffin, M. Labelle, Y.A. Lazebnik, N.A. Munday, S.M. Raju, M.E. Smulson, T.T. Yamin, V.L. Yu, and D.K. Miller. 1995. Identification and inhibition of the ICE/CED-3 protease necessary for mammalian apoptosis. *Nature* (Lond.) **376**, 37–43.

134. Chase, J.W., and K.R. Williams. 1986. Single-stranded DNA binding proteins required for DNA replication. *Annu. Rev. Biochem.* **55**, 103–136.

135. Georgaki, A., and U. Hubscher. 1993. DNA unwinding by replication protein A is a property of the 70 kDa subunit and is facilitated by phosphorylation of the 32 kDa subunit. *Nucleic Acids Res.* **21**, 3659–3665.

136. Showe, L.C., and C.M. Croce. 1987. The role of chromosomal translocations in B- and T-cell neoplasia. *Annu. Rev. Immunol.* **5**, 253–277.

137. Tsujimoto, Y., J. Cossman, E. Jaffe, and C.M. Croce. 1985. Involvement of the bcl-2 gene in human follicular lymphoma. *Science* (Wash. DC) **228**, 1440–1443.

138. DiCroce, P.A., and T.G. Krontiris. 1995. The BCL2 major breakpoint region is a sequence- and cell-cycle-specific binding site of the Ku antigen. *Proc. Natl. Acad. Sci. USA* **92**, 10137–10141.

139. Wyatt, R.T., R.A. Rudders, A. Zelenetz, R.A. Delellis, and T.G. Krontiris. 1992. BCL2 oncogene translocation is mediated by a chi-like consensus. *J. Exp. Med.* **175**, 1575–1588.

140. Mitsis, P.G., and P.C. Wensink. 1989. Identification of yolk protein factor 1, a sequence-specific DNA-binding protein from Drosophila melanogaster. *J. Biol. Chem.* **264**, 5188–5194.

141. Messier, H., T. Fuller, S. Mangal, H. Brickner, S. Igarashi, J. Gaikwad, R. Fotedar, and A. Fotedar. 1993. p70 lupus autoantigen binds the enhancer of the T cell receptor beta chain. *Proc. Natl. Acad. Sci. USA* **90**, 2685–2689.

142. Niu, H., J. Zhang, and S.T. Jacob. 1995. E1BF/Ku interacts physically and functionally with the core promoter binding factor CPBF and promotes basal transcription of rat and human ribosomal RNA genes. *Gene Expr.* **4**, 111–124.

143. Okumura, K., S. Takagi, G. Sakaguchi, K. Naito, N. Minoura Tada, H. Kobayashi, T. Mimori, Y. Hinuma, and H. Igarashi. 1994. Autoantigen Ku protein is involved in DNA binding proteins which recognize the U5 repressive element of human T-cell leukemia virus type I long terminal repeat. *FEBS Lett.* **356**, 94–100.

144. Logan, S.K., M.J. Garabedian, and P.C. Wensink. 1989. DNA regions that regulate the ovarian transcriptional specificity of Drosophila yolk protein genes. *Genes Dev.* **3**, 1453–1461.

145. Yaneva, M., and S. Jhiang. 1991. Expression of the Ku protein during cell proliferation. *Biochim. Biophys. Acta* **1090**, 181–187.

146. Bravo, R., and H. Macdonald-Bravo. 1987. Existence of two populations of cyclin/ proliferating cell nuclear antigen during the cell cycle: association with DNA replication sites. *J. Cell Biol.* **105**, 1549–1554.

147. Kleinberger, T., and T. Shenk. 1991. A protein kinase is present in a complex with adenovirus E1A proteins. *Proc. Natl. Acad. Sci. USA* **88**, 11143–11147.

148. Kuhn, A., T.M. Gottlieb, S.P. Jackson, and I. Grummt. 1995. DNA-dependent protein kinase: a potent inhibitor of transcription by RNA polymerase I. *Genes Dev.* **9**, 193–203.

149. Labhart, P. 1995. DNA-dependent protein kinase specfically represses promotor-directed transcription initation by RNA polymerase I. *Proc. Natl. Acad. Sci. USA* **92**, 2934–2938.

150. Comai, L., N. Tanese, and R. Tjian. 1992. The TATA-binding protein and associated factors are integral components of the RNA polymerase I transcription factor, SL1. *Cell* **68**, 965–976.

151. Kuhn, A., V. Stefanovsky, and I. Grummt. 1993. The nucleolar transcription activator UBF relieves Ku antigen-mediated repression of mouse ribosomal gene transcription. *Nucleic Acids Res.* **21**, 2057–2063.

152. Rodriguez-Sanchez, J., C. Gelpi, C. Juarez, and J.A. Hardin. 1987. A new autoantibody in scleroderma that recognizes a 90-kDa component of the nucleolus organizing region of chromatin. *J. Immunol.* **139**, 2579–2584.

153. Chan, E.K.L., H. Imai, J.C. Hamel, and E.M. Tan. 1991. Human autoantibody to RNA polymerase I transcription factor hUBF. Molecular identity of nucleolus organizer region autoantigen NOR-90 and ribosomal RNA transcription upstream binding factor. *J. Exp. Med.* **174**, 1239–1244.

154. Spanopoulou, E., P. Cortes, C. Shih, C.M. Huang, D.P. Silver, P. Svec, and D. Baltimore. 1995. Localization, interaction, and RNA binding properties of the V(D)J recombination-activating proteins RAG1 and RAG2. *Immunity* **3**, 715–726.

155. Blasquez, V.C., M. Xu, S.C. Moses, and W.T. Garrard. 1989. Immunoglobulin kappa gene expression after stable integration: I. role of the intronic MAR and enhancer in plasmacytoma cells. *J. Biol. Chem.* **264**, 21183–21189.

156. Berezney, R., and D.S. Coffey. 1975. Nuclear protein matrix: association with newly synthesized DNA. *Science* (Wash. DC) **189**, 291–293.

157. Hutchison, N., and H. Weintraub. 1985. Localization of DNase I-sensitive sequences to specific regions of interphase nuclei. *Cell* **43**, 471–482.

158. Maddison, P.J., and M. Reichlin. 1977. Quantitation of precipitating antibodies to certain soluble nuclear antigens in SLE. *Arthritis Rheum.* **20**, 819–824.

159. Elkon, K.B., E. Bonfa, and N. Brot. 1992. Antiribosomal antibodies in systemic lupus erythematosus. *Rheum. Dis. Clin. North Am.* **18**, 377–390.

160. Love, L.A., R.L. Leff, D.D. Fraser, I.N. Targoff, M. Dalakas, P.H. Plotz, and F.W. Miller. 1991. A new approach to the classification of idiopathic inflammatory myopathy: myositis-specific autoantibodies define a useful homogeneous patient group. *Medicine* **70**, 360–374.

161. Hardin, J.A. 1986. The lupus autoantigens and the pathogenesis of SLE. *Arthritis Rheum.* **29**, 457–460.

162. Reeves, W.H., Z.M. Sthoeger, and R.G. Lahita. 1989. Role of antigen-selectivity in autoimmune responses to the Ku (p70/p80) antigen. *J. Clin. Invest.* **84**, 562–567.

163. Shlomchik, M., M. Mascelli, H. Shan, M.Z. Radic, D. Pisetsky, A. Marshak-Rothstein, and M. Weigert. 1990. Anti-DNA antibodies from autoimmune mice arise by clonal expansion and somatic mutation. *J. Exp. Med.* **171**, 265–298.

164. Goodnow, C.C., J.G. Cyster, S.B. Hartley, S.E. Bell, M.P. Cooke, J.I. Healy, S. Akkaraju, J.C. Rathmell, S.L. Pogue, and K.P. Shokat. 1995. Self-tolerance checkpoints in B lymphocyte development. *Adv. Immunol.* **59**, 279–368.

165. Murakami, M., T. Tsubata, M. Okamoto, A. Shimizu, S. Kumagai, H. Imura, and T. Honjo. 1992. Antigen-induced apoptotic death of Ly-1 B cells responsible for autoimmune disease in transgenic mice. *Nature* (Lond.) **357**, 77–80.

166. Von Boehmer, H. 1990. Developmental biology of T cells in T cell receptor transgenic mice. *Annu. Rev. Immunol.* **8**, 531–556.

167. Harding, F.A., J.G. McArthur, J.A. Gross, D.H. Raulet, and J.P. Allison. 1992. CD28-mediated signalling co-stimulates murine T cells and prevents induction of anergy in T-cell clones. *Nature (Lond.)* **356**, 607–609.

168. Ashton Rickardt, P.G., A. Bandeira, J.R. Delaney, L. Van Kaer, H.P. Pircher, R.M. Zinkernagel, and S. Tonegawa. 1994. Evidence for a differential avidity model of T cell selection in the thymus. *Cell* **76**, 651–663.

169. Theofilopoulos, A.N. 1995. The basis of autoimmunity: Part I. Mechanisms of aberrant self-recognition. *Immunol. Today* **16**, 90–98.

170. Brett, S.J., K.B. Cease, and J.A. Berzofsky. 1988. Influences of antigen processing on the expression of the T cell repertoire. Evidence for MHC-specific hindering structures on the products of processing. *J. Exp. Med.* **168**, 357–373.

171. Finnegan, A., M.A. Smith, J.A. Smith, J.A. Berzofsky, D.H. Sachs, and R.J. Hodes. 1986. The T cell repertoire for recognition of a phylogenetically distant protein antigen. Peptide specificity and MHC restriction of staphylococcal nuclease-specific T cell clones. *J. Exp. Med.* **164**, 897–910.

172. Buus, S., A. Sette, S.M. Colon, C. Miles, and H.M. Grey. 1987. The relation between major histocompatibility complex (MHC) restriction and the capacity of Ia to bind immunogenic peptides. *Science* (Wash. DC) **235**, 1353–1358.

173. Shivakumar, S., E.E. Sercarz, and U. Krzych. 1989. The molecular context of determinants within the priming antigen establishes a hierarchy of T cell induction: T cell specificities induced by peptides of beta-galactosidase vs. the whole antigen. *Eur. J. Immunol.* **19**, 681–687.

174. Glimcher, L.H., J.A. Schroer, C. Chan, and E.M. Shevach. 1983. Fine specificity of cloned insulin-specific T cell hybridomas: evidence supporting a role for tertiary conformation. *J. Immunol.* **131**, 2868–2874.

175. Atassi, M.Z., M. Yoshioka, and G.S. Bixler. 1989. T cells specific for alpha-beta interface regions of hemoglobin recognize the isolated subunit but not the tetramer and indicate presentation without processing. *Proc. Natl. Acad. Sci. USA* **86**, 6729–6733.

176. Rouas, N., S. Christophe, F. Housseau, D. Bellet, J.G. Guillet, and J.M. Bidart. 1993. Influence of protein-quaternary structure on antigen processing. *J. Immunol.* **150**, 782–792.

177. Gammon, G., and E. Sercarz. 1989. How some T cells escape tolerance induction. *Nature* (Lond.) **342**, 183–185.

178. van Eden, W., J.E.R. Thole, R. van der Zee, A. Noordzij, J.D.A. van Embden, E.J. Hensen, and I.R. Cohen. 1988. Cloning of the mycobacterial epitope recognized by T lymphocytes in adjuvant arthritis. *Nature* (Lond.) **331**, 171–173.

179. Dong, X., K.J. Hamilton, M. Satoh, J. Wang, and W.H. Reeves. 1994. Initiation of autoimmunity to the p53 tumor suppressor protein by complexes of p53 and SV40 large T antigen. *J. Exp. Med.* **179**, 1243–1252.

180. Griem, P., and E. Gleichmann. 1995. Metal ion induced autoimmunity. *Curr. Opin. Immunol.* **7**, 831–838.

181. Cerottini, J.C., and H.R. MacDonald. 1989. The cellular basis of T-cell memory. *Annu. Rev. Immunol.* **7**, 77–89.

182. Oldstone, M.B.A. 1987. Molecular mimicry and autoimmune disease. *Cell* **50**, 819–820.

183. Fujinami, R.S., M.B.A. Oldstone, Z. Wroblewska, M.E. Frankel, and H. Koprowski. 1983. Molecular mimicry in virus infection: Crossreaction of measles virus phosphoprotein or of herpes simplex virus protein with human intermediate filaments. *Proc. Natl. Acad. Sci. USA* **80**, 2346–2350.

184. Query, C.C., and J.D. Keene. 1987. A human autoimmune protein associated with U1 RNA contains a region of homology that is cross-reactive with retroviral p30gag antigen. *Cell* **51**, 211–220.

185. Lin, R.H., M.J. Mamula, J.A. Hardin, and C.A. Janeway. 1991. Induction of autoreactive B cells allows priming of autoreactive T cells. *J. Exp. Med.* **173**, 1433–1439.

186. Lake, P., and N.A. Mitchison. 1976. Regulatory mechanisms in the immune response to cell-surface antigens. *Cold Spring Harbor Symp. Quant. Biol.* **41**, 589–595.

187. Russell, S.M., and F.Y. Liew. 1979. T cells primed by influenza virion internal components can cooperate in antibody response to haemagglutinin. *Nature* (Lond.) **280**, 147–148.

188. Russell, S.M., and F.Y. Liew. 1980. Cell cooperation in antibody responses to influenza virus: I. Priming of helper T cells by internal components of the virion. *Eur. J. Immunol.* **10**, 791–796.

189. Scherle, P.A., and W. Gerhard. 1986. Functional analysis of influenza-specific helper T cell clones in vivo: T cells specific for internal viral proteins provide cognate help for B cell responses to hemagglutinin. *J. Exp. Med.* **164**, 1114–1128.

190. Milich, D.R., A. McLachlan, G.B. Thornton, and J.L. Hughes. 1987. Antibody production to the nucleocapsid and envelope of the hepatitis B virus primed by a single synthetic T cell site. *Nature* (Lond.) **329**, 547–549.

191. Fatenejad, S., M.J. Mamula, and J. Craft. 1993. Role of intermolecular/intrastructural B- and T-cell determinants in the diversification of autoantibodies to ribonucleoprotein particles. *Proc. Natl. Acad. Sci. USA* **90**, 12010–12014.

192. Zinkernagel, R.M., S. Cooper, J. Chambers, R.A. Lazzarini, H. Hengartner, and H. Arnheiter. 1990. Virus-induced autoantibody response to a transgenic viral antigen. *Nature* (Lond.) **345**, 68–71.

193. James, J.A., T. Gross, R.H. Scofield, and J.B. Harley. 1995. Immunoglobulin epitope spreading and autoimmune disease after peptide immunization: Sm B/B'-derived PPPGMRPP and PPPGIRGP induce spliceosome autoimmunity. *J. Exp. Med.* **181**, 453–461.

194. Topfer, F., T. Gordon, and J. McCluskey. 1995. Intra- and intermolecular spreading of autoimmunity involving the nuclear self-antigens La (SS-B) and Ro (SS-A). *Proc. Natl. Acad. Sci. USA* **92**, 875–879.

195. Boire, G., and J. Craft. 1990. Human Ro ribonucleoprotein particles: characterization of native structure and stable association with the La polypeptide. *J. Clin. Invest.* **85**, 1182–1190.

196. Cibotti, R., J.M. Kanellopoulos, J.P. Cabaniols, O. Halle-Panenko, K. Kosmatopoulos, E. Sercarz, and P. Kourilsky. 1992. Tolerance to a self protein involves its immunodominant but does not involve its subdominant determinants. *Proc. Natl. Acad. Sci. USA* **89**, 416–420.

197. Lane, D.P., and L.V. Crawford. 1979. T antigen bound to a host protein in SV40-transformed cells. *Nature* (Lond.) **278**, 261–263.

198. Linzer, D.I.H., and A.J. Levine. 1979. Characterization of a 54K dalton cellular SV40 tumor antigen present in SV40-transformed cells and uninfected embryonal carcinoma cells. *Cell* **17**, 43–52.

199. Prives, C., and J.J. Manfredi. 1993. The p53 tumor suppressor protein: meeting review. *Genes Dev.* **7**, 529–534.

200. Scheffner, M., B.A. Werness, J.M. Huibregtse, A.J. Levine, and P.M. Howley. 1990. The E6 oncoprotein encoded by human papillomavirus types 16 and 18 promotes the degradation of p53. *Cell* **63**, 1129–1136.

201. Mohan, C., S. Adams, V. Stanik, and S.K. Datta. 1993. Nucleosome: a major immunogen for pathogenic autoantibody-inducing T cells of lupus. *J. Exp. Med.* **177**, 1367–1381.

202. Koffler, D., V. Agnello, R.I. Carr, and H.G. Kunkel. 1969. Anti-DNA antibodies and the renal lesions of patients with systemic lupus erythematosus. *Transplant. Proc.* **1**, 933–938.

203. Koffler, D., V. Agnello, and H.G. Kunkel. 1974. Polynucleotide immune complexes in serum and glomeruli of patients with systemic lupus erythematosus. *Am. J. Pathol.* **74**, 109–124.

204. Kalunian, K.C., N. Panosian-Sahakian, F.M. Ebling, A.H. Cohen, J.S. Louie, J. Kaine, and B.H. Hahn. 1989. Idiotypic characteristics of immunoglobulins associated with systemic lupus erythematosus. *Arthritis Rheum.* **32**, 513–522.

205. Gavalchin, J., and S.K. Datta. 1987. The NZB × SWR model of lupus nephritis. II. Autoantibodies deposited in renal lesions show a distinctive and restricted idiotypic diversity. *J. Immunol.* **138**, 138–148.

206. Solomon, G., J. Schiffenbauer, H.D. Keiser, and B. Diamond. 1983. Use of monoclonal antibodies to identify shared idiotypes on human antibodies to native DNA from patients with systemic lupus erythematosus. *Proc. Natl. Acad. Sci. USA* **80**, 850–854.

207. Tsao, B.P., F.M. Ebling, C. Roman, N. Panosian-Sahakian, K. Calame, and B.H. Hahn. 1990. Structural characteristics of the variable regions of immunoglobulin genes encoding a pathogenic autoantibody in murine lupus. *J. Clin. Invest.* **85**, 530–540.

208. Tsao, B.P., K. Ohnishi, H. Cheroutre, B. Mitchell, M. Teitell, P. Mixter, M. Kronenberg, and B. Hahn. 1992. Failed self-tolerance and autoimmunity in IgG anti-DNA transgenic mice. *J. Immunol.* **149**, 350–358.

209. Radic, M.Z., S.M. Inrahim, J. Rauch, S.A. Camper, and M. Weigert. 1995. Constitutive secretion of transgene-encoded IgG2b autoantibodies leads to symptoms of autoimmune disease. *J. Immunol.* **155**, 3213–3222.

210. Casali, P., S.E. Burastero, J.E. Balow, and A.L. Notkins. 1989. High-affinity antibodies to ssDNA are produced by CD-5 cells in systemic lupus erythematosus patients. *J. Immunol.* **143**, 3476–3483.

211. Casali, P., S.E. Burastero, M. Nakamura, G. Inghirami, and A.L. Notkins. 1987. Human lymphocytes making rheumatoid factor and antibody to ssDNA belong to Leu-1+ B cell subset. *Science* (Wash. DC) **236**, 77–81.

212. Reap, E.A., E.S. Sobel, P.L. Cohen, and R.A. Eisenberg. 1993. Conventional B cells, not B-1 cells, are responsible for producing autoantibodies in lpr mice. *J. Exp. Med.* **177**, 69–78.

213. Fisher, C.L., R.A. Eisenberg, and P.L. Cohen. 1988. Quantitation and IgG subclass distribution of antichromatin autoantibodies in SLE mice. *Clin. Immunol. Immunopathol.* **46**, 205–213.

214. Rothfield, N.F., and B.D. Stollar. 1967. The relation of immunoglobulin class, pattern of anti-nuclear antibody, and complement-fixing antibodies to DNA in sera from patients with systemic lupus erythematosus. *J. Clin. Invest.* **46**, 1785–1794.

215. Desai-Mehta, A., C. Mao, S. Rajagopalan, T. Robinson, and S.K. Datta. 1995. Structure and specificity of T cell receptors expressed by potentially pathogenic anti-DNA autoantibody-inducing T cells in human lupus. *J. Clin. Invest.* **95**, 531–541.

216. Monestier, M., and B.L. Kotzin. 1992. Antibodies to histones in systemic lupus erythematosus and drug-induced lupus syndromes. *Rheum. Dis. Clin. North Am.* **18**, 415–436.

217. Burlingame, R.W., and R.L. Rubin. 1991. Drug-induced anti-histone autoantibodies display two patterns of reactivity with substructures of chromatin. *J. Clin. Invest.* **88**, 680–690.

218. Fatenejad, S., W. Brooks, A. Schwartz, and J. Craft. 1994. Pattern of anti-small nuclear ribonucleoprotein antibodies in MRL/Mp-lpr/lpr mice suggests that the intact U1 snRNP particle is their autoimmunogenic target. *J. Immunol.* **152**, 5523–5531.

219. Hirakata, M., T. Mimori, M. Akizuki, J. Craft, J.A. Hardin, and M. Homma. 1992. Autoantibodies to small nuclear and cytoplasmic ribonucleoproteins in Japanese patients with inflammatory muscle disease. *Arthritis Rheum.* **35**, 449–456.

220. Suwa, A., T. Mimori, N. Hama, T. Fujii, M. Hirakata, Y. Ohosone, M. Akizuki, and M. Homma. 1992. Enzyme-linked immunosorbent assay of anti-Ku antibodies using purified recombinant Ku antigens. *Jpn. J. Clin. Immunol.* **15**, 337–345.

221. Satoh, M., J. Langdon, and W.H. Reeves. 1993. Clinical applications of an anti-Ku antigen capture ELISA. *Clin. Immunol. Newsletter* **13**, 23–31.

222. Yaneva, M., and F.C. Arnett. 1989. Antibodies against Ku protein in sera from patients with autoimmune diseases. *Clin. Exp. Immunol.* **76**, 366–372.

223. Isern, R.A., M. Yaneva, E. Weiner, A. Parke, N. Rothfield, D. Dantzker, S. Rich, and F.C. Arnett. 1992. Autoantibodies in patients with primary pulmonary hypertension: association with anti-Ku. *Am. J. Med.* **93**, 307–312.

224. Kuwana, M., Y. Okano, J. Kaburaki, T. Tojo, and T.A. Medsger. 1994. Racial differences in the distribution of systemic sclerosis-related serum antinuclear antibodies. *Arthritis Rheum.* **37**, 902–906.

225. Abu-Elheiga, L., and M. Yaneva. 1992. Antigenic determinants of the 70-kDa subunit of the Ku autoantigen. *Clin. Immunol. Immunopathol.* **64**, 145–152.

226. Suwa, A. 1990. Studies on the antigenic epitopes reactive with autoantibody in patients with PSS-PM overlap syndrome. *Keio Igaku* **67**, 865–879.

227. Chou, C.H., M. Satoh, J. Wang, and W.H. Reeves. 1992. B cell epitopes of autoantigenic DNA-binding proteins. *Mol. Biol. Rep.* **16**, 191–198.

228. Chan, E.K., and E.M. Tan. 1987. Human autoantibody-reactive epitopes of SS-B/La are highly conserved in comparison with epitopes recognized by murine monoclonal antibodies. *J. Exp. Med.* **166**, 1627–1640.

229. Davidson, H.W., and C. Watts. 1989. Epitope-directed processing of specific antigen by B lymphocytes. *J. Cell Biol.* **109**, 85–92.

230. Watts, C., and A. Lanzavecchia. 1993. Suppressive effect of antibody on processing of T cell epitopes. *J. Exp. Med.* **178**, 1459–1463.

231. Lanzavecchia, A. 1995. How can cryptic epitopes trigger autoimmunity? *J. Exp. Med.* **181**, 1945–1948.

232. Manca, F., A. Kunkl, D. Fenoglio, A. Fowler, E. Sercarz, and F. Celada. 1985. Constraints in T–B cooperation related to epitope topology on E. coli beta-galactosidase:

I. The fine specificity of T cells dictates the fine specificity of antibodies directed to conformation-dependent determinants. *Eur. J. Immunol.* **15**, 345–350.

233. Kuwana, M., T.A. Medsger Jr., and T.M. Wright. 1995. T and B cell collaboration is essential for the autoantibody response to DNA topoisomerase I in systemic sclerosis. *J. Immunol.* **155**, 2703–2714.

234. Lehmann, P.V., T. Forsthuber, A. Miller, and E.E. Sercarz. 1992. Spreading of T-cell autoimmunity to cryptic determinants of an autoantigen. *Nature1 (Lond.)* **358**, 155–157.

235. Tisch, R., X.D. Yang, S.M. Singer, R.S. Liblau, L. Fugger, and H.O. McDevitt. 1993. Immune response to glutamic acid decarboxylase correlates with insulitis in non-obese diabetic mice. *Nature* (Lond.) **366**, 72–75.

236. Satoh, M., A.K. Ajmani, T. Ogasawara, J.J. Langdon, M. Hirakata, J. Wang, and W.H. Reeves. 1994. Autoantibodies to RNA polymerase II are common in systemic lupus erythematosus and overlap syndrome. Specific recognition of the phosphorylated (IIO) form by a subset of human sera. *J. Clin. Invest.* **94**, 1981–1989.

237. Satoh, M., M. Kuwana, T. Ogasawara, A.K. Ajmani, J.J. Langdon, D. Kimpel, J. Wang, and W.H. Reeves. 1994. Association of autoantibodies to topoisomerase I and the phosphorylated (IIO) form of RNA polymerase II in Japanese scleroderma patients. *J. Immunol.* **153**, 5838–5848.

238. Satoh, M., J.J. Langdon, C.H. Chou, D.P. McCauliffe, E.L. Treadwell, T. Ogasawara, M. Hirakata, A. Suwa, P.L. Cohen, R.A. Eisenberg, and W.H. Reeves. 1994. Characterization of the Su antigen, a macromolecular complex of 100/102 and 200 kDa proteins recognized by autoantibodies in systemic rheumatic diseases. *Clin. Immunol. Immunopathol.* **73**, 132–141.

239. Zhang, J., and J.L. Corden. 1991. Phosphorylation causes a conformational change in the carboxyl-terminal domain of the mouse RNA polymerase II largest subunit. *J. Biol. Chem.* **266**, 2297–2302.

240. Garcia-Lozano, R., F. Gonzalez-Escribano, J. Sanchez-Roman, I. Wichmann, and A. Nunez-Roldan. 1995. Presence of antibodies to different subunits of replication protein A in autoimmune sera. *Proc. Natl. Acad. Sci. USA* **92**, 5116–5120.

241. Garcia-Lozano, R., I. Wichmann, A. Garcia, J. Sanchez-Roman, F. Gonzalez-Escribano, and A. Nunez-Roldan. 1996. Presence of antibodies to replication protein A in some patients with systemic lupus erythematosus (SLE). *Clin. Exp. Immunol.* **103**, 74–76.

242. Fuerst, T.R., E.G. Niles, F.W. Studier, and B. Moss. 1986. Eukaryotic transient-expression system based on recombinant vaccinia virus that synthesizes bacteriophage T7 RNA polymerase. *Proc. Natl. Acad. Sci. USA* **83**, 8122–8126.

243. Rio, D.C., and G.M. Rubin. 1988. Identification and purification of a Drosophila protein that binds to the terminal 31-base-pair inverted repeats of the P transposable element. *Proc. Natl. Acad. Sci. USA* **85**, 8929–8933.

Chapter

THREE

Differential Effects of Defective DNA-PK$_{cs}$ Expression: Equine and Murine SCID

KATHERYN MEEK,[†] RAY LEBER, RHONDA WILER and EUY KYUN SHIN

Harold C. Simmons Arthritis Research Center, Department of Internal Medicine, University of Texas Southwestern Medical Center, 5323 Harry Hines, Dallas, TX 75235, USA

I. INTRODUCTION

A near infinite array of diverse immune receptor molecules is central to the exquisite ability of the immune system to differentiate self from non-self. However, the genetic information which encodes immune receptor molecules does not exist in the genome as functional genes, but instead must be generated as a functional immune receptor gene by each lymphocyte during early lymphoid differentiation. In this process, distinct gene segments (V, D, and J) are joined to form the coding sequences of immunoglobulin (Ig) and T cell receptor (TCR) variable regions; thus, V(D)J rearrangement is the molecular mechanism by which the diverse array of specific immune receptors is generated ([1], reviewed in [2–4]). The centrality of this process to the development of the vertebrate immune system is demonstrated

Corresponding author: Phone (214) 648-3411, FAX (214) 648-7995. Abbreviations: DSBR = double strand break repair; DNA-PK = DNA dependent protein kinase; DNA-PK$_{cs}$ = catalytic subunit of DNA dependent protein kinase; V(D)J = variable (diversity) joining; Ig = immunoglobulin; RAG = recombinase activating gene; SCID = severe combined immunodeficiency.

in situations where V(D)J recombination is impaired [5–8]. In these situations, the development of both B and T lymphocytes is blocked resulting in the disease, severe combined immunodeficiency (SCID). Examples of this disease include murine SCID (C.B-17 mouse) and RAG1 or RAG2 (Recombinase Activating Genes) deficient mice.

V(D)J rearrangement has been the focus of intense research over the past two decades. It is now well understood that the rearrangement process depends upon a lymphoid specific site specific somatic recombinase which is targeted by simple DNA sequence elements found immediately adjacent to all functional immune receptor gene segments [9,10]. The DNA sequence elements which target the recombinase are called recombination signal sequences (RSS). Each RSS consists of a palindromic heptamer (5'CACAGTG3') and an A/C rich nonamer sequence. The heptamer is separated from the nonamer by a non-conserved spacer of either 12 (±1) or 23 (±1) base pairs (approximately one or two turns of the helix). Furthermore, efficient rearrangement only occurs between RSS having different spacer lengths: the 12/23 recombination rule [12,13]. The rearrangement process involves two double stranded DNA cuts and subsequent religations. This results in the formation of two new DNA joints: coding joints which contain the coding information and signal joints which contain the two recombination signal sequences [13, 14]. Two other joining reactions are possible following the initiation of V(D)J recombination. First, hybrid joints represent apparent errors by the recombinase machinery. These joints consist of ligations of the coding sequence from one gene segment to the RSS of another [15]. In addition, it has been demonstrated that the RSS of one gene segment can religate back to its own coding sequence: a so-called open and shut joint [16].

It has been appreciated for some time that the processing of coding and signal ends differs dramatically in that signal ends are precise ligations of the two heptamer sequences, whereas coding ends can be extensively modified through the actions of terminal deoxynucleotidyl transferase and as yet undefined exonucleases [17–19]. This differential processing appears associated with signal versus coding ends instead of signal versus coding ligations in that in hybrid joints, the signal end is almost always intact whereas the coding end is usually processed [15]. Furthermore, it has been suspected, and is now clear, that coding ends proceed first through a hairpinned intermediate prior to end modification and ligation ([20–24], see below).

The junctional region created during V(D)J recombination actually generates the part of the variable region exon that encodes the complementarity determining III (CDR3) region of either the antibody or T cell receptor molecule. Crystal structures of antigen specific antibody molecules demonstrate that CDR3 regions of the immunoglobulin heterodimer are often integral to antigen binding [25]; thus variations in these regions give rise to different antigen specificities. Thus, the consequence of the imprecisions of coding ligation is that infinitely greater diversity is achieved with a particular combination of V, (D), and J than if coding ligation were precise.

Until relatively recently, very little has been defined concerning the factors which mediate V(D)J recombination. In the last few years, important advances have been achieved in understanding the factors which participate in the V(D)J recombination reaction. In 1989 and 1990, two highly conserved genes were discovered,

RAG1 and RAG2 (recombinase activating genes 1 and 2) which are clearly central to this process [26,27]. These two genes are encoded within the same locus. Expression of these genes is, in general, coincident with expression of V(D)J recombinase activity. Furthermore, when these genes are transfected into fibroblasts, recombination of extrachromosomal recombination substrates occurs. Finally, gene targeting experiments have shown that disrupting expression of either RAG1 or RAG2 completely blocks the initiation of V(D)J recombination and results in a complete absence of both B and T cells and severe combined immunodeficiency [8,9].

Although it was presumed for some time that RAG1 and RAG2 were the key components of the recombinase, this was very difficult to establish experimentally. However, confirmation that RAG1 and RAG2 serve as the initiators of V(D)J recombination has recently been published [24]. It is now clear that RAG1 and RAG2 together direct DNA cleavage at the RSS coding juncture. This reaction occurs in a stepwise reaction where a nicked species precedes the appearance of the fully cleaved DNA products. The resulting DNA ends consist of blunt phosphorylated recombination signal end, and coding ends with hairpinned termini. Furthermore, under optimal experimental conditions, cleavage by RAG1 and RAG2 requires two RSS: one with a 12 base pair spacer and one with a 23 base pair spacer, reiterating in vitro the well accepted 12/23 recombination rule [28,29]. Thus, RAG1 and RAG2 together are both necessary and sufficient to direct the cleavage facet of V(D)J recombination.

II. SCID IN THE C.B-17 MOUSE

In 1983, Bosma and colleagues described a spontaneous mutation in C.B-17 mice which phenotypically resembled the human lymphoid deficiency disease, severe combined immunodeficiency (SCID) [5]. These animals are severely deficient in both B and T lymphocytes; whereas levels of NK cells are normal. In 1986, it became clear that the molecular mechanism which is deficient in C.B-17 mice is V(D)J recombination [6,7]. Thus, SCID mice lack both B and T lymphocytes because they are incapable of generating normal immunoglobulin and T cell receptors. In SCID mice, the only step in V(D)J recombination that appears to be impaired is resolution of coding ends (Figure 1). More specifically, it appears that hairpinned coding intermediates accumulate in developing SCID lymphocytes; whereas the blunt phosphorylated signal ends are resolved at a similar rate as in wild type lymphocytes. Thus, the mechanistic defect in C.B-17 SCID mice is fundamentally different from that found in RAG deficient mice. First, in C.B-17 mice, V(D)J recombination is not completely blocked; double strand breaks are initiated, signal ends are religated normally, and only coding end resolution is blocked. In fact, in SCID mice coding joint ligation is not completely blocked in that varying levels of relatively normal coding joints from a variety of different immune receptor loci are easily demonstrable (i.e., "leaky" SCID phenotype). These rearrangements often have large deletions and/or long P elements, consistent with the fact that broken coding ends with hairpinned termini accumulate in SCID lymphocytes. In addition, hybrid joints apparently occur more readily in SCID cells than in normal lymphocytes. In contrast, in either RAG1 or RAG2 deficient mice, the initial step of V(D)J recombination is blocked. Consequently, double strand breaks associated with V(D)J recombination are not generated and the immune receptor genes

V(D)J Recombination

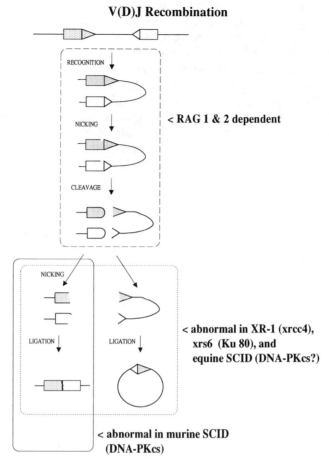

Figure 1. Depiction of V(D)J recombination and factors known to date that are involved in each step of the V(D)J recombination reaction.

remain in germline configuration. Another difference between SCID mice and RAG deficient mice is that the defect in SCID mice not only impairs V(D)J recombination, but also affects the more general process of double strand break repair (DSBR [30,31]). Thus, in C.B-17 SCID mice, cells of all lineages are impaired in their ability to rejoin double strand DNA breaks.

III. THE ASSOCIATION BETWEEN V(D)J RECOMBINATION AND DOUBLE STRAND BREAK REPAIR

The observation that cells from SCID mice are impaired in their capacity to repair double strand breaks was the first to link V(D)J recombination and DSBR. The connection between these two processes became more apparent when two other DSBR factors were implicated as being essential to both V(D)J recombination and DSBR [32,33]. These two factors were implicated by defining two cell lines (xrs6 and XR-1) which are defective in DSBR and are unable to support RAG induced

V(D)J recombination. The latter was shown by co-transfecting the cell lines with recombination substrates and RAG expression vectors. In both of these cell lines, both signal and coding ligation are severely depressed. The defective factor in the *xrs6* cell line is the 80 kD subunit of the Ku protein [34–36], a heterodimer that binds free DNA ends in a sequence independent manner [37,38]. Though it is clear that Ku80 is defective in the *xrs6* cell line, the nature of the mutation has not been defined.

The Ku heterodimer interacts with an ~450 kD protein to generate a protein kinase (DNA-PK) that is dependent on linear DNA for activation [39–41] Thus, Ku is the DNA binding component of DNA-PK and the 450 kD protein is the catalytic domain (DNA-PK$_{cs}$) of DNA-PK. Since DNA-PK requires free DNA ends for activation, it has been proposed that the role of this kinase may be to modulate the function and/or expression of other factors via phosphorylation in response to DNA damage. In fact it has become clear that not only does DNA-PK have the ability to phosphorylate a variety of different transcription factors, but also, that it can itself, modulate transcription in vitro [42–44].

Recently DNA-PK$_{cs}$ has been identified as the defective factor in C.B-17 SCID mice [45–47]. It is related to the phosphatidylinositol 3-kinase family whose members have such divergent functions as signal transduction by phosphorylation of phospholipids, control of cell cycle progression, and maintenance of telomere length [48,49]. Of note, the gene defective in the disease ataxia telangiectasia (ATM) is also a member of this family. As is the case with the Ku80 mutation in *xrs6*, the precise defect in the DNA-PK$_{cs}$ gene in C.B-17 mice has not been ascertained.

The defective factor in the XR-1 cell line has only recently been cloned (xrcc4). This factor has no homology to known proteins and its function is, to date, unknown [50]. The xrcc4 mutation is a complete deletion of both alleles in the XR-1 cell line. Impairment of V(D)J recombination in the XR-1 cell line is superficially analogous to that in the *xrs6* cell line in that both coding and signal ligation is impaired. It has been shown that rare signal joints in XR-1 cells are not precise, but are likely mediated by short sequence homologies, which can facilitate coding (but not signal) ligation in normal cells. Extremely rare coding joints in XR-1 cells appear relatively normal but, like signal joints in XR-1 cells, appear to have utilized short sequence homologies in resolving the ends. Also, as is the case in SCID rearrangements [51], hybrid joints make up a larger percentage of the rare joints in XR-1 cells than they do in normal rearrangements.

The radiation sensitivity in XR-1 differs significantly from both *xrs6* cells and SCID cells in that hypersensitivity to DNA damage is primarily limited to cells in G_0/G_1 [52,53]. This fits well with recent data suggesting that V(D)J recombination is limited to G_0/G_1 [54–56]. This evidence is two fold. First, RAG2 expression is limited to G_0/G_1 because of targeted degradation of the RAG2 protein mediated by *cdc2* phosphorylation [56]. Second, V(D)J recombination intermediates are only found in cells in G_0/G_1 [55,57]. Thus, the restriction of V(D)J recombination to G_0/G_1 is in agreement with what is understood about lack of cell/cycle progression in response to DNA damage, in this case the damage being RAG mediated double strand breaks.

In sum, it appears that the V(D)J recombinase is comprised of lymphoid specific factors (RAG1 and RAG2) and ubiquitously expressed components of the DSBR pathway. As noted above, it has been demonstrated that RAG1 and RAG2 are the

Table 1.

	SCID foals	C.B-17 SCID mice
B cells	Absent	Absent
T cells	Absent	Absent
NK cells	Normal activity	Normal numbers
Ig synthesis	Absent	Minimal
Inheritance	Autosomal recessive	Autosomal recessive

initiators of the recombination reaction [23,24]; whereas DNA-PK (i.e., Ku and DNA-PK$_{cs}$) and *xrcc4* are thought to be involved in the resolution of signal and coding ends [32,33]. Whether these three factors alone are sufficient for resolution of coding and signal ends is unclear, as is the precise roles each of these factors plays in both V(D)J recombination and double strand break repair.

IV. SCID IN ARABIAN FOALS

The occurrence of severe combined immunodeficiency (SCID) in Arabian foals was initially reported in 1973 by McGuire and Poppie [57]. This genetic defect has been shown to be an autosomal recessive mutation resulting in primary immunodeficiency [58]. The incidence of SCID in Arabian foals is approximately 2% and it has been estimated that approximately one forth of adult Arabian horses are silent carriers of the defective gene.

SCID in Arabian foals is characterized by a severe diminution of both B and T lymphocytes. There is no detectable antibody synthesis, though SCID foals have serum immunoglobulin derived from maternal colostrum. If colostrum is denied, the brief life span of SCID foals (up to 5 months) is markedly shortened. Unlike one form of SCID in humans, levels of adenosine deaminase are normal. As in C.B-17 mice, SCID in Arabian foals is characterized by a severe diminution of both B and T lymphocytes; furthermore the pathogenesis of equine SCID can be completely attributed to the absence of B and T cells. In fact, equine SCID is reversible by transplantation of lymphocyte precursor cells through the process of bone marrow transfer. The pathologic features of SCID in Arabian foals is compared to that in C.B-17 mice in Table 1.

We have recently demonstrated that as is the case in SCID mice, the disease in SCID foals is explained by a severe block in the generation of specific immune receptors by the process of V(D)J rearrangement [59,60]. Again, as is the case in murine SCID, equine SCID is characterized by severely diminished levels of the catalytic subunit of the DNA dependent protein kinase. However, these two genetic defects have important mechanistic differences. Here we describe what we currently understand about the equine SCID defect both mechanistically and genetically; and compare this information to the defect in C.B-17 SCID mice.

V. IMMUNE RECEPTOR REARRANGEMENT IN SCID MICE AND SCID FOALS

To assess V(D)J rearrangement in SCID foals, immunoglobulin light chain rearrangements were assessed by PCR analysis of spleen and bone marrow DNA. We have now assessed rearrangements from samples derived from five different SCID foals and found a consistent and severe diminution of endogenous $V_\kappa-J_\kappa$ coding joints, $V_\lambda-J_\lambda$ coding joints, and $V_\kappa-J_\kappa$ signal joints [59]. Representative experiments are depicted in Figure 2. Authenticity of signal ligation, as shown here, is normally demonstrated by susceptibility to the restriction endonuclease ApaL1 (perfect ligation of two RSS generates an ApaL1 site).

Lack of signal joint ligation in SCID foals was documented not only in assessing rearrangement of endogenous immune receptor genes, but also by assessing rearrangement of artificial recombination substrates in fibroblasts co-transfected with RAG expression vectors. These experiments are difficult in equine cell lines because the standard recombination substrates do not replicate in horse cells. Thus, rearrangement was assessed by PCR analysis (Figure 3). Though unrearranged substrate is easily detected in all transfected cell lines, rearrangements are apparent only in cell lines 0176 (derived from a normal horse) and 1826 (derived from an unaffected Arabian foal) which were co-transfected with RAG1 and RAG2 expression vectors. In one of six experiments, a very low level of rearrangement of the pJH201 substrate was detected in the 1863 cell line. In this case, the ligated signal ends were perfect ligations because they were sensitive to the enzyme ApaL1. The fact that V(D)J recombination remains impaired in SCID fibroblasts complemented with normal RAG1 and 2 rules out the possibility that RAG1 or RAG2 mutations are responsible for the equine SCID defect.

Though mice homozygous for the SCID mutation have severely depressed numbers of both B and T lymphocytes, coding joint ligation is not completely blocked. Some relatively normal immune receptor coding joints are present [61,62]. In fact, some animals (called leaky SCID mice) generate enough functional coding joints to have appreciable numbers of B and T cells. Using limiting dilution PCR analysis, we have compared the relative diminution of immunoglobulin light chain rearrangements in both normal and SCID mice as well as normal and SCID foals (Figure 4). Though the sensitivity of detecting $V_\lambda-J_\lambda$ rearrangements in normal horses (horses express >90% lambda light chains) is remarkably similar to the sensitivity of detecting $V_\kappa-J_\kappa$ rearrangements in normal mice, in SCID foals $V_\lambda-J_\lambda$ rearrangements are not detected using standard PCR analysis amplifying from as much as 5 µg DNA. In contrast, light chain rearrangements can easily be detected in as little as 50 ng spleen DNA from SCID mice. Similar results are consistently obtained from all SCID samples tested to date. Clearly, immune receptor rearrangement is more severely impaired in SCID foals than in SCID mice.

Because coding joint sequences isolated from SCID mice provided such important insight into the mechanistic defect in SCID mice, we decided to try to develop more sensitive PCR strategies to detect coding ligations from SCID foals. Our strategy was to use nested amplification primers as depicted in Figure 5. In this experiment, DNA from three SCID foals, one normal animal and an equine fibroblast cell line were subjected to a series of PCR amplifications. In panel A, an unrearranged V_H gene was amplified; as can be seen, all DNA samples were easily amplified. In panel B, the DNA samples were amplified for $V_\lambda J_\lambda$ rearrangements. As shown above, $V_\lambda J_\lambda$ rearrangements are easily detected in normal animals, however, even when utilizing 5 µg starting DNA, $V_\lambda J_\lambda$ rearrangements were not detected in the three SCID foals. As would be expected, no rearrangement was detected in the fibroblast cell line DNA. Panel C depicts secondary amplification

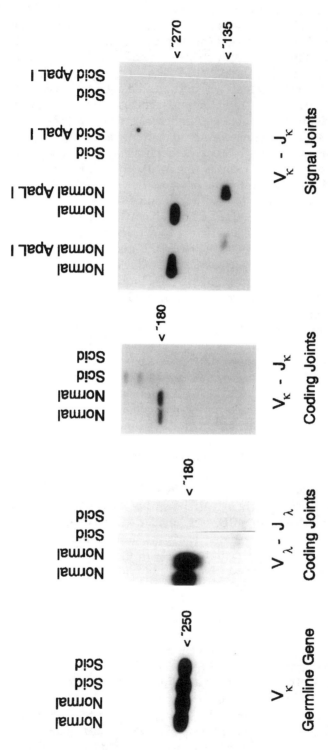

Figure 2. PCR analysis of light chain gene rearrangement in spleen DNA derived from two different SCID foals and two phenotypically normal horses. Amplification primers were based upon equine light chain sequences reported previously [63,64]. In each situation, 5 μg of spleen DNA was utilized. PCR products were separated on 1.8% agarose gels, transferred to nylon membranes and hybridized to ^{32}P labeled internal oligonucleotide probes. Unrearranged V_κ genes and V_λ–J_λ rearrangements were detectable after 40 cycles. V_κ–J_κ rearrangements required 50 cycles (horses overwhelmingly express λ light chains). Left panel: Unrearranged V_κ genes were amplified with primers within V_κ and 3′ of V_κ. Second panel: V_λ–J_λ rearrangements were amplified by primers within V_λ and J_λ. Third panel: V_κ–J_κ coding joints were amplified with primers within V_κ and 3′ of J_κ. Right panel: V_κ–J_κ signal joints were amplified with primers 3′ of V_κ and 5′ of J_κ. A portion of each amplification was digested with the restriction endonuclease Apa LI as indicated to confirm authenticity of the signal joints. From Wiler et al. [59].

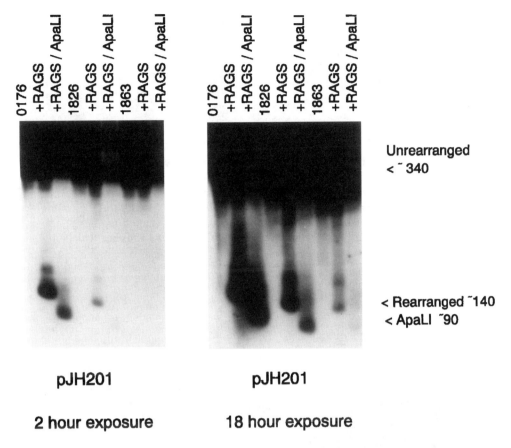

Figure 3. Assessment of pJH201 rearrangement in horse fibroblast cell lines: 0176: derived from normal horse; 1826: derived from an unaffected Arabian horse; 1863: derived from a homozygous SCID foal. Hirt fractionated DNA was recovered from substrate transfected cells (with or without cotransfection of RAG expression vectors). Unrearranged substrate generates a 340 nucleotide amplification product; rearranged plasmids generate a 140 nucleotide rearrangement product. 2 and 18 hour exposures are presented to demonstrate the occasional low level rearrangement in 1863 cells.

using internal $V_\lambda J_\lambda$ oligonucleotide primers. As can be seen, rearrangements were detected in two of the three SCID samples; importantly no rearrangement was detected in either the fibroblast cell line or the no DNA controls. Using this strategy several $V_\lambda J_\lambda$ rearrangements were isolated from three different SCID foals. The $V_\lambda J_\lambda$ junctional regions of these rearrangements are presented in Figure 6.

Eleven unique $V_\lambda J_\lambda$ sequences were isolated. Seven of the eleven rearrangements are in frame joins. Since the corresponding germline V_λ and J_λ germline genes are not available, it is impossible to precisely ascertain V_λ and J_λ contributed nucleotides. However, very long P nucleotides, as have been reported in SCID mice, should be apparent as palindromic sequences in the junctional regions in rearrangements that have no deletions in the gene segment in question. P elements are not apparent in any of the eleven rearrangements sequenced. Furthermore, we

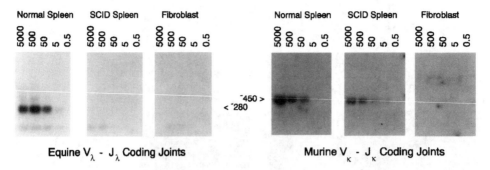

Figure 4. PCR analysis of light chain gene rearrangement in spleen DNA from normal and SCID foals (left panel) and normal and SCID mice (right panel). Limiting amounts of DNA were added to each amplification reaction as indicated. Amplification primers and experimental conditions are as in Figure 2. From Leber et al. [60].

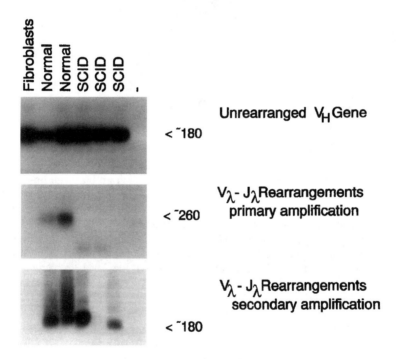

Figure 5. Nested PCR to detect rare coding joints in SCID foals. Primary PCR reactions were for 40 cycles in 100 μl amplification reactions. For nested amplifications, 10 μl of the initial reaction was amplified utilizing internal V_λ and J_λ oligonucleotides. Sequences of oligonucleotides used as PCR primers or as hybridization probes were based on published sequences [63,64] and are as follows: Eq5′V_λ outer: GGGCCAGACAGTCACCATG; Eq3′J_λ outer: ACCACCTGCGATGGTCAGGTG; Eq5′V_λ inner: CAACAGATCCCAGGAACAGCC; Eq3′J_λ inner: ACCACCTGCGATGGTCAGGTG; EqV_λ probe: TTCGGCGGAGGCACC.

```
Vλ2      TAT TAC TGT GGT ACC TAT TAC AGC AGT GAT GAT ATT GAT
Vλ3      TAT TAC TGT GGT ACC TCT AGC AGC AGT GGT ACA

8        TAT TAC TGT GGT TCC TAT TAC AAC AGT GAT AGT AGT GAT        GCT GTA TTC GGC CGA GGC ACC
3        TAT TAC TGT GGT ACG CTA GCG GCA GT                        GCT GCA TTC GGC CGA GGC ACC
12C      TAT TAC TGT GGT ACC TCC AGC ACT GGT GGT AGT A             GCT GTG TTC GGC GGA GGC ACC
4c       TAT TAC TGT GGT ACC TCT AGC AGC AGT GGT AAT                   GTA TTC GGC CGA GGC ACC
6c       TAT TAC TGT GGA ACA TTG TAC AGC AGT TGA GTA GTG AT        GTG GCA TTC GGC CGA GGC ACC
2D       TAT TAC TGT GGT ACG CAT GCG GCA GTG C                     ATG CTA TTC GGC CGA GGC ACC
10DM     TAT TAC TGT GTA CCT CTA AAG CAG TGT AGT                   ATA GTA TTC GGC CGA GGC ACC
10DR     TAT TAC TGT GGA ACA TTG TAC AGC AGT TGG AGT AGT GAT       GGT GCA TTC GGC CGA GGC ACC
3D       TAT TAC TGT GGT TCC TAT TAC AGC AGT GAT AGT AGT           GGT GCA TTC GGC CGA GGC ACC
12       TAT TAC TGT GGT ACC GCT AGC GGC AGT                       GCT GTA TTC GGC CGA GGC ACC
5        TAT TAC TGT GGT ACC TCT AAA AGC AGT GGT AGT ATA               GTA TTC GGC CGA GGC ACC
```

Figure 6. Fragments which hybridized to the internal V_λ hybridization probe were gel purified and cloned into SmaI digested PTZ19R. V_λJ_λ junctional sequences are presented. Assignment to V_λ or J_λ was as noted by Home et al. [64].

found no rearrangements with significant deletion of the coding segment — the other hallmark of murine SCID coding joints. The longest deletion in the equine V_λJ_λ rearrangements was only 4 codons. In sum, these CDR3 structures are not significantly different from those isolated from normal horses.

Finally, it has been reported that the rate of hybrid joint formation is higher in murine SCID lymphocytes than in wild type lymphocytes. Thus, we have also assessed hybrid joint formation in equine SCID bone marrow. Though it is very easy to detect hybrid V_λJ_λ joints from normal bone marrow, no hybrid rearrangements could be detected at all in SCID bone marrow samples.

Thus, the phenotypic characteristics of V(D)J recombination in equine SCID cells are different than in murine SCID cells:

1. In contrast to murine SCID, signal joint ligation is impaired in equine SCID as ascertained by endogenous rearrangements and rearrangement of extrachromosomal substrates in equine SCID fibroblasts.

2. The degree of coding ligation impairment is much more severe in equine SCID cells than in murine SCID cells.

3. Rare V_λ-J_λ coding joints in SCID foals do not have large deletions or long P elements like coding joints isolated from SCID mice. Furthermore, hybrid joints are not abundant in equine SCID lymphocytes as has been reported in murine SCID lymphocytes.

VI. SENSITIVITY TO DNA DAMAGE IN CELLS DERIVED FROM SCID FOALS

The finding that SCID fibroblasts complemented with RAG1 and RAG2 remain V(D)J recombinase negative supported the idea that the equine SCID defect might also be a ubiquitously expressed double strand break repair factor. Thus, relative sensitivity to various DNA damaging agents has also been analyzed. To illustrate, the hypersensitivity of equine SCID cells to ionizing radiation, normal and SCID fibroblasts were irradiated with varying doses of ionizing radiation and plated onto chamber slides as shown in Figure 7A. As can be seen, fibroblasts derived from normal horses can recover even after relatively high doses of ionizing radia-

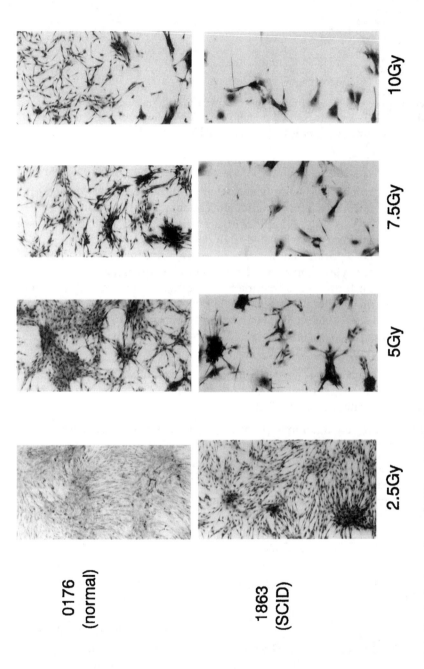

Figure 7. **A**: Equivalent numbers of 0176 and 1863 cells were exposed to varying amounts of ionizing radiation as indicated and cultured in chamber slides. 5 days later, the slides were fixed, stained, and photographed. **B** (opposite): 2×10^3 cells of cell lines 0176, 1826, and 1863 were cultured with increasing levels of bleomycin sulfate and then plated into 150 mm^2 tissue culture plates. 12 days later, cells were trypsinized and counted.

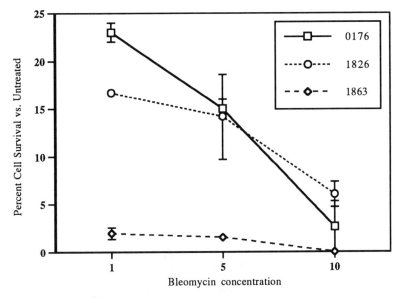

Figure 7B

tion (10 gray). In contrast, SCID fibroblasts are killed by relatively low levels of radiation (5 gray). Hypersensitivity to DNA damage can also be illustrated by exposure to such DNA cleaving agents as bleomycin sulfate. In fact, murine SCID cells have been shown to be hypersensitive to this agent. Thus, we assessed the relative sensitivity of these cell lines to bleomycin sulfate and found that equine SCID cell lines are also hypersensitive to bleomycin sulfate (Figure 7B). Thus, in this relatively crude assessment, in response to DNA damage, equine SCID cells behave very analogously to cells known to be defective in rejoining double stranded DNA breaks.

VII. ASSESSMENT OF DNA-PK IN SCID MICE AND SCID FOALS

The DNA-PK complex is an essential constituent in both double strand break repair and V(D)J recombination pathways. As noted above, this kinase consists of two components: the Ku heterodimer which targets the catalytic component, DNA-PK$_{cs}$ to DNA ends. DNA end binding activity is very easily assessed by electrophoretic mobility shift assays (EMSA). Thus, we assessed Ku activity in the fibroblast cell lines using this assay as depicted in Figure 8.

Nuclear extracts were prepared from the 1826, and 1863 cell lines. These extracts, as well as recombinant Ku [63], were incubated with a linear ^{32}P labelled DNA fragment in the presence of either circular DNA or dIdC as unlabelled competitor, and subsequently electrophoresed in a native acrylamide gel. As can be seen, the pattern of shifted DNA mobility is indistinguishable in the equine cell lines tested. Complexes with several different mobilities have been shown previously to represent DNA fragments with increasing numbers of Ku heterodimers bound [34]. The shifted pattern in the equine extracts is slightly different from that observed with

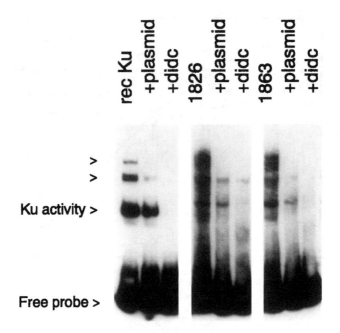

Figure 8. Nuclear extracts from cell lines 1863 and 1826 as well as recombinant Ku protein, were analyzed for DNA end binding activity. The linear probe utilized as well as recombinant Ku proteins have been described previously [34]. Briefly, labeled probe, and nuclear extracts were incubated for 30 minutes at room temperature alone or in the presence of plasmid or dIdC competitor as indicated and separated on a 4% native polyacrylamide gel. Positions of free probe as well as Ku/DNA complexes are indicated by arrows.

recombinant human Ku; this is likely a species specific variation as has been observed previously (i.e., hamster vs. human, [34]). Furthermore, the shifted bands are competitively inhibited by dIdC (which has abundant free DNA ends), but not by supercoiled plasmid DNA. Normal Ku binding activity is also observed in murine SCID cells [34]. In sum, the fact that end binding activity in equine SCID fibroblasts is indistinguishable from that of normal equine fibroblasts suggests that the molecular defect in equine SCID is not in the Ku heterodimer.

We next compared DNA-PK activity in normal and SCID equine cell lines as well as normal and SCID mouse cell lines (Figure 9). As has been observed previously, DNA-PK activity is very low in rodent cell lines (i.e., compare 3T3 and 0176 to ML1). Levels of DNA-PK activity in normal horse cell lines are more analogous to those observed in human cells. As can be seen neither the SF19 cells (derived from a SCID mouse) nor the 1863 cells have detectable DNA-PK activity when compared to their normal counterparts, 3T3 and 0176.

As noted above, it has now been formally demonstrated that the murine SCID factor is the catalytic subunit of DNA dependent protein kinase [44–47]. However, in all reports assessing DNA-PK$_{cs}$ expression in murine SCID cell lines, it is clear that some DNA-PK$_{cs}$ protein is present. We have recently shown that protein levels of DNA-PK$_{cs}$ are severely diminished; whereas mRNA levels of DNA-PK$_{cs}$ are

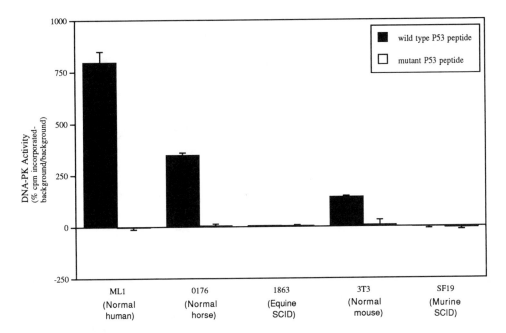

Figure 9. DNA-PK activity in various cell extracts was assessed by phosphorylation of wild type and mutant P53 peptides. In each case, relative phosphorylation was determined by comparing kinase reactions where no peptide, wild type peptide, or mutant peptide was added. Relative phosphorylation was determined as percent increase over no peptide. Standard deviations are based on a minimum of three separated experiments. (ML1, a human EBV transformed B cell line; 1776, fibroblast cell line derived from a normal horse; 1863, fibroblast cell line derived from a SCID foal; 3T3, fibroblast cell line derived from a normal mouse; SF19, fibroblast cell line derived from a SCID mouse). From Leber et al. [60].

consistently higher in equine SCID cells than in normals cells. In Figure 10, antibodies to human DNA-PK$_{cs}$ have been used in immunoblot analyses to compare the DNA-PK$_{cs}$ expression in these two animal models of SCID. The ~450 kD DNA-PK$_{cs}$ polypeptide is readily detected from both normal equine and murine fibroblasts. In addition, in mouse SCID fibroblasts, though the level is severely diminished, some DNA-PK$_{cs}$ is readily detected. In contrast, DNA-PK$_{cs}$ is not easily demonstrated in equine SCID fibroblasts. With long exposures, however, very small amounts of a protein with similar electrophoretic mobility can be detected. From recent reports, it is apparent that the DNA-PK$_{cs}$ gene is related to several other very large PI-like kinases (i.e., the product of the ataxia telangiectasia gene, ATM, 48). Thus, it is not possible to ascertain by western whether the weakly hybridizing protein detected in equine SCID cells is authentic DNA-PK$_{cs}$ or a related kinase. We conclude that the level of DNA-PK$_{cs}$ is virtually, if not completely absent in equine SCID cells.

VIII. IMPLICATIONS OF THE EQUINE SCID DEFECT

The role of DNA-PK in V(D)J recombination has yet to be delineated. Work from several laboratories has established a role for DNA-PK$_{cs}$ in coding joint ligation

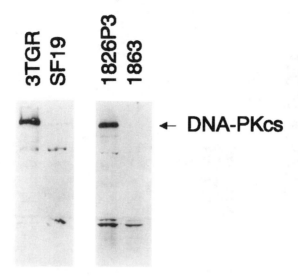

Figure 10. Immunoblot analysis of DNA-PK$_{cs}$. Equivalent amounts of extracts derived from the 1826P3, 1863, 3TGR, and SF19 cell lines were electrophoresed on a 5.5% SDS/polyacrylamide gel and transferred to PVDF paper. The filter was blocked in tris buffered saline with 0.5% Tween (TBS/Tween) and 1% powdered milk. Antibodies 42psc, 25-4, and 18-2 (the generous gift of T. Carter) were used in combination as primary antibody (1:1000 dilution of ascites). The membranes were washed three times for 10 minutes in TBS/Tween. The membranes were incubated for one hour with the secondary antibody (goat anti-mouse IgG conjugated to horseradish peroxidase; Capel, West Chester, PA) diluted 1:5000 in TBS/Tween with 1% powdered milk. The membranes were washed three times for 10 minutes as above. The membranes were then incubated with a chemiluminescent substrate (Renaissance, DuPont, Boston, MA) according to the manufacturer's recommendations. From Leber et al. [60].

[32,33]. These conclusions are based not only on the murine SCID defect, but also on another DSBR mutant CHO cell line, V3, which is also primarily defective in coding but not signal joint ligation [33]. The defect in SCID horses corroborates the role of DNA-PK$_{cs}$ in coding ligation. However, our data also implicates DNA-PK$_{cs}$ in signal joint ligation.

Table 2 compares the phenotype of cells defective in V(D)J recombination. As can be seen, with the exception of the RAG1 and RAG2 knockout cells, each defect is unique in its characteristics. Though it is clear that both the murine and equine SCID defects are characterized by defective DNA-PK$_{cs}$ expression, the two defects unquestionably have phenotypic differences. Since we find only subtle differences between the relative lack of DNA-PK$_{cs}$ in equine and murine SCID cells, one might predict that the degree of impairment of V(D)J recombination might also be similar. This is not the case. SCID mice have a block specifically in coding end resolution; SCID foals have a more dramatic block in coding end resolution as well as a severe block in signal joint resolution. Furthermore, very rare coding joints isolated from SCID foals do not have either excessive deletions or long P nucleotides — well established characteristics of coding joints in SCID mice.

Table 2. Comparison of Factors Implicated in V(D)J Recombination

	Equine SCID (DNA-PK$_{cs}$)	Murine SCID (DNA-PK$_{cs}$)	xrs6 (Ku 80)	XR-1 (xrcc4)	RAG1-/- (RAG1)	RAG2-/- (RAG2)
DSBR	→	→	→	→	ok	ok
CODING JOINTS						
Presence	→	→	→	→	absent	absent
Structure	ok	abnormal	abnormal	abnormal	–	–
SIGNAL JOINTS						
Presence	→	ok	→	→	absent	absent
Structure	ok	ok	abnormal	abnormal	–	–
DNA END BINDING	ok	ok	→	ok	ok	ok
IMMUNODEFICIENCY	+	+	?	?	+	+
DNA-PK activity	→	→	→	ok	ok	ok
DNA-PK$_{cs}$ expression	→	→	ok	ok	ok	ok

There are several explanations for the phenotypic differences between equine SCID and murine SCID/V3. First, it is possible that only low levels of DNA-PK$_{cs}$ are required to perform signal ligation; in this scenario a residual level of DNA-PK$_{cs}$ is able to facilitate signal ligation but not coding ligation. Thus, if the mutation in SCID foals completely blocks DNA-PK$_{cs}$ expression, this could explain a lack of both signal and coding ligation. At this point it is unclear whether there are very low levels of DNA-PK$_{cs}$ present in cells derived from SCID foals.

Another explanation is that the defect in SCID foals also allows some residual DNA-PK$_{cs}$, but the mutations in equine SCID and murine SCID are in different portions of the molecule. DNA-PK$_{cs}$ is a very large polypeptide and clearly has roles in a variety of cellular processes. It is possible that different mutations may lead to different phenotypes. An attractive hypothesis follows: Coding end ligation first requires resolution of hairpinned intermediates followed by ligation of the double strand breaks. In contrast, signal joint formation requires only ligation of broken ends. The murine SCID and V3 mutations could affect a portion of DNA-PK$_{cs}$ that deals with hairpin resolution — consistent with the fact that hairpinned coding ends accumulate in SCID mice [20,22]. In contrast, the defect in equine SCID could affect the portion of DNA-PK$_{cs}$ that facilitates ligation reactions. In fact, the characteristics of V(D)J joints in equine SCID cells more closely resemble those observed in the *xrs6* defect. Thus, it is possible that the defect in DNA-PK$_{cs}$ in SCID foals has to do with DNA-PK$_{cs}$ and Ku interactions. These possibilities are currently under investigation.

Finally, though our data most strongly support the conclusion that DNA-PK$_{cs}$ is the defective factor in equine SCID, this has not been formally proven. It is feasible that the mutation in equine SCID is not in DNA-PK$_{cs}$, but in a factor which affects the stability of DNA-PK$_{cs}$.

IX. SUMMARY

The pathologic features of the severe combined immunodeficiency of Arabian foals are explained by a severe defect in the process of V(D)J recombination, as is the case in the analogous syndrome in C.B-17 mice. Furthermore, cells from SCID mice and SCID horses 1) are hypersensitive to DNA damaging agents, 2) lack detectable DNA-PK activity, and 3) have diminished levels of DNA-PK$_{cs}$. However, equine SCID differs from murine SCID in the following ways: 1) both signal joint resolution and coding joint resolution are impaired in SCID horses whereas only coding joint resolution is impaired in SCID mice; 2) diminution of coding joint formation is more complete in SCID horses than in SCID mice, and rare V_λ–J_λ coding joints in SCID foals do not resemble those found in SCID mice.

REFERENCES

1. Tonegawa, S. 1993. Somatic generation of antibody diversity. *Nature* **302**, 575–581.
2. Lewis, S. 1994. The mechanism of V(D)J joining: lessons from molecular, immunological and comparative analyses. *Adv. Immunol.* **56**, 27–150.
3. Gellert, M. 1992. Molecular analysis of V(D)J recombination. *Annu. Rev. Genet.* **26**, 425–446.

4. Alt, F.W., E.M. Oltz, F. Young, J. Gorman, G. Taccioli, and J. Chen. 1992. VDJ recombination. *Immunol. Today* **13**, 306–314.

5. Bosma, G.C., R.P. Custer and M.J. Bosma. 1983. A severe combined immunodeficiency mutation in the mouse. *Nature* **301**, 527–530.

6. Lieber, M.R., J.E. Hesse, S. Lewis, G.C. Bosma, N. Rosenberg, K. Mizuuchi, M.J. Bosma, and M. Gellert. 1988. The defect in murine severe combined immune deficiency: joining of signal sequences but not coding segments in V(D)J recombination. *Cell* **55**, 7–16.

7. Schuler, W., I.J. Weiler, A. Schuler, R.A. Phillips, N. Rosenberg, T.W. Mak, J.F. Kearney, R.P. Perry, and M. Bosma. 1986. *Cell* **46**, 963–972.

8. Mombaerts, P., J. Iacomini, R.S. Johnson, K. Herrup, S. Tonegawa, and V.E. Papaioannou. 1992. RAG-1 deficient mice have no mature B and T lymphocytes. *Cell* **68**, 129–140.

9. Shinkai, Y., G. Rathbun, K.-P. Lam, E.M. Oltz, V. Stewart, M. Mendelsohn, J. Charron, M. Datta, F. Young, A.M. Stall, and F.W. Alt. 1992. RAG-2 deficient mice lack mature lymphocytes owing to inability to initiate V(D)J rearrangement. *Cell* **68**, 855–867.

10. Hesse, J.E., M.R. Lieber, K. Mizuuchi, and M. Gellert. 1989. V(D)J recombination: a functional definition of the joining signals. *Genes and Devel.* **3**, 1053–1061.

11. Honjo, T. 1983. Immunoglobulin genes. *Annu. Rev. Immunol.* **1**, 499–518.

12. Hesse, J.E., M.R. Lieber, M. Gellert, and K. Mizuuchi. 1987. Extrachromosomal DNA in pre-B cells undergo inversion or deletion at immunoglobulin V–(D)–J joining signals. *Cell* **49**, 775–783.

13. Desiderio, S.V., and K.R. Wolff. 1988. Rearrangement of exogenous immunoglobulin VH and DJH gene segments after retroviral transduction into immature lymphoid cell lines. *J. Exp. Med.* **167**, 372–388.

14. Lewis, S.M., A. Gifford, and D. Baltimore. 1985. DNA elements are asymmetrically joined during the site-specific recombination of kappa immunoglobulin genes. *Science* **228**, 677–685.

15. Lewis, S.M., J.E. Hesse, K. Mizuuchi, and M. Gellert. 1988. Novel strand exchanges in V(D)J recombination. *Cell* **55**, 1099–1107.

16. Lewis, S.M., and J.E. Hesse. 1991. Cutting and closing without recombination in V(D)J joining. 1991. *EMBO J.* **10**, 3631–3639.

17. Alt, F.W., and D. Baltimore. 1982. Joining of immunoglobulin heavy chain gene segments. Implications from a chromosome with evidence of three D–JH fusions. *Proc. Natn. Acad. Sci. USA* **79**, 4118–4122.

18. Gilfillan, S., A. Dierich, M. Lemeur, C. Benoist, and D. Mathis. 1993. Mice lacking TdT: mature animals with an immature lymphocyte repertoire. *Science* **261**, 1175–1178.

19. Komor, T., A. Okada, V. Stewart, and F.W. Alt. 1993. Lack of N regions in antigen receptor variable region genes of TdT-deficient lymphocytes. *Science* **261**, 1171–1175.

20. Roth, D.B., J.P. Menetski, P.B. Nakajima, M.J. Bosma, and M. Gellert. 1992. V(D)J recombination: broken DNA molecules with covalently sealed (hairpin) coding ends in scid mouse thymocytes. *Cell* **70**, 983–991.

21. Roth, D.B., C. Zhu, and M. Gellert. 1993. Characterization of broken DNA molecules associated with V(D)J recombination. *Proc. Natl. Acad. Sci. USA* **90**, 10788–10792.

22. Zhu, C., and D.B. Roth. 1995. Characterization of coding ends in thymocytes of scid mice: implications for the mechanism of V(D)J recombination. *Immunity* **2**, 101–112.

23. van Gent, D.C., J.F. McBlane, D.A. Ramsden, M.J. Sadofsky, J.E. Hesse, and M. Gellert. 1995. Initiation of V(D)J recombination in a cell-free system. *Cell* **81**, 925–934.

24. McBlane, J.F., D.C. van Gent, D.A. Ramsden, C. Romeo, C.A. Cuomo, M. Gellert, and M.A. Oettinger. 1996. Cleavage at a V(D)J recombination signal requires only RAG1 and RAG2 proteins and occurs in two steps. *Cell* **83**, 387–395.

25. Davies, D. D., S. Sheriff, and E.A. Padlan. 1988. Antibody–antigen complexes. *J. Biol. Chem.* **263**, 10541–10544.

26. Schatz, D.G., M.A. Oettinger, and D. Baltimore. 1989. The V(D)J Recombination activating gene, RAG-1. *Cell* **59**, 1035–1048.

27. Oettinger, M.A., D.G. Schatz, C. Gorka, and D. Baltimore. 1990. RAG-1 and RAG-2, adjacent genes that synergistically activate V(D)J recombination. *Science* **248**, 1517–1523.

28. Eastman, Q.M., T.M.J. Leu, and D.G. Schatz. 1996. Initiation of V(D)J recombination *in vitro* obeying the 12/23 rule. *Science* **380**, 85–88.

29. van Gent, D.C., Ramsden, D.A., and Gellert, M. 1996. The RAG1 and RAG2 proteins establish the 12/23 rule in V(D)J recombination. *Cell*, in press.

30. Fulop, G.M., and R.A. Phillips. 1990. The scid mutation in mice causes a general defect in DNA repair. *Nature* **347**, 479–482.

31. Biedermann, K.A., J. Sun, A.J. Giaccia, L.M. Tosto, and M. Brown. 1991. SCID mutation in mice confers hypersensitivity to ionizing radiation and a deficiency in DNA double-strand break repair. *Proc. Natl. Acad. Sci. USA* **88**, 1394–1397.

32. Taccioli, G.E., G. Rathbun, E. Oltz, T. Stamato, P.A. Jeggo, and F.W. Alt. 1993. Impairment of V(D)J recombination in double-strand break repair mutants. *Science* **260**, 207–210.

33. Pergola, F., M.Z. Zdzienicka, and M.R. Lieber. 1993. V(D)J recombination in mammalian cell mutants defective in DNA double-strand break repair. *Mol. Cell. Biol.* **13**, 3464–3470.

34. Getts, R.C., and T.D. Stamato. 1994. Absence of a Ku-like DNA end binding activity in the xrs double-strand DNA repair-deficient mutant. *J. Biol. Chem.* **269**, 15981–15984.

35. Rathmell, W.K., and G. Chu. 1994. A DNA end-binding factor involved in double strand break repair and V(D)J recombination. *Mol. Cell Biol.* **14**, 4741–4748.

36. Taccioli, G.E., T.M. Gottlieb, T. Blunt, A. Priestley, J. Demengeot, R. Mizuta, A.R. Lehmann, F.W. Alt, S.P. Jackson, P.A. Jeggo. 1994. Ku80: product of the *xrcc5* gene and its role in DNA repair and V(D)J recombination. *Science* **265**, 1442–1445.

37. Mimori, T., and J.A. Hardin. 1986. Mechanism of interaction between Ku protein and DNA. *J. Biol. Chem.* **261**, 10375–10379.

38. Ono, M., P.W. Tucker, and J.D. Capra. 1994. Production and characterization of recombinant human Ku antigen. *Nuc. Acids Res.* **22**, 3918–3924.

39. Jackson, S.P., J.J. MacDonald, S. Lees-Miller, and R. Tjian. 1990. GC box binding induces phosphorylation of Sp1 by a DNA-dependent protein kinase. *Cell* **63**, 155–165.

40. Carter, T., I. Vancurova, I. Sun, W. Lou, and S. DeLeon. 1990. A DNA-activated protein kinase from HeLa cell nuclei. *Mol. Cell. Biol.* **10**, 6460–6471.

41. Gottlieb, T.M., and S.P. Jackson. 1993. The DNA-dependent protein kinase: requirement for DNA ends and association with Ku antigen. *Cell* **72**, 131–142.

42. Tuteja, N., R. Tuteja, A. Ochem, P. Taneja, N.W. Huang, A. Simoncsits, S. Susic, K. Rahman, L. Marusic, J. Chen, J. Zhang, S. Wang, S. Pongor, and A. Falaschi. 1994. *EMBO J.* **13**, 4991–5001.

43. Kuhn, A., T.M. Gottlieb, S.P. Jackson, and I. Grummt. 1995. DNA-dependent protein kinase: a potent inhibitor of transcription by RNA polymerase I. *Genes and Devel.* **9**, 193–203.

44. Ono, M., P.W. Tucker, and J.D. Capra. 1996. Ku is a general inhibitor of DNA-protein complex formation and transcription, submitted.

45. Kirchgessner, C.U., C.K. Patil, J.W. Evans, C.A. Cuomo, L.M. Fried, T. Carter, M.A. Oettinger, and J.M. Brown. 1995. *Science* **267**, 1178–1182.

46. Blunt, T., N.J. Finnie, G.E. Taccioli, G.C.M. Smith, J. Demengeot, T.M. Gottlieb, R. Mizuta, A.J. Varghese, F.W. Alt, P.A. Jeggo, and S.P. Jackson. 1995. Defective DNA-dependent protein kinase activity is linked to V(D)J recombination and DNA repair defects associated with the murine scid mutation. *Cell* **80**, 813–823.

47. Hartley, K.O., D. Gell, G.C.M. Smith, H. Zhang, N. Divecha, M.A. Connelly, A. Admon, S.P. Lees-Miller, C.W. Anderson, and S. Jackson. DNA-dependent protein kinase catalytic subunit: a relative of phosphatidylinositol 3-kinase and the ataxia telangiectasia gene product. *Cell* **82**, 849–856.

48. Savitsky, K., A. Bar-Shira, S. Gilad, G. Rotman, Y. Ziv, L. Vanagaite, D. A. Tagle, S. Smith, T. Uziel, S. Stez, M. Ashkenazi, I. Peckaer, M. Frydman, R. Harnik, S. R. Patanjali, A. Simmons, G. A. Clines, A. Sartiel, R.A. Gatti, L. Chessa, O. Sanal, M.F. Lavin, N.G.J. Jaspers, M.R. Taylor, C.F. Arlett, T. Miki, S.M. Weissman, M. Lovett, F.S. Collins, and Y. Shiloh. 1995. A single ataxia telangiectasia gene with a product similar to PI-3 kinase. *Science* **268**, 1749–1753.

49. Hunter, T. 1995. When is a lipid kinase not a lipid kinase? When it is a protein kinase. *Cell* **83**, 1–4.

50. Li, Z., T. Otevrel, Y. Gao, H.-L. Cheng, B. Seed, T.D. Stamato, G.E. Taccioli, and F.W. Alt. The *xrcc4* gene encodes a novel protein involved in DNA double-strand break repair and V(D)J recombination. *Cell* **83**, 1079–1090.

51. Hendrickson, E.A., M.S. Schlissel, and D.T. Weaver. 1990. Wild type V(D)J recombination in scid pre-B cells. *Mol. Cell. Biol.* **10**, 5397–5407.

52. Stamato, T.D., R. Weinstein, A. Giaccia, and L. Mackenzie. 1983. Isolation of cell cycle-dependent γ-ray sensitive Chinese hamster ovary cell. *Somat. Cell Mol. Genet.* **9**, 165–173.

53. Giaccia, A., R. Weinstein, J. Hu, and T.D. Stamato. 1985. Cell cycle-dependent repair of double-strand DNA breaks in a γ-ray sensitive Chinese hamster cell. *Somat. Cell Mol. Genet.* **11**, 485–491.

54. Lin, W., and S. Desiderio. 1994. Cell cycle regulation of V(D)J recombination activating protein RAG-2. *Proc. Natl. Acad. Sci. USA* **91**, 2733–2737.

55. Schlissel, M. Al Constantinescu, T. Morrow, M. Baxter, and A. Peng. 1993. Double strand signal sequence breaks in V(D)J recombination are blunt, 5' phosphorylated, RAG dependent, and cell cycle regulated. *Genes Dev.* **7**, 2523–2532.

56. Lin, W., and S. Desiderio. 1993. Regulation of V(D)J recombination activator protein RAG-2 by phosphorylation. *Science* **260**, 953–959.

57. McGuire, T.C., and M.J. Poppie. 1973. Hypogammaglobulinemia and thymic hypoplasia in horses: a primary combined immunodeficiency. *Infect. Immunity* **8**, 272–277.

58. Perryman, L.E. 1982. Domestic animal models of severe combined immunodeficiency: canine x-linked severe combined immunodeficiency and severe combined immunodeficiency in horses. *Immunodeficiency Reviews* **3**, 277–303.

59. Wiler, R., R. Leber, B.B. Moore, L.F. VanDyk, L.E. Perryman, and K. Meek. 1995. Equine severe combined immunodeficiency: a defect in V(D)J recombination and DNA-dependent protein kinase activity. *Proc. Natl. Acad. Sci. USA* **92**, 11485–11489.

60. Leber, R., R. Wiler, L.E. Perryman, and K.D. Meek. Equine SCID: Mechanistic analysis and comparison to murine SCID, in press.

61. Schuler, W., N.R. Ruetsch, J. Amster, and M.J. Bosma. 1991. Coding joint formation of endogenous T cell receptor genes in lymphoid cells from scid mice: unusual P nucleotide additions in VJ coding joints. *Eur. J. Immunol.* **21**, 589–596.

62. Kienker, L.J., W.A. Kuziel, and P.A. Tucker. 1991. T cell receptor γ and δ gene junctional sequences in SCID mice: excessive P nucleotide insertion. *J. Exp. Med.* **174**, 769–773.

63. Ford, J.E., W.A. Home, and D.M. Gibson. 1994. Light chain isotype regulation in the horse: characterization of Ig λ genes. *J. Immunol.* **153**, 1099–1111.

64. Home, W.A., J.E. Ford, and D.M. Gibson. 1992. Light chain isotype regulation in the horse: characterization of Ig κ genes. *J. Immunol.* **149**, 3927–3936.

Chapter

FOUR

Phylogenetic Diversification of Antibody Genes

MICHELE K. ANDERSON,* JONATHAN P. RAST
and GARY W. LITMAN [†]

Department of Pediatrics, University of South Florida, All Children's Hospital, 801
Sixth Street South, St. Petersburg, FL 33701, USA

I. INTRODUCTION

Antibodies are present in representatives of all of the major radiations of the jawed
vertebrates which have been investigated (a detailed cladogram defining the inter-
relationships of the various vertebrate taxa is provided below in a different context). Detailed molecular analyses of the structure and organization of the genes
encoding the Igs (immunoglobulins) and other molecules involved in immune
recognition in a wide variety of vertebrate taxa provide a basis for exploring the
evolutionary origins of these complex gene systems. Studies on the phylogenetic
diversity of antibody genes also allow inferences to be drawn regarding the relationships of gene structure to antibody function and diversity. The vast amounts of
information that have been acquired concerning the mammalian Ig gene system
are beyond the scope of this chapter and are addressed comprehensively elsewhere
in this series; however, it is important to recognize that the observations obtained
from phylogenetic studies of other groups are usually placed within the context of
mammalian immunity. This chapter will focus on the more divergent vertebrate
radiations relative to mammals, beginning with the most divergent group known
to possess Ig genes, the chondrichthyans (cartilaginous fishes), continuing through
the teleosts (bony fishes), Crossopterygii (coelacanth), Dipnoi (lungfishes),

*Present address: California Institute of Technology, Division of Biology, 156-29, 1201 East
California Boulevard, Pasadena, CA 91125. [†]Corresponding author.

amphibians, and finally will address basic aspects of these genes in the avian systems. Ig heavy and light chain genes are easily distinguished in all jawed vertebrates, and emerged before the divergence of the cartilaginous and bony fishes. Therefore, they will be discussed separately and a discussion of immunity in the jawless vertebrates will follow.

Although extensive information is accumulating regarding the Ig genes of the "lower" (i.e., non-mammalian) vertebrates, such studies have been limited by practical considerations. Routine approaches, such as cell lines, monoclonal antibodies for the detection of specific cell types, and inbred lines, which have facilitated studies in mammalian systems, have not been available for studies in the more phylogenetically distant species. However, several laboratories are now making progress in short term culturing of leukocytes from lower vertebrates (Miller et al., 1994; C. Luer and C. Walsh, personal communication). Molecular genetic analyses of lower vertebrate Ig genes have revealed highly complex genetic loci which resemble mammalian Ig genes closely in their segmental structure, rearrangement mechanisms, and in the higher order structures of their protein products. However, there is a major division between the chondrichthyans (cartilaginous fishes) and the osteichthyans-tetrapods (bony fishes, amphibians, reptiles, avians, and mammals) in terms of the chromosomal organization of the segmental elements, the control of transcriptional activity, and the mechanisms which are available for the generation of variable (V) region diversity. In addition, within the osteichthyan-tetrapod groups, extraordinary degrees of phylogenetic variability are evident in the mechanisms used to diversify their antigen-binding repertoires. A careful examination of the distribution of these features allows hypotheses to be formulated and tested concerning the evolutionary origins of these genes and the mechanisms driving their divergence.

II. Ig HEAVY CHAIN GENES

The Chondrichthyans

Heterodontus as prototypical chondrichthyan

The chondrichthyans, which include the elasmobranchs (sharks, skates, and rays) and the holocephalans (chimeras), are the most phylogenetically divergent vertebrates from mammals known to possess Igs. Early studies in sharks established the ability of these animals to reject allografts in an accelerated manner, implying the presence of a T cell–major histocompatibility complex (MHC) like self/nonself discrimination (Borysenko and Hildemann, 1970). The existence of such a genetic system is supported by observations of extensive polymorphisms in shark MHC class II genes (Kasahara et al., 1993), evidence for class I-like genes (Hashimoto et al., 1992), and the recent identification of T cell antigen receptors (TCRs; Rast and Litman, 1994; Rast et al., 1995) in these species. The primary humoral antibody response of sharks is characterized by low affinity antibodies which fail to exhibit affinity maturation even after long periods of hyperimmunization (Mäkelä and Litman, 1980; Clem and Leslie, 1982). However, nonimmune shark serum protein consists of up to 50% secretory Ig (Rosenshein and Marchalonis, 1987), which exists in both pentameric and monomeric forms (Small et al., 1970). Many "natural" antibodies are found in the serum of cartilaginous fish and appear to be autoreactive and multispecific (Marchalonis et al., 1993). Their presence suggests that the mechanisms of B cell activation operating in these animals may be different from those seen typically in mammals. It is possible that the autoreactivity of the antibodies is involved in the maintenance of B cell activation, which helps to compensate for the lack of a mammalian-like secondary response, while the low affinities of the antibodies prevent significant autoimmune damage (Marchalonis et al., 1993).

The most intensively studied chondrichthyan, *Heterodontus francisci* (horned shark), has been the subject of considerable effort on our part. A gene encoding a shark V_H element was isolated originally from a genomic DNA library by cross-hybridization with a mouse variable region heavy chain (V_H) probe (Litman et al., 1985a). The shark V_H probe, which exhibited ~60% nucleotide identity to mammalian V_H genes (Litman et al., 1985a), was used in turn to recover an Ig heavy chain cDNA from a spleen cDNA library. The heavy chain was shown to consist of six constant region heavy chain exons (C_H1, C_H2, C_H3, C_H4/secretory [SEC], transmembrane 1 [TM1], and TM2), and to resemble a mammalian μ chain transcript. Subsequent isolation and sequence analyses of genomic clones revealed the presence of segmental V region elements (V_H, D_H1, D_H2, J_H) which each are separated by ~350 bp (average), and are flanked by mammalian-like recombination signal sequences (RSSs; Hinds and Litman, 1986; Kokubu et al., 1988b). However, in contrast to the tandem distribution of segmental V region elements found in all osteichthyan and tetrapod vertebrates, the majority of *Heterodontus* genes exist in ~18 kb clusters: $V_H–D_H1–D_H2–J_H–C_{H1-4/SEC}–TM1–2$ (Figure 1A; Hinds and Litman, 1986; Kokubu et al., 1988a; Kokubu et al., 1988b). Mapping and partial sequencing of multiple genomic clones suggest that there are a large number of Ig gene clusters present in the *Heterodontus* genome. Fluorescence in situ hybridization analyses indicate that these clusters are chromosomally dispersed (Amemiya and Litman, 1991; C. Amemiya, unpublished observations).

Although hundreds of clusters are estimated to be present in the genome, relatively little sequence diversity is encoded in the V_H regions of different clusters. All but one of the known V_H genes in *Heterodontus* belong to a single family, whose members are ~90% related to each other at the nucleotide level (Kokubu et al., 1988b). The single V_HII family member is ~60% related to the V_HI family members and reflects an apparent inversion in the $D_H1–D_H2$ region. The orientation of the RSSs in the V_HI genes is such that either D_H1 and D_H2 or D_H2 only can be utilized in rearrangement. The inversion of the $D_H1–D_H2$ region in the V_HII gene allows both D_H1 and D_H2 or only D_H1 to be used in recombination. This unique gene provides an opportunity to characterize transcription products without encountering the problems distinguishing genes stemming from the high degree of similarity among the V_HI gene family members. Specifically, it enabled us to determine levels of somatic variation produced after rearrangement of this locus, and along with other findings, demonstrated that segmental rearrangement is restricted to a single cluster, as discussed below (Kokubu et al., 1988b; Hinds-Frey et al., 1993). Efforts to detect other V_H families by screening for $C_H^+/V_HI^-/V_HII^-$ clones were uniformly unsuccessful, as were similar differential screening efforts to detect additional C_H types. However, there are significant sequence differences between C_H exons obtained from different clusters, most notably in the C_H1 exon (Kokubu et al., 1987). The functional significance of these differences, if any, remains unclear.

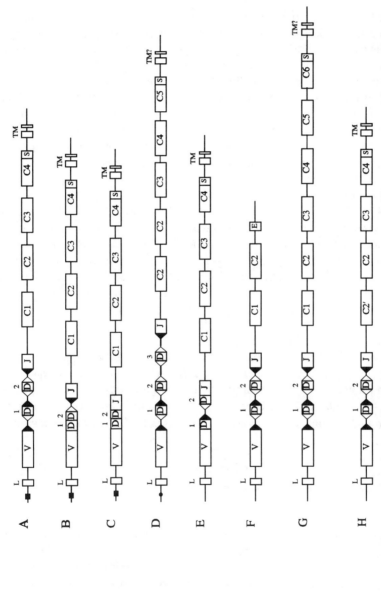

Figure 1. The organization of chondrichthyan Ig heavy chains and related genes. **A:** Unrearranged V–D$_1$–D$_2$–J–C cluster arrangement found in *Hydrolagus, Heterodontus,* and *Raja.* **B:** Partially rearranged VDD–J–C cluster found in *Heterodontus* and *Raja.* **C:** Fully rearranged VDDJ–C arrangement found in *Heterodontus* and *Hydrolagus.* **D:** The nurse shark antigen receptor (NAR) chain described from *Ginglymostoma cirratum.* **E:** Partially joined VD–DJ–C cluster type found in *Raja.* **F:** IgX cluster found in *Raja.* **G:** Long chain IgX-related gene found in *Ginglymostoma, Carcharhinus,* and *Raja.* **H:** Ig heavy chain-type from *Hydrolagus,* where C$_H$1 is replaced by an exon related to C$_H$2. L = hydrophobic leader sequence; V = variable segment; D = diversity segment; J = joining segment; C1–C6 = constant region exons; S = secretory exon; TM = transmembrane exons; E = terminal exon of unknown affinities that may function as a secretory exon. ■ = decamer-nonamer TCR CRE promoter element (found in *Heterodontus*); ● = Ig octamer promoter element found upstream of NAR V region. RSS spacer lengths are indicated by triangles: open triangles = 12 bp, solid triangles = 23 bp.

Several characteristics of the *Heterodontus* gene loci are more reminiscent of mammalian TCR loci than mammalian Ig loci, supporting the hypothesis that the chondrichthyan Ig genes retain characteristics of the putative Ig/TCR common ancestor. The close proximity of the D_H, J_H, and C_H segments are characteristic of TCRβ and TCRγ, and the closely linked V_H, J_H, and C_H segments are reminiscent of murine TCRγ. Two closely linked D_H segments are found in TCRδ. The regulatory octamer found in the 5' regions of all osteichthyan and higher vertebrate Ig V regions is missing and a decamer–nonamer cyclic AMP reactive element is located upstream of both the *Heterodontus* Ig V regions (Kokubu et al., 1988b; Litman et al., 1993) and mammalian TCRβ V region (Anderson et al., 1989). The low affinity binding of *Heterodontus* IgM antibodies (Mäkelä and Litman, 1980) also resembles the low affinity binding of TCRs, which are not believed to undergo somatic hypermutation and characteristic antibody-type affinity maturation, although a recent study provides evidence for somatic mutation of TCRs in a specialized microenvironment (Zheng et al., 1994). In spite of this, it must be emphasized that the organization of the μ-type heavy chain exons and predicted amino acid sequences are distinctive Ig properties. The identification of TCR genes in cartilaginous fish (see below) provides a further basis for defining genetic mechanisms involved in the divergence of Ig and TCR systems.

The cluster-type genomic organization of Ig genes seen in *Heterodontus* is present throughout the chondrichthyan lineage but is confined within this lineage for the heavy chain genes. Cluster-type genomic organization also is characteristic of chondrichthyan light chain genes (see below). A second characteristic which is unique to the chondrichthyans is the presence of V_H region segments which are joined in the nonlymphoid ("germline") genome. Approximately half of the germline heavy chain genes examined thus far in *Heterodontus* are either partially (VD–J; Figure 1B) or fully (VDJ; Figure 1C) joined (Kokubu et al., 1988b). The V_H coding sequences of these genes closely resemble unjoined genes at the nucleotide and predicted amino acid levels, with the exception of the D_H segments, which are notably different. These differences may be due to the typical deletions and N (nontemplated) additions which accompany the joining process. Alternatively, these D_H segments may have diversified either by typical evolutionary mechanisms, or they may have originated as different types of D_H elements. The intact leader and J_H–C_H intervening sequences (IVSs), typical J_H–C_H splice sites, correct reading frame, absence of internal stop codons, and presence of 5' and 3' sequence identity with unjoined genes strongly suggest that these genes are not processed, reintegrated pseudogenes (Kokubu et al., 1988b). It is unlikely that the observation of germline-joined genes is an artifact of B cell contamination from other tissues owing to the high relative frequency of these genes and because identical germline-joined genes have been isolated from both liver and gonadal DNA of unrelated animals (Kokubu et al., 1988b). In addition, the germline-joined state has been observed in both the heavy and light chains genes of not only *Heterodontus*, but also *Raja* and *Hydrolagus* (ratfish), as will be described below.

There are several reasons to believe that germline-joined genes are not derived from ancestral unsegmented genes, but instead originated from unjoined genes. First, the integration of the elements enabling somatic recombination of V_H elements probably occurred prior to the divergence of the Ig and TCR genes, since both types of genes carry essentially identical RSS. Second, only half of the heavy chain genes are joined, and it seems more likely that these were joined at some point in evolution, perhaps mediated by a recombinase activating gene (RAG)-like mechanism, rather than through the integration of multiple RSSs in equivalent positions in each cluster. Alternatively, it is possible that the joined genes could be a monophyletic diversification of a single secondary integration event. Third, the presence of both unjoined and germline-joined light chain genes in different chondrichthyan groups (see below) provides further evidence that in this case this state is derived and not primordial.

The high incidence of germline-joined genes combined with the relatively low amount of diversity encoded in V_H genes raises questions as to how the chondrichthyans generate sufficient diversity in order to accommodate the wide range of antigenic challenges to which they presumably are exposed. In mammals, antibody diversity is accomplished by a variety of means, including combinatorial usage of different V_H, D_H, and J_H segments, imprecise joining and fusions of multiple elements (Sanz, 1991; Pascual and Capra, 1991), which are subject to both deletions and N additions at the junctional boundaries, and post-rearrangement hypermutation events confined to the VDJ region (for review, see Desiderio, 1993). The lack of intercluster recombination effectively rules out combinatorial diversification in *Heterodontus* as does the high degree of nucleotide identity among the different elements (e.g., near identity of D segments) which would introduce very little (germline) sequence diversity even if a combinatorial system did exist. This contrasts with the Ig heavy chain locus of most tetrapods and bony fishes in which significant differences exist between segmental elements. While the multiplicity of clusters, which at first appears to create additional sources of diversity, are likewise limited to some degree by their similarity to one another, studies comparing unjoined parental clusters (both V_H1- and V_HII-types) to their corresponding cDNA sequences indicate that extensive deletions and N additions accompany the rearrangement process in the heavy chain gene loci of *Heterodontus*. These loci also appear to undergo at least limited somatic mutation following rearrangement (Hinds-Frey et al., 1993). The joined genes, which (depending on the degree of joining) undergo reduced or no junctional diversification owing to the decrease in or absence of somatic rearrangement could still be subject to somatic mutation. Somatic (hyper) mutation in mammals appears to be activated after rearrangement of the locus and activation of the lymphocyte, during subsequent rounds of replication. In the case of fully joined genes, it is unclear what events would be necessary to (1) trigger the transcription of these genes and (2) provide accessibility to mutational machinery, since rearrangement per se does not occur. However, if somatic hypermutation is linked to transcription-coupled DNA repair in the cartilaginous fishes, as it appears to be in mice (Peters and Storb, 1996), then there may be a unique rearrangement-independent process in this system which initiates mutation of both joined and unjoined loci. Alternatively, the genetic distances that are eliminated between some segments through rearrangement in cluster organization are several orders of magnitude shorter than in the mammalian extended locus. Thus, it is unclear whether the effects of such processes (e.g., bringing the enhancer sequences into close proximity to the promoter sequences) are operating in either the unjoined or the joined clusters in *Heterodontus*, especially given the lack of conservation of linear relationships of homologous regulatory sequence motifs between the J_H–C_H IVSs of the chondrichthyan and mammalian loci (Anderson et al., 1994; Litman et al., 1996).

Maintenance of germline-joined genes in the genome suggests a functional role in immunity. However, extensive searches for transcripts arising from these genes in *Heterodontus* have been unsuccessful (Hinds-Frey et al., 1993; Litman et al., 1996). In contrast, studies of both *Hydrolagus* IgM heavy chain genes (Rast et al, 1996, in preparation) and *Raja* light chain genes (Anderson et al., 1995) have shown that joined genes are expressed. Germline-joined genes also could be templates for gene conversion, or could serve as substrates for secondary recombination events. Furthermore, germline-joined genes have fixed specificities which may be selected for entirely by conventional, direct evolutionary processes, and could provide antigen-binding motifs for specialized needs. The restriction of germline-joining to the chondrichthyan lineage could be a function of the multiple cluster-type organization in these species, since joining of some clusters in order to create predetermined specificities would leave other clusters free for generating a more diverse repertoire. Moreover, joining of one cluster does not disrupt the integrity of other clusters, since the V region segments are not tandemly arrayed in close linkage as in mammals.

It has been proposed that the lack of affinity maturation in both *Heterodontus* (Hinds-Frey et al., 1993) and other lower vertebrates which exhibit somatic hyper-mutation (Wilson et al., 1992) is attributable to an absence of germinal centers which would result in inefficient cellular selection. An alternative, though not incompatible, explanation is that the B cells involved in the primary response are terminally differentiated, and thus, after the first exposure to antigen, are unable to persist long enough to initiate a typical secondary response or simply are unable to be restimulated upon subsequent exposures. In this scenario, somatic (hyper) mutation would occur in the small number of cells selected during the primary response in subsequent rounds of cell replication. However, these cells would not be competent to undergo a subsequent expansion and further rounds of mutation, resulting in levels of affinity maturation below detection. The "memory" cell phenotype may have evolved after the divergence of the cartilaginous fishes and is only represented in contemporary forms of other lower vertebrate species such as teleosts and amphibians. This phenotype, of either long-lived or clonally persistent B cells, may have become more advantageous with the evolution of multiple constant regions isotypes, which are associated with the complex mammalian-type secondary responses. This hypothesis remains to be tested, and is complicated by our lack of full understanding of the character of mammalian memory lymphocytes. It also should be noted that a second Ig-like antigen receptor (NAR; Figure 1D) from the nurse shark appears to undergo unprecedented levels of somatic mutation and thus may require a highly competent selection mechanism (Greenberg et al., 1995). In summary, studies in *Heterodontus* have revealed that while the segmental building blocks of Ig genes have been highly conserved throughout evolution, the chromosomal architecture and thus the mechanisms available for generating antibody diversity are flexible and divergent.

Raja as developmental model

The skates and rays diverged from the lineage leading to *Heterodontus* approximately 220 million years ago, and as such, provide an important group for assessing diversification of the Ig genes in the chondrichthyans (by way of comparison) over an extended evolutionary time period. Furthermore, *Raja* (skate) possesses a distinct advantage over *Heterodontus* in that staged embryos are available for developmental studies of antigen receptor gene expression (Luer, 1989). These advantages have led us to focus our more recent efforts on defining Ig gene structure and expression in *Raja*. Serum protein analyses first indicated the presence of IgM-like molecules in two species of stingray and in several skate species (Marchalonis and Schonfeld, 1970; Kobayashi et al., 1984; Kobayashi et al., 1985). IgM heavy chain genes were isolated from *Raja* by cross-hybridization with *Heterodontus* V_H and C_H probes. *Raja* V_H segments exhibit ~78% nucleotide identity with *Heterodontus* V_H segments, and share 60% overall amino acid identity. Like *Heterodontus* μ-chain genes, the *Raja* μ-chain genes exist as V_H–D_H1–D_H2–J_H–C_{H1-4}/SEC–TM1–2 (Figure 1A) clusters. In addition, 50% of the clusters are found in a partially germline-joined configuration (VD–DJ [Figure 1E]) or VD-J [Figure 1B]; Harding et al., 1990a). The fully joined configuration (VDJ) seen in *Heterodontus*, has not been identified in the *Raja* IgM heavy chain clones examined thus far. The minimal variability of D_H segments in *Raja* is similar to that seen in *Heterodontus*, but greater variation is seen in J_H segments in *Raja*, than is observed in *Heterodontus*. As in *Heterodontus*, there is no octamer present in the region upstream of V_H, but there also is no nonamer–decamer sequence such as was identified in *Heterodontus* (Harding et al., 1990b). *Raja* μ-type clusters are present at different chromosomal locations (Anderson et al., 1994).

As indicated above, analyses of *Heterodontus* Ig genes have established that only one constant region type (μ) is found in association with the V_H segments, and there currently is no molecular evidence to suggest the presence of other types in this species. However, a second heavy chain type has been identified in *Raja*. Serum protein analyses reveal two antigenically distinct Igs in two species of *Raja*. The higher molecular weight form is believed to be IgM, and the lower molecular weight form was initially designated IgR (Kobayashi et al., 1984; Kobayashi et al., 1985). IgR, which forms dimers, is coexpressed early in development with IgM on individual spleen cells, whereas adult spleen cells express only IgM or IgR (Kobayashi et al., 1985). There also is evidence from protein studies for a second heavy chain isotype in the frill shark, a member of a basal elasmobranch lineage (Kobayashi et al., 1992), suggesting that multiple heavy chain types may occur throughout the elasmobranchs.

In order to identify the genes encoding the IgR-type heavy chains, a *Raja* cDNA library was screened for the presence of V_H^+/C_H1^- (μ-type) clones and a second heavy chain gene, IgX was identified (Harding et al., 1990a, 1990b). The size of the predicted peptide encoded by the IgX heavy chain gene corresponds approximately to the size of IgR. The *Raja* V_x elements are approximately 60% related in nucleotide sequence to the V_H elements of *Raja* IgM-type. Based on the lack of predicted peptide and nucleotide sequence identity with constant regions of higher vertebrate Ig the IgX heavy chain gene(s) appears to be an isotype that is unique to the chondrichthyans rather than an evolutionary forerunner to other isotypes seen in other vertebrates (Harding et al., 1990a). The one IgX gene locus that has been mapped and fully sequenced exists as a cluster consisting of V_x, D_x1, D_x2, J_x, C_x1, C_x2, and a cysteine-rich exon which may have a secretory function(s) (Anderson et al., 1994; Figure 1F). The V_x, D_x, and J_x segments are flanked by typical RSSs. The existence and/or extent of germline-joining in IgX clusters has yet to be determined. As in *Heterodontus* and *Raja* IgM (type) clusters, there is neither an octamer within ~1500 bp upstream of the start codon nor is there a decamer–nonamer CRE-like sequence(s) found 5' of the *Raja* IgX clusters. The chromosomal distribution of IgX heavy chain genes, as revealed by fluorescence in situ hybridization, suggests that, as with IgM, there are multiple dispersed IgX loci, and that the clusters of IgM and IgX are not chromosomally linked (Anderson et al., 1994).

This unique case of two different types of noncontiguous cluster-type Ig heavy chain loci raises questions about the regulation of Ig gene expression in this species. The coexpression of IgM and IgR on embryonic spleen cells suggests that these loci are not subject to isotypic exclusion during at least one stage of development. Furthermore, the lack of conventional mammalian-type switch sequences in either *Heterodontus* J_H–C_H1 or *Raja* J_x–C_x1 IVS (Anderson et al., 1994; Litman et al., 1996) and the absence of detectable linear arrangements of constant region types are inconsistent with mammalian-type class switching. At this point there is no molecular or biochemical evidence for or against the presence of an allelic exclusion mechanism in chondrichthyan Ig loci; however, trans-acting diffusible factors, such have been postulated to regulate allelic exclusion in higher vertebrates, could in principle act on multiple clusters as they do on two alleles and thus play a role in regulation either at the levels of rearrangement or transcription. Any model suggesting regulation at the level of rearrangement must take into account the presence of fully germline-joined genes, as discussed above.

In order to identify potential cis-acting regulatory elements, the J_x–C_x1 IVS of an IgX genomic clone was searched for regions with significant identity to regulatory motifs shown to be important in mammalian Ig and TCR genes. Although many short sequence stretches in the *Raja* J_x–C_x1 IVS exhibit significant extended identity with these motifs, their arrangements differ considerably between the mammalian and *Heterodontus* J_H–C_H1 IVS. The functional significance of these motifs remains unclear, although recent studies of catfish Ig regulatory regions (see below) indicate that these types of motifs may operate cooperatively in different organizational contexts. Both the *Heterodontus* IgM (type) and the *Raja* IgX J–C IVS sequences were obtained from unjoined clusters. It would be of considerable interest to determine their relationship to the J–C IVSs of joined clusters as it is entirely possible that joined genes are under a different form of transcriptional regulation.

Like mammalian IgM, *Raja* IgM-type gene loci generate either SEC or TM forms of heavy chains through alternative splicing and polyadenylation (Harding et al., 1990a). However, the IgX gene cluster does not appear to include either typical SEC or TM exons. IgX gene loci give rise instead to three different types of transcripts, as determined by Northern blotting (Harding et al., 1990a) and cDNA sequencing (Anderson et al., 1994). One type of cDNA contains the V_x region sequence from an unrearranged or partially rearranged IgX locus with J_x correctly spliced to the first constant region exon, followed by a C_x1–C_x2 intron-like sequence, without any apparent polyadenylation signals. One of these transcripts exhibits apparent elimination of the D_x2 element, the RSS 5' of D_x2, and most of the RSS 3' of D_x2. This transcript presumably arose from an IgX heavy chain cluster lacking a D_x2 element, or may be the result of an aberrant joining event. The unrearranged, incompletely spliced nature of these transcripts suggest that they represent a class of developmentally early transcripts which function in facilitating accessibility of the Ig loci to recombinational machinery (Yancopoulos and Alt, 1985). A second type of IgX heavy chain cDNA contains a fully rearranged $V_xD_xJ_x$ region with two constant region exons followed by the cysteine-rich putative terminal exon. In the third type of cDNA, the terminal exon is replaced by ~1250 bp of sequence containing a number of putative Ig domains. This type of transcript contains rearranged and unrearranged or partially rearranged V_x regions. The putative extra Ig domains of this third type are especially intriguing, as they lack significant nucleotide or amino acid identity with any known Ig superfamily members, but possess the characteristic spacing of certain residues which are conserved in these family members (Williams and Barclay, 1988). The constant region of this gene type possesses six Ig domains and terminates in an SEC-type sequence (Figure 1G). Although only pseudogenes of this type have been identified thus far in the skate, similar, presumably functional genes have been isolated recently from the nurse and sandbar sharks (Greenberg et al., 1996; M. Flajnik, personal communication).

Hydrolagus: an independent chondrichthyan lineage

The holocephalans, or chimeras and ratfishes, are a group of predominantly deep-sea chondrichthyans that are thought to form a outgroup to the extant elasmobranchs and probably diverged from them approximately 350 million years ago (Maisey, 1984). As such this group affords an opportunity to elucidate the origin of the cluster-type Ig system. Heavy chain gene organization in a representative species, the spotted ratfish (Hydrolagus colliei), is generally of the elasmobranch cluster type of which three varieties have been identified. The first and most abundant type is comprised of V–D–D–J unjoined genes, similar to those found in the sharks and skates. These genes are related closely to the most abundant immunoglobulin heavy chain transcripts (cDNAs) identified in spleen and exhibit greater than 90% sequence identity to each other. Although each cDNA of this type which has been analyzed thus far has a unique constant region, it has not been possible to identify corresponding recombinant bacteriophage lambda genomic clones in which V_H and C_H regions are linked, implying a greater linkage distance between these elements than has been observed in Heterodontus or Raja. A second cluster organization has been identified in cosmid clones. V_H regions in this gene subset form a family that exhibits ~85% nucleotide identity to the V_H genes of the first type. In these clusters, a C_H1-type exon is replaced by a second C_H2-like exon, which appears to be the result of a relatively recent exon duplication (Figure 1H). Although transcripts arising from this cluster type have not been recovered in direct cDNA library screening, they have been detected using a reverse transcriptase–polymerase chain reaction (RT–PCR) approach. A third cluster type is represented by a monotypic VDJ-joined gene. The V_H region and first exon of the constant region in this cluster are only about 80% and 75% related, respectively to those of the first type. Linkage distances between V_H and C_H region exons in this cluster are equivalent to those in Heterodontus heavy chain gene clusters. Transcripts of both the transmembrane and secretory form of this gene have been identified using RT–PCR employing second complementarity determining region

(CDR2)- and constant region-specific primers. Only ~10% of V_H region clones in a *Hydrolagus* genomic lambda library can be identified with an oligonucleotide probe complementing J_H. Although appreciable J_H diversity offers one possible explanation for the paucity of V_H^+/J_H^+ clones, sequencing and PCR analyses have demonstrated that the remaining 90% of V_H^+ clones are truncated V_H pseudogenes which are nearly identical to each other as well as to the V_H region of the monotypic joined heavy chain gene cluster. Whether or not these genes play any role in the generation of V_H region diversity is not understood; however, the near identity between these pseudogenes makes this possibility unlikely. The presence of a cluster type gene arrangement (and variants thereof) in a holocephalan implies that this form of segmental organization is present throughout the entire vertebrate class Chondrichthyes and that it emerged at least 350 million years ago. Extensive heavy chain cluster divergence appears to have occurred in this holocephalan, as has been reported in *Raja* and likely will be the case in *Heterodontus*.

The Osteichthyans

The osteichthyan lineage, which diverged from the chondrichthyan lineage early in vertebrate evolution, includes both the Actinopterygians (ray-finned fishes), which includes the teleost fishes as well as the Sarcopterygians (lobed-finned fishes), which includes the lungfishes and the coelacanth (*Latimeria*). Among the living sarcopterygians, Ig gene structure has been studied most closely extensively in the coelacanth, *Latimeria chalumnae*. The coelacanth is of particular interest because it and the lungfish are considered to be close relatives of the tetrapods. In *Latimeria*, the V_H region genes are linked within ~190 bp upstream of D_H elements; multiple copies of V_H–D_H have been identified in this species. Each of these V_H elements is associated with a typical upstream octamer and a RSS with a 23 bp spacer, and the D_H elements are flanked on their 5' and 3' ends by RSSs with 12 bp spacers (Figure 2A). A large number of V_H pseudogene elements have been identified which are not linked to D_H elements (Amemiya et al., 1993). Further investigations into this unique organization have been hindered by the difficulties in obtaining lymphoid tissue suitable for RNA extraction. The atypical, somewhat chondrichthyan-like arrangement of the V_H and D_H elements is consistent with a number of other chondrichthyan-like characters found in the coelacanth (Amemiya et al., 1993).

Another sarcopterygian, the African lungfish (*Protopterus aethiopicus*) is of great interest owing to its unique phylogenetic position, high haploid cellular DNA content (~37 times the genome size of humans), and its evolutionary relationship to the coelacanth. Protein studies reveal that *Protopterus* has at least three Ig heavy chain constant region isotypes (Litman et al., 1971). cDNAs encoding two of the three isotypes have been sequenced to date. Preliminary results indicate that two different V_H families may associate with specific constant region isotypes in a mutually exclusive manner (T. Ota, J. Rast, G. Litman, and C. Amemiya, unpublished observations). These results differ from those typically seen in other tetrapods in which different V_H families associate with different C_H isotypes through conventional class switching, suggesting that the Ig heavy chain locus is complex in lungfish. Unfortunately the extraordinarily large genome size in lungfish will complicate investigations of the genomic organization of these genes.

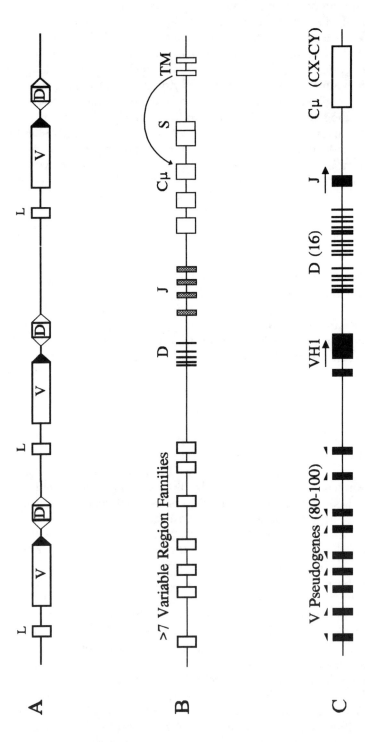

Figure 2. Heavy chain gene organization of osteichthyans and avians. **A:** Tandem repeating V–D organization found in the living coelacanth *Latimeria chalumnae*. **B:** Tandem Ig heavy chain gene organization of teleosts. Arrow indicates unusual splicing of transmembrane exons to C_H3 instead of C_H4. **C:** Chicken Ig heavy chain gene organization. Arrows and wedges indicate transcriptional polarity. The IgX- and IgY-type constant regions are located downstream from IgM. L = hydrophobic leader sequence; V = variable segment; D = diversity segment; J = joining segment; C = constant region exons; S = secretory exon; TM = transmembrane exons. Octamer promoter elements are found upstream of V_H genes in these groups. RSS spacer lengths are indicated by triangles: open triangles = 12 bp, solid triangles = 23 bp and also are present in teleost and avian genes.

A major division in the organization of the Ig heavy chain locus was firmly established with the emergence of the osteichthyans. The extended locus form, maintained and expanded in later tetrapod radiations, is composed of multiple V_H region elements arrayed tandemly along a single locus, followed by one or more sets of constant region exons. Teleost V_H genes (Figure 2B) closely resemble those of other tetrapods (with the exception of avians, which will be discussed later) in both primary structure and chromosomal arrangement. Early descriptions of V_H genes in the ladyfish, *Elops saurus*, revealed the presence of multiple, putative functional gene segments within one genomic clone, each possessing a leader split by a short intron, typical RSSs and upstream octamers. Numerous pseudogenes also were identified in other species of teleost fishes (Amemiya and Litman, 1990; Wilson et al., 1988). Subsequently, the extended locus motif was identified in additional teleost species (Matsunaga et al., 1990; Ventura-Holman et al., 1994; Bengten et al., 1994). Field inversion gel electrophoretic mapping in the ladyfish indicated that V_H elements are found within ~100 kb of C_H (Amemiya and Litman, 1990). V_H intergenic distances range from ~3 kb (Ventura-Holman et al., 1994) to >9 kb (Bengten et al., 1994). Earlier analyses of ladyfish genomic clones are consistent with values between these two lengths (Amemiya and Litman, 1990). V_H genes from different families are interspersed in the catfish and the Atlantic cod, like in man (Kodaira et al., 1986) and *Xenopus* (Haire et al., 1991) but are not interspersed in an equivalent manner in mouse (Rathbun et al., 1987). Interspersion of different families may minimize positional effects of V_H usage (Walter et al., 1991).

Teleost V_H gene diversity is extensive, as shown by a number of studies in different species. There are at least nine V_H families expressed in the rainbow trout (Roman and Charlemagne, 1994; Matsunaga et al., 1990; Andersson et al., 1991; Lee et al., 1996; Andersson and Matsunaga, 1993), at least seven V_H families in the channel catfish (Ghaffari and Lobb, 1991), and at least three V_H families in the Atlantic cod (Bengten et al., 1994). DNA sequencing of isolated clones reveals the existence of at least three V_H families in the pufferfish, *Spheroides nephulus* (M. Margittai, C. Amemiya, G. Litman, unpublished observations), which possesses a relatively small genome size. Most of these V_H families are comprised of at least 20 members each, and sequence diversity among the members of each family is substantial. Diversity among V_H segments both within and between families is highest in the CDRs.

A combination of phylogenetic analyses of sequence data (Ghaffari and Lobb, 1991; Roman and Charlemagne, 1994; Ota and Nei, 1994) and Southern blot analyses (Jones et al., 1993) have been used to evaluate the relationships of these teleost V_H family members to each other and to other vertebrate V_H genes. Both types of analyses support an early emergence of two major V_H groups in the vertebrate lineage, detectable in a wide array of diverse teleost lineages. Furthermore, these two major V_H groups appear to have diverged prior to the divergence of the cartilaginous and bony fishes.

In addition to extensive V_H family diversity, several other findings indicate that teleosts have the ability to generate a large repertoire of antigen-binding specificities. Specifically, multiple J_H segments have been described in the ladyfish (Amemiya and Litman, 1990), the channel catfish (Ghaffari and Lobb, 1991), and the rainbow trout (Roman and Charlemagne, 1994). Although D_H segments have not yet been characterized at the genomic level, the types of RSSs present 3' of the

V_H segments and 5' of the J_H segments as well as the recognition of regions in cDNAs with high identity to known D_H core sequences suggest that D_H elements are present and are used in mammalian-like VDJ recombination. It is apparent from cDNA sequencing that different V_H and J_H segments are recombined, and that diversity is contributed in the CDR3 region through the use of D_H regions and most likely N- and P-type junctional diversification processes. Furthermore, in the Atlantic cod, multiple, sometimes overlapping D motifs are present and there is evidence that these are functional in several reading frames (Bengten et al., 1994).

The linkage distances between the most C_H-proximal J_H segment and the $C_H 1$ exon range from ~3.6 kb in the ladyfish (Amemiya and Litman, 1990) to ~825 bp in the rainbow trout (Roman and Charlemagne, 1994). The J_H–$C_H 1$ introns of both the catfish and the rainbow trout contain regions with identity to mammalian enhancer motifs. Although no enhancer activity has been detected in these regions, strong enhancer activity is present in a region beginning downstream of TM1 and extending downstream of TM2 (Magor et al., 1994a). This enhancer extends over a ~1.8 kb region, and does not appear to have a defined core, since progressive deletions cause progressive loss of activity. This enhancer region which functions in a B cell specific manner in both catfish and mammalian cells, contains multiple copies of motifs similar or identical to mammalian octamer and $\mu E5$ enhancer motifs, but lacks extended regions of identity with mammalian Ig heavy chain 3' enhancers. These results suggest that the J_H–C_H intronic enhancer developed later in evolution, possibly accompanying expansion of multiple C_H region isotypes, of which some are deleted in isotype switching.

Only the μ heavy chain isotype has been established unequivocally in teleosts. Although there are reports of multiple antigenically distinct isotypes in teleosts, it is likely that the antigenic differences are due to different V_H families rather than to different C_H isotypes (Lobb and Olson, 1988). Furthermore, Southern blotting and quantitative genomic titration analyses indicate that only one constant region gene is present in most teleosts (Amemiya and Litman, 1990; Ghaffari and Lobb, 1989a; Ghaffari and Lobb, 1989b; Andersson and Matsunaga, 1993). In the Atlantic salmon, *Salmo salmar* L., two IgM heavy chain genes, $C_H A$ and $C_H B$ have been defined, which are approximately 96% identical at the amino acid level. This unique situation is believed to have resulted from the duplication of the entire Ig heavy chain locus during a proposed tetraploidization event in a salmonid ancestor (Hordvik et al., 1992).

With the above exceptions noted, it appears that the teleosts and presumably the other osteichthyans are the most divergent group from mammals to have evolved a single Ig heavy chain locus with multiple tandemly repeating V_H, D_H, and J_H elements. These genes undergo combinatorial rearrangement and junctional diversification, although the antibody response in teleost fishes more closely resemble that of the chondrichthyans than it does the mammalian response (Espelid et al., 1991). Like all other vertebrate IgM heavy chains genes, both SEC and TM transcript forms can be identified. However, transmembrane forms in teleosts lack $C_H 4$, and splice from $C_H 3$ directly to TM1. The typical consensus 5' splice site found embedded in the $C_H 4$ exon of all other jawed vertebrate species is absent in all teleost species investigated thus far (Wilson et al., 1990; Bengten et al., 1991; Hordvik et al., 1992). The loss of the $C_H 4$ exon in membrane-bound IgM does not appear to alter its function, suggesting that $C_H 4$ function is specific to the secretory form of IgM, possibly through the formation of covalent structures (Wilson et al., 1990).

The Amphibians

The amphibian Ig heavy chain genes are present in a single extended locus of tandemly arranged elements, consisting of multiple V_H families and multiple C_H isotypes. Antigenic stimulation of the immune system in the most extensively studied amphibian, *Xenopus laevis* (African clawed toad), results in a weak secondary response which is intermediate between chondrichthyan and mammalian levels. As in teleosts, it appears that the limitations in affinity maturation are not due to a lack of potential for somatically recombining and diversifying segmental elements. Eleven highly diversified V_H families, at least 17 D_H elements, and at least 10 J_H elements are present in the *Xenopus* genome, a level of complexity which may exceed the possibilities for combinatorial diversity found in the Ig heavy chain loci of most mammals (Haire et al., 1990). The framework regions (FR) of the different V_H families exhibit ~35–70% nucleotide identity with each other, and the V_H family members, with some exceptions, are interspersed within the locus (Haire et al., 1991). Several amino acid positions, which are highly conserved in FR1 and FR2 of human, mouse, shark, caiman, chicken, and ladyfish genes, are altered in some *Xenopus* V_H families (Haire et al., 1990). In addition, *Xenopus* D_H segments are used in different reading frames and may be truncated, inverted, or fused (Schwager et al., 1991a). The level of junctional diversity, possible combinations of V_H, D_H, and J_H segments, and the rate of somatic mutation (Haire et al., 1990; Wilson et al., 1992) in *Xenopus* are comparable to that found in mammalian systems. Since highly developed germinal centers have not been reported in these animals, it is possible that, as in the shark (Hinds-Frey et al., 1993), the deficit in affinity maturation has more to do with cellular selection microenvironments than with Ig gene diversity (Wilson et al., 1992) or with the capacity of the lymphocytes for restimulation.

Xenopus possesses three constant region isotype genes, designated IgM (Schwager et al., 1988b; Schwager et al., 1988a), IgY (Amemiya et al., 1989), and IgX (Haire et al., 1989). The *Xenopus* IgM is a homolog of other vertebrate IgM heavy chains. IgX is not homologous to the *Raja* IgX heavy chain gene and does not have any other known vertebrate homologs. Although IgY lacks a mammalian counterpart, it is homologous to an avian heavy chain gene bearing the same designation. Homologs of IgM and IgY heavy chain genes also have been described in a urodele amphibian, the Mexican axolotl (*Ambystoma mexicanum*; Fellah et al., 1992; Fellah et al., 1993). However, the physiological function of axolotl IgY resembles that of *Xenopus* IgX and mammalian IgA in that it appears in the intestinal mucosa of young animals in close association with secretory component-like molecules up to the seventh month, after which it disappears from the intestine and appears in the serum (Fellah et al., 1992). Evidence for class switching between IgM and IgY includes observations of IgM and IgY heavy chain cDNAs sharing a common J_H or V_H sequences (Wilson et al., 1992). However, this type of class switching differs from mammalian class switching, which occurs typically after antigenic stimulation, in that the IgM levels remain high after the appearance of IgY.

The Reptiles

Little information is available on the reptilian Ig genes, perhaps because they appear to be very similar in their chromosomal organization and segmental structure to the genes in amphibians and mammals. However, the first nonmammalian Ig V_H gene to be characterized at the molecular level was identified in caiman (*Caiman crocodylus*) by cross-hybridization to a mouse V_H probe (Litman et al., 1983). The caiman V_H gene segment, has 65–70% overall nucleotide and 60–65% overall amino acid sequence identity to mammalian V_H genes, most of which is in the FRs. One caiman V_H gene has several unusual features including a RSS at the split leader intron (Litman et al., 1985b). The presence of the RSS in this site suggests that the RSSs may be derived from mobile repeat elements, which would provide a mechanism for the introduction of recombining segmental elements during the emergence of the rearranging gene families. In addition, this gene exhibits a RSS spacer which could allow potential joining of J_H directly to V_H, bypassing rearrangement of D_H. Extremely large numbers of V_H genes were identified in another reptilian species, the snapping turtle (*Chelydra serpentina*; G. Litman, unpublished observation). Furthermore, in situ hybridization studies have demonstrated the presence of multiple, chromosomally dispersed loci in this species (C. Amemiya, J. Bickham, and G. Litman, unpublished observation). Further investigations into these unique situations may provide important clues as to the evolution of these complex systems.

The Avians

The avian Ig gene loci are unique in several ways from other higher vertebrate systems. Although most of the studies conducted thus far have focused on the chicken, *Gallus gallus*, other studies seem to indicate that the general phenomena extend to other avian species as well (McCormack et al., 1989a). The chicken Ig loci provide striking examples of the conservation of certain structural features and the diversification of functional features as compared to the mammalian system. The chicken Ig heavy chain locus contains multiple V_H segments, tandemly arrayed along a single chromosomal region, and only the most C_H proximal V_H gene, designated V_H1, is functional. The remainder of the 60–80 kb V_H locus is comprised of V_H pseudogenes, which lack RSSs and leader sequences, exhibit 5′ truncation, and vary in transcriptional polarity (Figure 2C). Some of the V_H pseudogenes are fused to sequences which are related closely to D_H segments, and some of these contain putative J_H codons at their respective 3′ ends (Reynaud et al., 1989). The D_H segments exhibit a high level of sequence similarity to each other, and there appears to be only one J_H segment located 3′ of the D_H region (Reynaud et al., 1991b). Therefore, combinatorial diversity is limited to variable usage of D_H and junctional diversity does not appear to play a large role in creating the antibody repertoire of most avian species, although exceptions have been noted (McCormack et al., 1989b; McCormack et al., 1989a). Instead, it appears that the Ig heavy chain genes are diversified primarily by gene conversion between the rearranged allele and upstream pseudogenes, which donate blocks of sequence to the rearranged V_H1 gene. This process may be mediated partially by the sequence identity between the rearranged D_H and J_H segments and the regions at the ends of the pseudogenes. The use of different pseudogenes as donors is associated with some preferred exchanges. Furthermore, multiple gene conversion exchanges gradually increase the diversification of the rearranged gene. The greatest diversity accumulates in the D_H region with increasing cell divisions (Reynaud et al., 1989). The homology of the pseudogene elements to D_H regions and in at least one case to a J_H region suggests that either germline V–D joining occurred at some time in evolution, as in the chondrichthyans, or that a reverse transcription of a message derived from a somatically rearranged VD(J) gene has been inserted into the genome and then duplicated. Alternatively, selection may have preserved pseudogenes with identity in this area, if the gene conversion process were augmented.

The V_H genes in higher vertebrates have been classified into three groups (A, B, and C; Ota and Nei, 1994) using the minimum evolution method of phylogenetic analysis. All of the chicken V_H pseudogenes and the V_H1 gene are descended from an ancestral gene belonging to the vertebrate group C, from which other tetrapod group C genes, also are descended. Estimates of divergence times of the pseudogenes indicate that they evolved much later than the time of the emergence of the avians (Ota and Nei, 1995). These results indicate that group A, B, and C genes, other than V_H1, have been lost from the avian genome, and that the pseudogenes have arisen recently by tandem duplication, regardless of which mechanism(s) generated the first VD-fused pseudogene. The loss of all V_H genes, other than V_H1, could have been caused by population bottlenecks, or from accumulations of deleterious mutations during an extended time of population size reduction. It currently is unclear whether gene conversion evolved as a compensatory mechanism before or after these genes became nonfunctional, thus allowing the loss of fully functional genes and accumulation of pseudogenes to occur without extreme deleterious effects (Ota and Nei, 1995).

The development of B cells in the chicken takes place in a specialized organ, the bursa, in which all Ig gene rearrangement occurs during a restricted time in ontogeny (Weill and Reynaud, 1987). After this ontogenic time point, a high rate of B cell division persists in the bursa of juvenile chickens. However, most of these cells undergo programmed cell death, and only ~5% emigrate to the periphery. Surface Ig expression is lost shortly before cell death in the bursa. The chicken *bcl-2* gene, which is expressed at high levels in the embryonic bursa and juvenile thymus, but at low levels in the juvenile bursa, may be instrumental in protecting developing B cells from apoptosis during the stage-specific program of gene rearrangement and diversification via gene conversion (Vainio and Imhof, 1995). This differs from the mammalian system in which B cell development occurs in the bone marrow continuously throughout the lifetime of the animal. It is intriguing that the rabbit uses a similar system of gene conversion in the diversification of its Ig heavy chain gene employing intact upstream V_H genes instead of pseudogenes in the process. This could represent a functional (although of course not phylogenetic) intermediate between the typical tetrapod locus and that of the avians (Becker and Knight, 1990; Knight, 1992). In another mammalian species, the sheep, light chain V region rearrangement events are restricted to one ontogenetic stage, and point mutation is used as a primary means for generating diversity (Reynaud et al., 1991a). Clearly, a variety of different strategies are employed for generating sequence diversity and expanding the potential antibody repertoire.

Three constant region isotypes — IgM, IgY, and IgA — are located downstream of the J_H locus in the chicken. The first antibody produced in the serum in response to antigenic challenge is IgM, which subsequently is replaced by IgY, the major constituent serum antibody in birds, reptiles, and amphibians. The evolutionary relationships between these isotypes and those similarly denoted in other vertebrate species is at this time unclear, with the exception of IgM that appears to be orthologous throughout the jawed vertebrates. Chicken IgA appears to be functionally equivalent to mammalian IgA in that it is most abundantly expressed in epithelial associated lymphoid tissue, and has the ability to bind to purified human secretory component (Mansikka, 1992). IgY of the white Peking duck, *Anas platyrhynchos*, is expressed in two secreted forms, one of which is truncated. These two forms also are present in two other avian species, but not in the chicken (Magor et al., 1994b; Parham, 1995). The full length form, IgY, appears to function normally, while the shorter form, IgY(ΔFc), binds antigen effectively but is defective in certain immunological effector mechanisms such as complement fixation and skin sensitization (Magor et al., 1992). A transmembrane form also is expressed. These three forms result from alternative splicing of a single gene, which is unique in its organization, in that it has two constant region exons followed by an exon termed "T," which encodes two amino acids and a polyadenylation signal sequence. Splicing of the second C_H exon to T results in the expression of IgY(ΔFc). C_v3 and C_v4/SEC are located downstream of the T exon, followed by two putative TM exons which are similar in both length and amino acid sequence to both IgG and IgE TM exons. IgY has been proposed to represent an evolutionary precursor isotype of mammalian IgG and IgE (Parvari et al., 1988; Magor et al., 1994b).

III. Ig LIGHT CHAIN GENES

Ig light chain gene structure exhibits a high degree of interspecies variation. In mammals the two light chain gene loci (Igκ and Igλ) are found on separate chromosomes and each locus exhibits differential relative ordering of the segmental elements. $V_κ$ and $J_κ$ segments are arrayed upstream of a single $C_κ$ exon, as in the heavy chains, whereas the human Igλ locus consists of a $V_λ$ locus containing many $V_λ$ elements upstream of seven sets of closely linked $J_λ$–$C_λ$ elements (Combriato and Klobeck, 1991). This basic form of a V_L locus, upstream of relatively closely linked J_L–C_L exons, is found throughout the mammals, but the number of V_L segments and J_L–C_L structures varies considerably among species (Steen et al., 1987; Desiderio, 1993). The question of the timing of the divergence of heavy and light chain gene loci is unresolved, since no intermediate forms of these genes have been identified in extant species. However, studies in primitive vertebrates provide strong evidence that the complexity of structure and organizational variability of light chain gene loci in these species exceeds that found in higher vertebrates. It is clear that light chain genes diversified early in vertebrate evolution.

Chondrichthyan Light Chain Genes

The Ig light chain genes found in the chondrichthyans are arranged in multiple clusters, consisting of closely linked V, J, and C elements (Figure 3A). This type of organization parallels that described above for heavy chain gene loci. Three

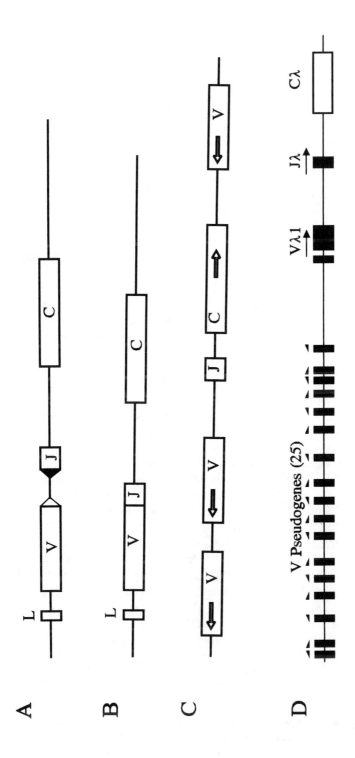

Figure 3. Non-mammalian Ig light chain gene organizations. **A:** Unjoined cluster found in *Heterodontus* type-I, and nurse shark (*Gingly-mostoma*) and possibly *Heterodontus* type-III (κ) clusters. **B:** Germline rearranged cluster arrangement of *Raja* type-I clusters and all known chondrichthyan type-II clusters. **C:** Catfish (*Ictalurus*) light chain genes cluster organization. Open arrows indicate transcriptional orientation (Ghaffari and Lobb, 1993). **D:** Chicken Igλ light chain gene organization. Wedges and arrows indicate transcriptional polarity. L = hydrophobic leader sequence; V = variable segment; J = joining segment; C = constant region exon; Octamer promoter element is present upstream of all light chain genes. RSS spacer lengths are indicated by triangles: open triangles = 12 bp, solid triangles = 23 bp. Presumably RSSs are present in *Ictalurus* but have not been defined.

distinct light chain isotypes have been described in the cartilaginous fishes and are designated type I, type II, and type III (or κ-type). All three types are present in the genome of *Heterodontus* (Rast et al., 1994). Type I light chain genes were described first in *Heterodontus* (Shamblott and Litman, 1989a; Shamblott and Litman, 1989b) and subsequently were identified in *Raja* (Rast et al., 1994; Anderson et al., 1995), but as of yet, have not been isolated from *Hydrolagus* (Rast et al., 1994). Although there is a high degree of identity between the type I light chain and the mammalian TCRβ chain, the amino acid sequences and general domain structure of the type I genes demonstrate unequivocally that these sequences encode Ig light chains. Inverse octamer sequences, as found in both mammalian light and heavy chain genes, occur upstream of the *Heterodontus* type I V_L genes. This observation is contrasted with an absence of 5' octamers in chondrichthyan heavy chains. Out of the forty *Heterodontus* type I light chain clusters isolated and characterized, none were germline-joined. However, extensive analyses of over fifty different type I light chain gene loci in *Raja* have established that all of the type I loci in this species are V–J joined in the germline (Figure 3B). Most of the variability between different gene clusters is present in the CDRs. The majority of differences are concentrated in CDR3, which, by analogy to the mammalian antibody combining site, most likely contains residues involved in actual contact with the antigen. Furthermore, there is strong evidence that at least some of these joined genes are expressed in *Raja*. As with joined heavy chain genes, the germline-joined state of these genes imparts heritability to a specificity, which is more subject to direct evolutionary pressures than those in which specificities are derived in part through somatic mechanisms (Anderson et al., 1995).

Type II genes have been identified at the genomic level in all of the chondrichthyans studied thus far (Hohman et al., 1993; Rast et al., 1994). Actual transcription of these genes has been demonstrated in *Raja*, *Carcharhinus*, and *Hydrolagus*. At present, the type II light chain gene is the only light chain isotype that has been identified in *Hydrolagus*. The *Hydrolagus* type II light chain genes exhibit strong identity with peptide sequences of Ig isolated from another species of holocephalan (De Ioannes and Aguila, 1989), suggesting that they are a major expressed form of antibody in this order of cartilaginous fish. The type II light chain gene loci observed in *Heterodontus* and *Raja* possess an inverse octamer upstream of their V region segments, as do type I genes. Different type II genes of the sandbar shark contain either direct or inverse octamer sequences (Hohman et al., 1995). All of the type II light chain gene loci that have been characterized thus far are germline-joined (Rast et al., 1994; Hohman et al., 1993). The type II genes of the sandbar shark appear to be diversified and are comprised of at least two families which share less than 60% identity. Variations in J–C intron length as well as a high level of diversity in the CDR3 regions are apparent (Hohman et al., 1993).

The V regions of chondrichthyan type III light chains in the nurse shark, *Ginglymostoma cirratum*, exhibit relatively high amino acid sequence identity (57–60%) with mammalian κ light chains. The constant regions of type III light chain genes are less related (39–47%; Greenberg et al., 1993). This light chain class has also been identified in *Heterodontus* (Rast et al., 1994) and is not germline-joined in either species. The configuration of RSSs in type III genes resembles mammalian κ light chain genes, although it should be noted that the type I light chain genes also have this RSS spacer configuration but otherwise share relatively little sequence identity with mammalian κ light chain genes. Type III genes, like other chondrichthyan light and heavy chain genes, exist in multiple clusters in the genome. Thus far, only one type III V_L and one type I V_L family have been described in each species. However, in *Hydrolagus*, type II light chain cDNAs have been identified which share nearly identical constant regions but exhibit only ~70% nucleotide identity in V regions (Rast et al., 1994). In addition, the 3' untranslated regions of the cDNAs encoding the two V_L families are almost identical, suggesting that constant region identity is the result of recent duplication, unequal crossing over, or gene conversion, and not merely purifying selection. Both type II V_L families exhibit characteristic cluster organization. A second type II V_L family also has been identified in *Raja* (M. Anderson, unpublished observation).

Interestingly, the *Heterodontus* type I light chain genes share considerable nucleotide sequence identity with mammalian TCRβ chain (Shamblott and Litman, 1989a). Furthermore, when V_H and C_H4 exons sequences are used as outgroups in phylogenetic analyses, the elasmobranch type I genes form a basal assemblage to all other vertebrate light chain types, including the chondrichthyan type II and III light chain genes (Rast et al., 1994). These observations suggest that the type I light chain genes diverged very early from the common light chain ancestor. Preliminary results from in situ hybridization studies in *Raja* suggest that the expression patterns of type I light chain mRNAs resemble the TCRβ and/or TCRδ expression patterns more closely than the expression patterns of the heavy chains (Anderson, Rast, Luer, Walsh, and Litman, unpublished observations).

The absence of germline-joined type I light chain genes in *Heterodontus* in contrast to their unjoined state in *Raja* raises questions as to the evolutionary timing of the joining of these genes. Along with other considerations discussed above, this discrepancy in joining status suggests that type I joining occurred after the divergence of the sharks and skates. Conversely, type II genes are joined in both *Raja* and *Heterodontus*, suggesting that these genes may have been joined prior to the divergence of these two species. A scenario in which joining occurred multiple times in these loci, independent of the joining which occurred in the heavy chains, seems more likely than a scenario requiring multiple RSS integration events. In the former case, the machinery for rearrangement is present and requires only atopic activation for germline-joining to occur. Furthermore, variations in the lengths of the CDR3 regions of different type II light chain genes in the sandbar shark (Hohman et al., 1993) contrast with the same length CDR3s in type I light chain gene in *Raja* (Anderson et al., 1995). This observation is most consistent with a germline-joining effect.

Teleost Light Chain Genes

Ig light chain genes have been described thus far in three species of teleost fishes: the channel catfish (*Ictalurus punctatus*; Ghaffari and Lobb, 1993), the cod (*Gadus morhua*), and the rainbow trout (*Oncorhynchus mykiss*; Daggfeldt et al., 1993). These light chain genes are organized into multiple, cluster-type loci resembling the Ig heavy and light chain genes of the chondrichthyans, although this resemblance is probably superficial (Figure 3C). One Ig light chain isotype has been described thus far in the teleosts and both its V_L and C_L genes exhibit moderate affinities with mammalian κ light chain genes. Furthermore, the V_L elements in these loci are in opposite transcriptional orientation to the J_L regions, consistent with rearrangement by inversion rather than by deletion. In this regard it is interesting to note that several different types of aberrant light chain cDNAs have been identified from spleen and kidney, including an unspliced cDNA, which contains a C_L preceded by what presumably represents J_L–C_L IVS. Another transcript (cDNA) contains a portion of presumably V_L–J_L IVS, followed by J_L correctly spliced to C_L. These transcripts, reminiscent of the IgX heavy chain transcripts found in *Raja* spleen (Harding et al., 1990a; Anderson et al., 1994), resemble transcription products of pre-B cells, as have been described in mammals.

Amphibian Light Chain Genes

Xenopus laevis represents the only amphibian species for which there is comprehensive molecular genetic information concerning light chains. Protein studies indicate that *Xenopus* possesses at least three different light chain isotypes (Hsu et al., 1991). Light chain gene sequences corresponding to the three isotypes, are designated σ, ρ (Schwager et al., 1991b), and type III. The type III gene shares considerable identity with mammalian λ chains (Haire et al., 1996). The σ light chain isotype may associate preferentially with a heavy chain class, which would be exceptional among vertebrate Igs (Hsu and Du Pasquier, 1984). From analyses of cDNAs, the σ locus has been inferred to be comprised of multiple $V_σ1$, a few $V_σ2$, and two $J_σ$ segments as well as two $C_σ$ segments. Several features of the $V_σ$ and $C_σ$ elements differ from V_L and C_L segments found in other vertebrates, including differences in canonical tryptophan residues, different spacing between cysteines, and predicted variations in secondary structures which could factor in heavy and light chain interactions (Schwager et al., 1991b). The expressed $V_σ$ sequences are highly conserved and exhibit little divergence in the CDR regions in outbred animals. There are two ρ families, one of which appears to have several members.

The type III light chain in *Xenopus* consists of six highly diverse V_LIII families (V_LIII.1-V_LIII.6), two J_LIII segments, and two closely related C_LIII regions (Haire et al., 1996). In the cDNAs thus far characterized, J_LIII.1 and C_LIII.1 as well as J_LIII.2 and C_LIII.2 are exclusively associated. Furthermore, there is a preferential but not invariant association of V_LIII.1-V_LIII.3 family members with J_LIII.1/C_LIII.1 and of V_LIII.4-V_LIII.6 with J_LIII.2/C_LIII.2. The differences between the coding regions of the two constant regions are minor; more pronounced differences are present in the 3′ untranslated regions. The C_LIII regions share approximately 38% and 33% amino acid identity, respectively with the μ and σ constant regions, and share ~50% amino acid identity with mammalian λ constant regions. Phylogenetic tree analyses using either V_L or C_L strongly group the type III genes with λ light chains. Transcription of the type III constant region exon(s) appears to occur very early in development. As with the heavy chains, the findings for light chain genes are inconsistent with restricted genetic diversity. These studies of the type III genes in *Xenopus* place the divergence of the λ light chain at the earliest point in vertebrate phylogeny thus far reported.

Avian Light Chain Genes

The one light chain type that has been identified in avians is a homolog of the mammalian λ isotype. The avian light chain locus consists of 25 $V_λ$ pseudogenes, a single functional V_λ segment ($V_\lambda 1$), a J_λ segment, and a C_λ segment (Figure 3D; Reynaud et al., 1985; Reynaud et al., 1987). Rearrangement occurs by deletion of the intervening DNA between the $V_\lambda 1$ and the J_λ segments. This single rearrangement event, coupled with subsequent diversification of the rearranged gene, accounts for the diversity in the chicken light chain repertoire. Three distinct mechanisms diversify the rearranged light chain gene. First, imprecise joining of the segments, leads to junctional diversity. In some cases, deletions occur 3' of the V segment and/or 5' of the J segment. However, in the absence of base loss 3' of the V segment, there is almost always an additional cytosine added to the V segment, and in the absence of base loss 5' of the J segment, an additional adenosine is added. These observations have led to the hypothesis that the recombinase may exchange a cytosine for the RSS of the V segment, and an adenosine for the RSS of the J segment, thus leaving the coding ends susceptible to exonuclease activity while protecting the signal sequence joints. Conversely, when the recombinase does not use these nucleotides, the coding ends remain intact (McCormack et al., 1989b). Additionally, as in the avian heavy chain locus, the V_λ pseudogenes of the chicken donate blocks of sequence to the rearranged V_λ gene, resulting in diversification by gene conversion (Reynaud et al., 1987; Carlson et al., 1990). Although rearrangements of both heavy and light chain genes occur concomitantly in the embryonic spleen, gene conversion takes place in the bursa (Pickel et al., 1993).

The process of somatic conversion of Ig genes in avians is distinct from meiotic gene conversion in several ways. It occurs only between genes on the same chromosome, and prior to DNA replication during the cell cycle. Furthermore, the gene conversion is specific to the rearranged $V_\lambda 1$ gene; interconversion does not occur among the pseudogenes at the somatic level. This contrasts with the high incidence of meiotic gene conversion among the V pseudogenes (Carlson et al., 1990; McCormack et al., 1993). The use of different pseudo V_λ segments as donors is not random. Instead, preferred donors tend to be more proximal to the $V_\lambda 1$ segment, have higher identity with $V_\lambda 1$, and have an inverted orientation to $V_\lambda 1$ (McCormack and Thompson, 1990). Finally, the preimmune repertoire is diversified by somatic point mutations, which exhibit a distribution pattern and frequency equivalent to that seen in the mouse. These mutations occur more frequently in the spleen than in the bursa. In mice, a matrix association region (MAR) located in the J–C intron is believed to allow for selective somatic modification of the VJ region by physically separating it from the C region (Betz et al., 1994). The identification of sequence with the structural features of an MAR (Parvari et al., 1990) in the chicken J_λ–C_λ intron is consistent with a role for point mutation in diversification, which takes place after exposure to antigen and results in affinity maturation.

Insights into the evolution of this unique form of an Ig locus have been facilitated by studies of two closely related chicken strains as well as different avian species. The relatedness of the different pseudo V_λ segments indicates that the cluster of pseudogenes probably arose from repeated duplications of a single primordial V_λ gene. The studies of closely related strains suggest that germline polymorphisms have arisen through both homologous recombination and gene conversion events. Meiotic gene conversion appears to function both in removing random mutations, which preserves the pseudogene V_λ character, and in diversifying the pseudogene sequence pool by shuffling blocks of sequence between genes. The alternating orientation of most of the pseudogenes appears to be essential in maintaining the number of pseudogenes and avoiding losses due to homologous recombination (McCormack et al., 1993).

The organization of the Ig light chain locus described in the chicken has been observed in four additional taxonomic orders of avians. An Ig light chain locus with multiple functional V_λ segments has been identified in the Muscovy duck, indicating that combinatorial diversity has evolved independently in at least one avian species. Nevertheless, the widespread occurrence of the pseudogene cluster, indicates that this organizational form evolved before or early in the evolution of the birds (McCormack et al., 1989a). Inquiries into the organization of reptilian light chain genes will help discern the origins of this system.

IV. IMMUNITY IN THE AGNATHANS: THE JAWLESS VERTEBRATES

The extant jawed vertebrates, which have been addressed extensively in this chapter, diverged from the jawless vertebrates at least 500 million years ago (Forey and Janvier, 1993). The jawless vertebrates, which at one time formed a vast assemblage, are represented today only by hagfish and lampreys. These two species are highly divergent forms and it remains controversial whether they diverged from each other prior to or after their divergence from a common ancestor with the jawed vertebrates (Stock and Whitt, 1992; Forey and Javier, 1993). Considerable amounts of peptide sequence information have been obtained for the putative, inducible lamprey recognition molecule (Litman et al., 1970; Pollara et al., 1970), and have shown little appreciable sequence identity with higher vertebrate Ig or TCR genes (A. Zilch, G. Litman, unpublished observations). A hagfish molecule resembling this lamprey factor has been shown to possess a heterodimeric structure with very limited peptide identity to Ig. However, molecular genetic analyses revealed that the structural resemblance is coincidental, and that the Ig-like molecule is a complement component homolog (Ishiguro et al., 1992). Extensive screening of both lamprey and hagfish genomic and cDNA libraries from various tissues with a wide variety of Ig gene probes and various PCR amplification strategies, including those which proved instrumental in identifying TCR genes in the chondrichthyans, as of yet, have failed to produce recognizable Ig or TCR gene homologs in these species. These findings and the similar failures of attempts to isolate MHC and RAG genes suggest that authentic rearranging homologs may not exist or that they are highly divergent. It may be that inducible humoral recognition of foreign antigens in the Agnathans involves genes which are only distantly related, if at all, to Igs.

V. CONCLUSIONS

This chapter has outlined the similarities and differences between Ig genes of species representing divergent points in vertebrate evolution. The diversity of characters of the adaptive immune system is superimposed on a cladogram relating the major vertebrate taxa that have been discussed in this chapter (Figure 4). It is apparent that the genetic elements encoding Ig heavy and light chains, which have nearly parallel structures and functions, exhibit particularly varied chromosomal arrangements throughout vertebrate phylogeny. Comparisons of divergence rates between orthologous mouse and human proteins have suggested that those

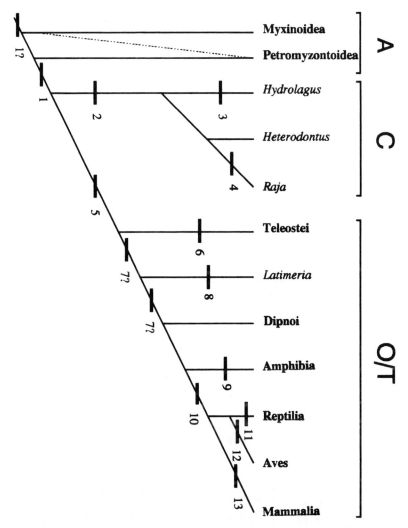

Figure 4. Summary of vertebrate Ig associated characteristics superimposed on a hypothetical vertebrate phylogeny. A = Agnatha; C = Chondrichthyes; O/T = Osteichthyes/Tetrapod. Bold represents taxonomic class, order, or suborder; italics represents genus. **1**: Humoral immunity; MHC class I and II proteins, RAG mediated rearranging TCR, μ-type Ig heavy and Ig light chain, somatic mutation of Ig V region genes, isotypic diversification of light chains and divergence of κ-type variable regions. **2**: Cluster-type Ig gene arrangement, some intercluster diversification and emergence of new constant region isotypes. **3**: Ig heavy chain constant region formed by replacement of C_H1 by a duplicated and divergent C_H2 exon. **4**: All type I light chain genes joined. **5**: Tandem Ig heavy chain gene organization, V_H family diversification, significant affinity maturation. **6**: Transmembrane exons spliced to C_H3. **7**: Constant region isotype diversification (class switching). **8**: V–D-tandem heavy chain organization. **9**: More extensive V_H family diversification. **10**: Enhanced affinity maturation. **11**: Multiple heavy chain loci dispersed on separate chromosomes. **12**: Single copy (limited copy number) V_H and V_L pseudogene gene conversion diversification system. **13**: Further expansion of Ig diversifying mechanisms such as gene conversion in the rabbit and pre-antigen stimulated somatic hypermutation of IgV regions in sheep. Placement of traits is inferred from the phylogenetic distribution of where they have been established and in some cases (e.g., MHC and TCR) may be present in more primitive taxa. The position of character 7 is ambiguous in the absence of a complete data set. Placement of the sarcopterygians (*Latimeria* and the Dipnoi) relative to the tetrapods is uncertain, as is the relationship between the living Agnatha relative to the jawed vertebrates (this uncertainty is indicated by a dotted line).

associated with the immune system evolve at a higher rate than other protein types. This adaptation may serve to avoid molecular mimicry and other mechanisms of subversion of the immune system by pathogenic organisms (Murphy, 1993). This accelerated rate of evolution within the immune system potentially relates to its interaction with foreign organisms which are able to counteradapt in response, unlike the typical factors to which living systems must adapt (e.g., changes in the physical environment). Clearly, the anticipatory capacities of the Ig and TCR somatic diversification systems are well-suited for this requirement. Knowledge of the molecular genetics of antigen-binding molecules from widely divergent species has important implications in understanding the overall nature and developmental regulation of adaptive immunity and the relationships between gene organization and the generation of antibody diversity.

ACKNOWLEDGMENTS

We would like to thank Barbara Pryor for editorial assistance. This work was supported by a grant from the National Institutes of Health R37-AI23338.

REFERENCES

Amemiya, C.T., and G.W. Litman. 1990. The complete nucleotide sequence of an immunoglobulin heavy chain gene and analysis of immunoglobulin gene organization in a primitive teleost species. *Proc. Natl. Acad. Sci. USA* **87**, 811–815.

Amemiya, C.T., and G.W. Litman. 1991. Early evolution of immunoglobulin genes. *Am. Zool.* **31**, 558–564.

Amemiya, C.T., R.N. Haire, and G.W. Litman. 1989. Nucleotide sequence of a cDNA encoding a third distinct *Xenopus* immunoglobulin heavy chain isotype. *Nucleic Acids Res.* **17**, 5388.

Amemiya, C.T., Y. Ohta, R.T. Litman, J.P. Rast, R.N. Haire, and G.W. Litman. 1993. V_H gene organization in a relict species, the coelacanth *Latimeria chalumnae*: evolutionary implications. *Proc. Natl. Acad. Sci. USA* **90**, 6661–6665.

Anderson, M., C. Amemiya, C. Luer, R. Litman, J. Rast, Y. Niimura, and G. Litman. 1994. Complete genomic sequence and patterns of transcription of a member of an unusual family of closely related, chromosomally dispersed immunoglobulin gene clusters in *Raja*. *International Immunol.* **6**, 1661–1670.

Anderson, M.K., M.J. Shamblott, R.T. Litman, and G.W. Litman. 1995. The generation of immunoglobulin light chain gene diversity in *Raja erinacea* is not associated with somatic rearrangement, an exception to a central paradigm of B cell immunity. *J. Exp. Med.* **181**, 109–119.

Anderson, S.J., S. Miyake, and D.Y. Loh. 1989. Transcription from a murine T-cell receptor VB promoter depends on a conserved decamer motif similar to the cyclic AMP response element. *Mol. Cell. Biol.* **9**, 4835–4845.

Andersson, E., and T. Matsunaga. 1993. Complete cDNA sequence of a rainbow trout IgM gene and evolution of vertebrate IgM constant domains. *Immunogenetics* **38**, 243–250.

Andersson, E., V. Törmänen, and T. Matsunaga. 1991. Evolution of a V_H gene family in low vertebrates. *Int. Immunol.* **3**, 527–533.

Becker, R.S., and K.L. Knight. 1990. Somatic diversification of immunoglobulin heavy chain VDJ genes: evidence for somatic gene conversion in rabbits. *Cell* **63**, 987–997.

Bengten, E., T. Leanderson, and L. Pilstrom. 1991. Immunoglobulin heavy chain cDNA from the teleost Atlantic cod (*Gadus morhua* L.): nucleotide sequence of secretory and membrane form show an unusual splicing pattern. *Eur. J. Immunol.* **21**, 3027–3033.

Bengten, E., S. Stromberg, and L. Pilstrom. 1994. Immunoglobulin V_H regions in Atlantic cod (*Gadus morhua* L.): their diversity and relationship to V_H families from other species. *Dev. Comp. Immunol.* **18**, 109–122.

Betz, A.G., C. Milstein, A. Gonzalez-Fernandez, R. Pannell, T. Larson, and M.S. Neuberger. 1994. Elements regulating somatic hypermutation of an immunoglobulin kappa gene: Critical role for the intron enhancer/matrix attachment region. *Cell* **77**, 239–248.

Borysenko, M., and W.H. Hildemann. 1970. Reactions to skin allografts in the horn shark, *Heterodontus francisci. Transplantation* **10**, 545–551.

Carlson, L.M., W.T. McCormack, C.E. Postema, E.H. Humphries, and C.B. Thompson. 1990. Templated insertions in the rearranged chicken Ig_L V gene segment arise by intrachromosomal gene conversion. *Genes and Development* **4**, 536–547.

Clem, L.W., and G.A. Leslie. 1982. Phylogeny of immunoglobulin structure and function. XIV. Peptide map and amino acid composition studies of shark antibody light chains. *Dev. Comp. Immunol.* **6**, 263–269.

Combriato, G., and H.-G. Klobeck. 1991. $V\lambda$ and $J\lambda$–$C\lambda$ gene segments of the human immunoglobulin lambda light chain locus are separated by 14 kb and rearrange by a deletion mechanism. *Eur. J. Immunol.* **21**, 1513–1522.

Daggfeldt, A., E. Bengten, and L. Pilström. 1993. A cluster type organization of the loci of the immunoglobulin light chain in Atlantic cod (*Gadus morhua* L.) and rainbow trout (*Oncorhynchus mykiss Walbaum*) indicated by nucleotide sequences of cDNAs and hybridization analysis. *Immunogenetics* **38**, 199–209.

De Ioannes, A.E., and H.L. Aguila. 1989. Amino terminal sequence of heavy and light chains from ratfish immunoglobulin. *Immunogenetics* **30**, 175–180.

Desiderio, S.V. Organization and Assembly of Immunoglobulin Genes. 1993. In *Developmental Immunology*. Edited by E. Cooper and E. Nisbet-Brown. New York: Oxford Univ. Press, p. 129.

Espelid, S., O.-M. Rodseth, and T.O. Jorgensen. 1991. Vaccination experiments and studies of the humoral immune response in cod, *Gadus morhua*, to four monoclonal-defined *Vibrio guillarum. J. Fish Dis.* **10**, 85–90.

Fellah, J.S., M.V. Wiles, J. Charlemagne, and J. Schwager. 1992. Evolution of vertebrate IgM: complete amino acid sequence of the constant region of *Ambystoma mexicanum* μ chain deduced from cDNA sequence. *Eur. J. Immunol.* **22**, 2595–2601.

Fellah, J.S., F. Kerfourn, M.V. Wiles, J. Schwager, and J. Charlemagne. 1993. Phylogeny of immunoglobulin heavy chain isotypes: structure of the constant region of *Ambystoma mexicanum* upsilon chain deduced from cDNA sequence. *Immunogenetics* **38**, 311–317.

Forey, P., and P. Janvier. 1993. Agnathans and the origin of jawed vertebrates. *Nature* **361**, 129–134.

Ghaffari, S.H., and C.J. Lobb. 1989a. Cloning and sequence analysis of channel catfish heavy chain cDNA indicate phylogenetic diversity within the IgM immunoglobulin family. *J. Immunol.* **142**, 1356–1365.

Ghaffari, S.H., and C.J. Lobb. 1989b. Nucleotide sequence of channel catfish heavy chain cDNA and genomic blot analyses: implications for the phylogeny of immunoglobulin heavy chains. *J. Immunol.* **143**, 2730–2739.

Ghaffari, S.H., and C.J. Lobb. 1991. Heavy chain variable region gene families evolved early in phylogeny: Ig complexity in fish. *J. Immunol.* **146**, 1037–1046.

Ghaffari, S.H., and C.J. Lobb. 1993. Structure and genomic organization of immunoglobulin light chain in the channel catfish. *J. Immunol.* **151**, 6900–6912.

Greenberg, A.S., L. Steiner, M. Kasahara, and M.F. Flajnik. 1993. Isolation of a shark immunoglobulin light chain cDNA clone encoding a protein resembling mammalian type kappa light chains: implications for the evolution of light chains. *Proc. Natl. Acad. Sci. USA* **90**, 10603–10607.

Greenberg, A.S., D. Avila, M. Hughes, A. Hughes, E.C. McKinney, and M.F. Flajnik. 1995. A new antigen receptor gene family that undergoes rearrangement and extensive somatic diversification in sharks. *Nature* **374**, 168–173.

Greenberg, A.S., A.L. Hughes, J. Guo, D. Avila, E.C. McKinney, and M.F. Flajnik. 1996. A novel chimeric antibody class in cartilaginous fish: IgM may not be the primordial immunoglobulin. *Eur. J. Immunol.*, in press.

Haire, R., M.J. Shamblott, C.T. Amemiya, and G.W. Litman. 1989. A second *Xenopus* immunoglobulin heavy chain constant region isotype gene. *Nucleic Acids Res.* **17**, 1776.

Haire, R.N., C.T. Amemiya, D. Suzuki, and G.W. Litman. 1990. Eleven distinct V_H gene families and additional patterns of sequence variation suggest a high degree of immunoglobulin gene complexity in a lower vertebrate, *Xenopus laevis*. *J. Exp. Med.* **171**, 1721–1737.

Haire, R.N., Y. Ohta, R.T. Litman, C.T. Amemiya, and G.W. Litman. 1991. The genomic organization of immunoglobulin V_H genes in *Xenopus laevis* shows evidence for interspersion of families. *Nucleic Acids Res.* **19**, 3061–3066.

Haire, R.N., T. Ota, J.P. Rast, R.T. Litman, F.Y. Chan, L.I. Zon, and G.W. Litman. 1996. A third immunoglobulin light chain gene isotype in *Xenopus laevis* consists of six distinct V_L families and is related to mammalian lambda genes. *J. Immunol.*, submitted.

Harding, F.A., C.T. Amemiya, R.T. Litman, N. Cohen, and G.W. Litman. 1990a. Two distinct immunoglobulin heavy chain isotypes in a primitive, cartilaginous fish, *Raja erinacea*. *Nucleic Acids Res.* **18**, 6369–6376.

Harding, F.A., N. Cohen, and G.W. Litman. 1990b. Immunoglobulin heavy chain gene organization and complexity in the skate, *Raja erinacea*. *Nucleic Acids Res.* **18**, 1015–1020.

Hashimoto, K., T. Nakanishi, and Y. Kurosawa. 1992. Identification of a shark sequence resembling the major histocompatibility complex class I $\alpha 3$ domain. *Proc. Natl. Acad. Sci. USA* **89**, 2209–2212.

Hinds, K.R., and G.W. Litman. 1986. Major reorganization of immunoglobulin V_H segmental elements during vertebrate evolution. *Nature* **320**, 546–549.

Hinds-Frey, K.R., H. Nishikata, R.T. Litman, and G.W. Litman. 1993. Somatic variation precedes extensive diversification of germline sequences and combinatorial joining in the evolution of immunoglobulin heavy chain diversity. *J. Exp. Med.* **178**, 825–834.

Hohman, V.S., D.B. Schuchman, S.F. Schluter, and J.J. Marchalonis. 1993. Genomic clone for the sandbar shark lambda light chain: generation of diversity in the absence of gene rearrangement. *Proc. Natl. Acad. Sci. USA* **90**, 9882–9886.

Hohman, V.S., S.F. Schluter, and J.J. Marchalonis. 1995. Diversity of Ig light chain clusters in the sandbar shark (*Carcharhinus plumbeus*). *J. Immunol.* **155**, 3922–3928.

Hordvik, I., A.M. Voie, J. Glette, R. Male, and C. Endresen. 1992. Cloning and sequence analysis of two isotypic IgM heavy chain genes from Atlantic salmon, *Salmo salar* L. *Eur. J. Immunol.* **22**, 2957–2962.

Hsu, E., I. Lefkovits, M. Flajnik, and L. Du Pasquier. 1991. Light chain heterogeneity in the amphibian *Xenopus*. *Mol. Immunol.* **28**, 985–994.

Hsu, E., and L. Du Pasquier. 1984. Studies on *Xenopus* immunoglobulins using monoclonal antibodies. *Mol. Immunol.* **21**, 257–270.

Ishiguro, H., K. Kobayashi, M. Suzuki, K. Titani, S. Tomonaga, and Y. Kurosawa. 1992. Isolation of a hagfish gene that encodes a complement component. *EMBO J.* **11**, 829–837.

Jones, J.C., S.H. Ghaffari, and C.J. Lobb. 1993. Immunoglobulin heavy chain constant and heavy chain variable region genes in phylogenetically diverse species of bony fish. *J. Mol. Evol.* **36**, 417–428.

Kasahara, M., E.C. McKinney, M.F. Flajnik, and T. Ishibashi. 1993. The evolutionary origin of the major histocompatibility complex: polymorphism of class II alpha-chain genes in the cartilaginous fish. *Eur. J. Immunol.* **23**, 2160–2165.

Knight, K.L. 1992. Restricted V_H gene usage and generation of antibody diversity in rabbit. *Ann. Rev. Immunol.* **10**, 593–616.

Kobayashi, K., S. Tomonaga, and T. Kajii. 1984. A second class of immunoglobulin other than IgM present in the serum of a cartilaginous fish, the skate, *Raja Kenojei*: isolation and characterization. *Mol. Immunol.* **21**, 397–404.

Kobayashi, K., S. Tomonaga, K. Teshima, and T. Kajii. 1985. Ontogenetic studies on the appearance of two classes of immunoglobulin-forming cells in the spleen of the Aleutian skate, *Bathyraja aleutica*, a cartilaginous fish. *Eur. J. Immunol.* **15**, 952–956.

Kobayashi, K., S. Tomonaga, and S. Tanaka. 1992. Identification of a second immunoglobulin in the most primitive shark, the frill shark. *Dev. Comp. Immunol.* **16**, 295–299.

Kodaira, M., T. Kinashi, I. Umemura, F. Matsuda, T. Noma, Y. Ono, and T. Honjo. 1986. Organization and evolution of variable region genes of the human immunoglobulin heavy chain. *J. Mol. Biol.* **190**, 529–541.

Kokubu, F., K. Hinds, R. Litman, M.J. Shamblott, and G.W. Litman. 1987. Extensive families of constant region genes in a phylogenetically primitive vertebrate indicate an additional level of immunoglobulin complexity. *Proc. Natl. Acad. Sci. USA* **84**, 5868–5872.

Kokubu, F., K. Hinds, R. Litman, M.J. Shamblott, and G.W. Litman. 1988a. Complete structure and organization of immunoglobulin heavy chain constant region genes in a phylogenetically primitive vertebrate. *EMBO J.* **7**, 1979–1988.

Kokubu, F., R. Litman, M.J. Shamblott, K. Hinds, and G.W. Litman. 1988b. Diverse organization of immunoglobulin V_H gene loci in a primitive vertebrate. *EMBO J.* **7**, 3413–3422.

Lee, M.A., E. Bengten, A. Daggfeldt, A.-S. Rytting, and L. Pilström. 1993. Characterisation of rainbow trout cDNAs encoding a secreted and membrane-bound Ig heavy chain and the genomic intron upstream of the first constant region. *Mol. Immunol.* **30**, 641–648.

Litman, G.W., D. Frommel, J. Finstad, J. Howell, B.W. Pollara, and R.A. Good. 1970. The evolution of the immune response. VIII. Structural studies of the lamprey immunoglobulin. *J. Immunol.* **105**, 1278–1285.

Litman, G.W., A.C. Wang, H.H. Fudenberg, and R.A. Good. 1971. N-terminal amino-acid sequence of African lungfish immunoglobulin light chains. *Proc. Natl. Acad. Sci. USA* **68**, 2321–2324.

Litman, G.W., L. Berger, K. Murphy, R.T. Litman, K.R. Hinds, C.L. Jahn, and B.W. Erickson. 1983. Complete nucleotide sequence of an immunoglobulin V_H gene homologue from *Caiman*, a phylogenetically ancient reptile. *Nature* **303**, 349–352.

Litman, G.W., L. Berger, K. Murphy, R. Litman, K.R. Hinds, and B.W. Erickson. 1985a. Immunoglobulin V_H gene structure and diversity in *Heterodontus*, a phylogenetically primitive shark. *Proc. Natl. Acad. Sci. USA* **82**, 2082–2086.

Litman, G.W., K. Murphy, L. Berger, R.T. Litman, K.R. Hinds, and B.W. Erickson. 1985b. Complete nucleotide sequences of three V_H genes in *Caiman*, a phylogenetically ancient reptile: evolutionary diversification in coding segments and variation in the structure and organization of recombination elements. *Proc. Natl. Acad. Sci. USA* **82**, 844–848.

Litman, G.W., J.P. Rast, M.J. Shamblott, R.N. Haire, M. Hulst, W. Roess, R.T. Litman, K.R. Hinds-Frey, A. Zilch, and C.T. Amemiya. 1993. Phylogenetic diversification of immunoglobulin genes and the antibody repertoire. *Mol. Biol. Evol.* **10**, 60–72.

Litman, G.W., M.K. Anderson, J.P. Rast, and C.T. Amemiya. 1996. Organization and mechanism of rearrangement of immunoglobulin genes in lower vertebrates. In *Handbook of Experimental Immunology*. Edited by D.M. Weir, L.A. Herzenberg, and L.A. Herzenberg. Blackwell Scientific, in press.

Lobb, C.J., and M.O.J. Olson. 1988. Immunoglobulin heavy chain isotypes in a teleost fish. *J. Immunol.* **141**, 1236–1245.

Luer, C.A. 1989. Elasmobranchs (sharks, skates, and rays) as animal models for biomedical research. In *Nonmammalian Animal Models for Biomedical Research*. Edited by A.D. Woodhead. Boca Raton: CRC Press, p. 121.

Magor, K.E., G.W. Warr, D. Middleton, M.R. Wilson, and D.A. Higgins. 1992. Structural relationship between the two IgY of the duck, Anas platyrhynchos: molecular genetic evidence. *J. Immunol.* **149**, 2627–2633.

Magor, B.G., M.R. Wilson, N.W. Miller, L.W. Clem, D.L. Middleton, and G.W. Warr. 1994a. An Ig heavy chain enhancer of the channel catfish Ictalurus punctatus: evolutionary conservation of function but not structure. *J. Immunol.* **153**, 5556–5563.

Magor, K.E., D.A. Higgins, D.L. Middleton, and G.W. Warr. 1994b. One gene encodes the heavy chains for three different forms of IgY in the duck. *J. Immunol.* **153**, 5549–5555.

Maisey, J.G. 1984. Chondrichthyan phylogeny: a look at the evidence. *J. Vert. Paleont.* **4**, 359–371.

Mansikka, A. 1992. Chicken IgA H chains: implications concerning the evolution of H chain genes. *J. Immunol.* **149**, 855–861.

Marchalonis, J.J., and S.A. Schonfeld. 1970. Polypeptide chain structure of stingray immunoglobulin. *Biochimica et Biophysica Acta* **221**, 604–611.

Marchalonis, J.J., V.S. Hohman, C. Thomas, and S.F. Schluter. 1993. Antibody production in sharks and humans: a role for natural antibodies. *Dev. Comp. Immunol.* **17**, 41–53.

Matsunaga, T., T. Chen, and V. Tormanen. 1990. Characterization of a complete immunoglobulin heavy-chain variable region germ-line gene of rainbow trout. *Proc. Natl. Acad. Sci. USA* **87**, 7767–7771.

Mäkelä, O., and G.W. Litman. 1990. Lack of heterogeneity in anti-hapten antibodies of a phylogenetically primitive shark. *Nature* **287**, 639–640.

McCormack, W.T., and C.B. Thompson. 1990. Chicken IgL variable region gene conversions display pseudogene donor preference and 5′ to 3′ polarity. *Genes and Development* **4**, 548.

McCormack, W.T., L.M. Carlson, L.W. Tjoelker, and C.B. Thompson. 1989a. Evolutionary comparison of the avian IgL locus: combinatorial diversity plays a role in the generation of the antibody repertoire in some avian species. *International Immunol.* **1**, 332–341.

McCormack, W.T., L.W. Tjoelker, L.M. Carlson, B. Petryniak, C.F. Barth, E.H. Humphries, and C.B. Thompson. 1989b. Chicken IgL gene rearrangement involves deletion of a circular episome and addition of single nonrandom nucleotides to both coding segments. *Cell* **56**, 785–791.

McCormack, W.T., E.A. Hurley, and C.B. Thompson. 1993. Germ line maintenance of the pseudogene donor pool for somatic immunoglobulin gene conversion in chickens. *Mol. Cell. Biol.* **13**, 821–830.

Miller, N.W., M.A. Rycyzyn, M.R. Wilson, G.W. Warr, J.P. Naftel, and L.W. Clem. 1994. Development and characterization of channel catfish long term B cell lines. *J. Immunol.* **152**, 2180–2189.

Murphy, P.M. 1993. Molecular mimicry and the generation of host defense protein diversity. *Cell* **72**, 823–826.

Ota, T., and M. Nei. 1994. Divergent evolution and evolution by the birth-and-death process in the immunoglobulin V_H gene family. *Mol. Biol. Evol.* **11**, 469–482.

Ota, T., and M. Nei. 1995. Evolution of immunoglobulin V_H pseudogenes in chickens. *Mol. Biol. Evol.* **12**, 94–102.

Parham, P. 1995. Antibody structure. The duck's dilemma. *Nature* **374**, 16–17.

Parvari, R., A. Avivi, F. Lentner, E. Ziv, S. Tel-Or, Y. Burstein, and I. Schechter. 1988. Chicken immunoglobulin γ-heavy chains: limited V_H gene repertoire, combinatorial diversification by D gene segments and evolution of the heavy chain locus. *EMBO J.* **7**, 739–744.

Parvari, R., E. Ziv, F. Lantner, D. Heller, and I. Schechter. 1990. Somatic diversification of chicken immunoglobulin light chains by point mutations. *Proc. Natl. Acad. Sci. USA* **87**, 3072–3076.

Pascual, V., and J.D. Capra. 1991. Human immunoglobulin heavy-chain variable region genes: organization, polymorphism, and expression. *Adv. Immunol.* **49**, 1–74.

Peters, A., and U. Storb. 1996. Somatic hypermutation of immunoglobulin genes is linked to transcription initiation. *Immunity* **4**, 57–65.

Pickel, J.M., W.T. McCormack, C.-L.H. Chen, M.D. Cooper, and C.B. Thompson. 1993. Differential regulation of V(D)J recombination during development of avian B and T cells. *International Immunol.* **5**, 919–927.

Pollara, B., G.W. Litman, J. Finstad, J. Howell, and R.A. Good. 1970. The evolution of the immune response. VII. Antibody to human "O" cells and properties of the immunoglobulin in lamprey. *J. Immunol.* **105**, 738–745.

Rast, J.P., and G.W. Litman. 1994. T cell receptor gene homologs are present in the most primitive jawed vertebrates. *Proc. Natl. Acad. Sci. USA* **91**, 9248–9252.

Rast, J.P., M.K. Anderson, T. Ota, R.T. Litman, M. Margittai, M.J. Shamblott, and G.W. Litman. 1994. Immunoglobulin light chain class multiplicity and alternative organizational forms in early vertebrate phylogeny. *Immunogenetics* **40**, 83–99.

Rast, J.P., R.N. Haire, R.T. Litman, S. Pross, and G.W. Litman. 1995. Identification and characterization of T-cell antigen receptor related genes in phylogenetically diverse vertebrate species. *Immunogenetics* **42**, 204–212.

Rathbun, G.A., J.D. Capra, and P.W. Tucker. 1987. Organization of the murine immunoglobulin V_H complex in the inbred strains. *EMBO J.* **6**, 2931–2937.

Reynaud, C.-A., V. Anquez, A. Dahan, and J.-C. Weill. 1985. A single rearrangement event generates most of the chicken immunoglobulin light chain diversity. *Cell* **40**, 283–291.

Reynaud, C.-A., V. Anquez, H. Grimal, and J.-C. Weill. 1987. A hyperconversion mechanism generates the chicken light chain preimmune repertoire. *Cell* **48**, 379–388.

Reynaud, C.-A., A. Dahan, V. Anquez, and J.-C. Weill. 1989. Somatic hyperconversion diversifies the single V_H gene of the chicken with a high incidence in the D region. *Cell* **59**, 171–183.

Reynaud, C.-A., C.R. Mackay, R.G. Muller, and J.-C. Weill. 1991a. Somatic generation of diversity in a mammalian primary lymphoid organ: the sheep ileal Peyer's patches. *Cell* **64**, 995–1005.

Reynaud, C.-A., V. Anquez, and J.-C. Weill. 1991b. The chicken D locus and its contribution to the immunoglobulin heavy chain repertoire. *Eur. J. Immunol.* **21**, 2661–2670.

Rogers, J., P. Early, C. Carter, K. Calame, M. Bond, L. Hood, and R. Wall. 1980. Two mRNAs with different 3′ ends encode membrane-bound and secreted forms of immunoglobulin μ chain. *Cell* **20**, 303–312.

Roman, T., and J. Charlemagne. 1994. The immunoglobulin repertoire of the rainbow trout (*Oncorhynchus mykiss*): definition of nine IgH–V families. *Immunogenetics* **40**, 210–216.

Rosenshein, I.L., and J.J. Marchalonis. 1987. The immunoglobulins of carcharhine sharks: a comparison of serological and biochemical properties. *Comp. Biochem. Physiol.* **86b**, 737–747.

Sanz, I. 1991. Multiple mechanisms participate in the generation of diversity of human H chain CDR3 regions. *J. Immunol.* **147**, 1720–1729.

Schwager, J., D. Grossberger, and L. Du Pasquier. 1998a. Organization and rearrangement of immunoglobulin M genes in the amphibian *Xenopus*. *EMBO J.* **7**, 2409–2415.

Schwager, J., C.A. Mikoryak, and L.A. Steiner. 1988b. Amino acid sequence of heavy chain from *Xenopus laevis* IgM deduced from cDNA sequence: implications for evolution of immunoglobulin domains. *Proc. Natl. Acad. Sci. USA* **85**, 2245–2249.

Schwager, J., N. Burckert, M. Courtet, and L. Du Pasquier. 1991a. The ontogeny of diversification at the immunoglobulin heavy chain locus in *Xenopus*. *EMBO J.* **10**, 2461–2470.

Schwager, J., N. Burckert, M. Schwager, and M. Wilson. 1991b. Evolution of immunoglobulin light chain genes: analysis of *Xenopus* IgL isotypes and their contribution to antibody diversity. *EMBO J.* **10**, 505–511.

Shamblott, M.J., and G.W. Litman. 1989a. Complete nucleotide sequence of primitive vertebrate immunoglobulin light chain genes. *Proc. Natl. Acad. Sci. USA* **86**, 4684–4688.

Shamblott, M.J., and G.W. Litman. 1989b. Genomic organization and sequences of immunoglobulin light chain genes in a primitive vertebrate suggest coevolution of immunoglobulin gene organization. *EMBO J.* **8**, 3733–3739.

Small, P.A., D.G. Klapper, and L.W. Clem. 1987. Half-lives, body distribution and lack of interconversion of serum 19S and 7S IgM of sharks. *J. Immunol.* **105**(1970), 29–37.

Steen, M.-L., L. Hellman, and U. Pettersson. The immunoglobulin lambda locus in rat consists of two C_x genes and a single Vx gene. *Gene* **55**, 75–84.

Stock, D.W., and G.S. Whitt. 1992. Evidence from 18S ribosomal RNA sequences that lampreys and hagfishes form a natural group. *Science* **257**, 787–789.

Vainio, O., and B.A. Imhof. 1995. The immunology and developmental biology of the chicken. *Immunol. Today* **16**, 365–370.

Ventura-Holman, T., J.C. Jones, S.H. Ghaffari, and C.J. Lobb. 1994. Structure and genomic organization of V_H gene segments in the channel catfish: members of different V_H gene families are interspersed and closely linked. *Mol. Immunol.* **31**, 823–832.

Walter, M.A., H.M. Dosch, and D.W. Cox. 1991. A deletion map of the human immunoglobulin heavy chain variable region. *J. Exp. Med.* **174**, 335–349.

Weill, J.-C., and C.-A. Reynaud. 1987. The chicken B cell compartment. *Science* **238**, 1094–1098.

Williams, A.F., and A.N. Barclay. 1988. The immunoglobulin superfamily-domains for cell surface recognition. *Ann. Rev. Immunol.* **6**, 381–405.

Wilson, M., E. Hsu, A. Marcuz, M. Courtet, L. Du Pasquier, and C. Steinberg. 1992. What limits affinity maturation of antibodies in *Xenopus* — the rate of somatic mutation or the ability to select mutants? *EMBO J.* **11**, 4337–4347.

Wilson, M.R., D. Middleton, and G.W. Warr. 1988. Immunoglobulin heavy chain variable region gene evolution: structure and family relationships of two genes and a pseudogene in a teleost fish. *Proc. Natl. Acad. Sci. USA* **85**, 1566–1570.

Wilson, M.R., A. Marcuz, F. van Ginkel, N.W. Miller, L.W. Clem, D. Middleton, and G.W. Warr. 1990. The immunoglobulin M heavy chain constant region gene of the channel catfish, *Ictalurus punctatus*: an unusual mRNA splice pattern produces the membrane form of the molecule. *Nucleic Acids Res.* **18**, 5227–5233.

Yancopoulos, G.D., and F.W. Alt. 1985. Developmentally controlled and tissue-specific expression of unrearranged V_H gene segments. *Cell* **40**, 271–281.

Zheng, B., W. Xue, and G. Kelsoe. 1994. Locus-specific somatic hypermutation in germinal centre T cells. *Nature* **372**, 556–559.

Chapter

FIVE

Therapeutic Immunomodulation with Normal Polyspecific Immunoglobulin G (Intravenous Immunoglobulin, IVIg)

MICHEL D. KAZATCHKINE and SRINI V. KAVERI

INSERM U430 and Université Pierre et Marie Curie, Hôpital Broussais, Paris, France

The last ten years have witnessed major changes in paradigms on self-reactivity and significant advances in the understanding of the genetic, molecular and cellular basis of autoimmune responses and their control (Coutinho and Kazatchkine, 1994). The structure and functions of "natural" antibodies, i.e., antibodies circulating in normal individuals and produced in the absence of overt specific antigenic stimulation, within and outside the immune system have been extensively studied (Coutinho et al., 1996). Natural antibodies have been shown to prevent autoimmune manifestations in animal models of autoimmunity. Normal polyspecific IgG prepared from plasma of healthy donors has been shown to be beneficial in the treatment of patients with autoimmune disorders. In this chapter, we wish to review the available information on mechanisms by which pooled normal human IgG for therapeutic use (intravenous immunoglobulin, IVIg) exerts its immunomodulatory effects in autoimmune and inflammatory conditions.

I. INTRAVENOUS IMMUNOGLOBULIN

Intravenous immunoglobulin (IVIg) for therapeutic use is normal polyspecific immunoglobulin G prepared from plasma pools of large numbers of healthy donors. The number of donors in the pools often exceeds 10,000, so that, for conceptual purposes, IVIg may be considered as containing the entire spectrum of antibody reactivities that may be expressed by IgG in normal human serum. These reactivities comprise antibodies to foreign antigens, including viral and bacterial antigens and superantigens, as well as self-antigens that are targets for natural IgG autoantibodies in serum. Natural IgG antibodies in serum react with a variety of self-antigens, including membrane-associated self molecules, intracellular components, and extracellular autoantigens. Self-reactivities have recently been shown to be primarily directed toward a conserved and limited set of dominant antigens, as shown in mouse and in man, by the analysis of densitometric patterns of immunoblots of normal serum IgG with solubilized extracts of normal homologous tissues (Lacroix-Desmazes et al., 1995; Mouthon et al., 1995a; Nobrega et al., 1993). Self-reactive antibodies in IVIg are representative of the self-reactivities expressed by IgG of individual healthy donors contributing to the IVIg pool (Figure 1). Self-antigens recognized by normal IgG include idiotypes of immunoglobulins. The network of complementary interactions occurring between antibody molecules and between antibodies and variable regions of antigen receptors on lymphocytes is essential for the selection of immune repertoires and establishment of tolerance to self (Varela and Coutinho, 1991).

Available preparations of IVIg for clinical use almost exclusively contain intact IgG molecules, with small amounts of contaminating IgA and IgM. IVIg also contains trace amounts of $F(ab')_2$ fragments of IgG, soluble CD4, CD8 and HLA molecules (Blasczyk et al., 1993). Removal of aggregates is achieved by enzymatic hydrolysis of IgG (e.g., with pepsin), reduction and alkylation, reductive sulfonation of disulfide bonds, or treatment with beta-propiolactone. Methods have been developed for processing conditions of Cohn-Oncley fraction II or Kistler-Nitschmann precipitated IgG to remove impurities and to ensure viral inactivation of the preparations, in addition to removal of potentially contaminating virus particles by physical partitioning. The distribution of IgG subclasses in IVIg preparations is similar or close to that of IgG in normal serum. The half life of infused IVIg is three weeks in the case of IgG1, IgG2 and IgG4, and one week in the case of IgG3.

II. THE USE OF INTRAVENOUS IMMUNOGLOBULIN IN THE TREATMENT OF AUTOIMMUNE AND INFLAMMATORY DISEASES

Intravenous immunoglobulin has proven effective and safe in the long-term treatment of antibody deficiencies (Eibl and Wedgwood, 1993). In the early 1980s, the use of IVIg in autoimmune disorders began with the treatment of idiopathic thrombocytopenic purpura (ITP) (Imbach et al., 1981). The list of disorders reportedly responding to IVIg has then continuously grown. It now includes a wide spectrum of diseases mediated by pathogenic autoantibodies or believed to be primarily dependent on autoaggressive T cells, e.g., autoimmune cytopenias (Blanchette et al., 1994; Imbach et al., 1981; Lalezari et al., 1986; McGuire et al., 1987; McIntyre et al., 1985; Oda et al., 1985), the acute Guillain Barré syndrome (Hughes, 1996; van der Meché et al., 1992), myasthenia gravis (Gajdos et al., 1984), anti-Factor VIII autoimmune disease (Sultan et al., 1984), dermatomyositis (Dalakas et al., 1993), anti-neutrophil cytoplasmic antigens (ANCA)-associated systemic vasculitis (Jayne et al., 1991) and autoimmune uveitis (LeHoang et al., 1996). More recently, the use of IVIg has been suggested in chronic inflammatory conditions with the goal of reducing the needs for prolonged systemic steroid treatment (Gelfand et al.,

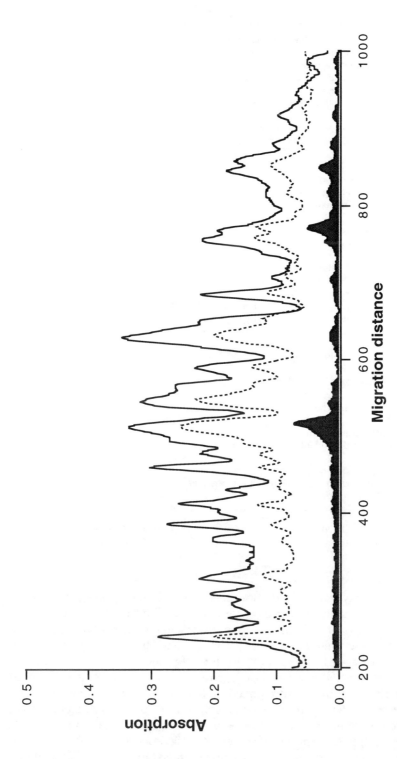

Figure 1. Densitometric profile of reactivity of IVIg (full line) and mean reactivity profile of purified IgG from 18 healthy adult male donors (dotted line) with antigens in normal human liver. IgG was tested at 200 µg/ml. Migration distance on the abscissa and light absorption on the ordinate are expressed as arbitrary units. For details of the immunoblotting technique see Mouthon et al., 1995a. Adapted from Mouthon et al., 1995a, with permission.

Table 1. Immune-Mediated Diseases in which a
Beneficial Effect of IVIg Has Been Reported

Idiopathic thrombocytopenic purpura (ITP)*
Acquired immune thrombocytopenias
Autoimmune neutropenia
Autoimmune hemolytic anemia
Autoimmune erythroblastopenia
Parvovirus B19-associated red cell aplasia

Anti-factor VIII autoimmune disease
Acquired von Willebrand's disease

Guillain-Barré syndrome*
Chronic inflammatory demyelinating polyneuropathy (CIDP)*
Myasthenia gravis*
Multifocal neuropathy

Polymyositis
Dermatomyositis*

Kawasaki disease*
ANCA-positive systemic vasculitis
Antiphospholipid syndrome
Recurrent spontaneous abortions
Rheumatoid arthritis and Felty's syndrome
JRA
SLE
Thyroid ophthalmopathy

Birdshot retinochoroidopathy*

Graft versus host disease*

Multiple sclerosis
Insulin-dependent diabetes mellitus

Steroid-dependent asthma
Steroid-dependent severe atopic dermatitis
Crohn's disease

*Disease in which evidence for the effect of IVIg has been obtained
in controlled trials.

1994) (Table 1). In only few of the diseases listed in Table 1, has the beneficial effect of IVIg been established in prospective randomized clinical trials; in many other conditions, the effects of IVIg have only been documented in small and uncontrolled studies. Our current knowledge is clearly insufficient as to which diseases represent the most appropriate indications for IVIg therapy, how should IVIg be administered for immunomodulation, e.g., aiming at keeping high serum concentrations of immunoglobulin for prolonged periods of time or, alternatively, "spiking" the immune system with intermittent high doses of immunoglobulin, and which are the mechanisms of action of IVIg. The regimen initially proven to be efficacious for the treatment of acute ITP, i.e., 0.4 g/kg body weight/day given over five consecutive days, has been used as starting point in most attempts of treatment

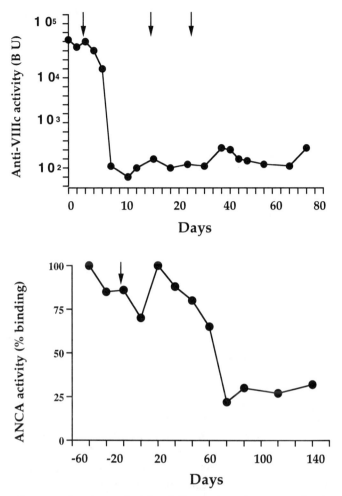

Figure 2. Decrease in plasma levels of disease-specific autoantibodies following treatment with IVIg. Upper panel: kinetics of decrease in anti-factor VIII antibodies in a patient with anti-factor VIII autoimmune disease. Autoantibody activity is expressed as Bethesda Units (BU). Adapted from Sultan et al., 1984. Lower panel: kinetics of decrease in ANCA activity in a patient with systemic vasculitis. ANCA activity is expressed as percent binding as compared to a reference high titer ANCA-containing serum. Adapted from Jayne et al., 1991. Arrows denote infusions of IVIg.

of autoimmune diseases with IVIg. More recently, alternative schedules of administration, e.g., 0.8 to 1.0 g/kg body weight/day over two consecutive days have often been preferred. Figure 2 depicts the decrease in autoantibody titers that is seen in patients with autoantibody-mediated autoimmune disease following infusion of IVIg.

Emphasis will be given in this chapter on data that has accumulated in the last ten years, including our own work, on the mechanisms by which IVIg exerts its immunoregulatory and anti-inflammatory functions. We believe that elucidating these mechanisms should allow to define appropriate indications and schedules of

Table 2. Proposed Mechanisms of Action of IVIg in Autoimmune
and Inflammatory Disorders

Fc receptor blockade

Anti-inflammatory effects:
    attenuation of complement-mediated tissue damage
    alteration of the structure and solubility of immune complexes
    induction of anti-inflammatory cytokines
    decreased production of proinflammatory cytokines
    neutralization of microbial toxins

Neutralization of pathogenic autoantibodies by anti-idiotypes

Neutralization of superantigens

V region and Fc-dependent selection of immune repertoires:
    control of emergent repertoires of bone marrow B cells and thymocytes
    modulation of immunoglobulin production and long term modifications in antibody repertoires
    modulation of cytokine production by monocytes and T cells
    regulation of expansion and activation of lymphocyte subsets

---

administration of IVIg, and to design "second generation" IVIg preparations targeted for immunomodulation of autoimmune disease, at a time when human monoclonal antibodies and recombinant antibodies may provide alternative therapeutic approaches for immunomodulation. In addition, comprehending the basis for the immunoregulatory effects of IVIg should provide a better understanding of the functions of natural antibodies that are relevant to the maintenance of tolerance to self and of immune homeostasis in healthy individuals.

Proposed mechanisms of action of IVIg are summarized in Table 2. Each of these mechanisms may be operative to some extent in the treatment of different diseases, which could affect the choice of IVIg preparations that are to be considered for clinical use. Some of the mechanisms are dependent on the interaction between the Fc portion of infused immunoglobulin and Fcγ receptors on target cells (e.g., Fc receptor blockade by IVIg in patients treated for autoimmune cytopenias); other mechanisms, including the capacity of IVIg to select immune repertoires, are primarily dependent on the spectrum of variable regions of antibodies administered to the patients. The distinction between Fc- and variable region-dependent mechanisms remains however artificial in that functions of IVIg are amplified or indeed made possible at all, by cooperative Fc binding to Fc receptors on cells targeted by the relevant V regions. In addition, integrity of the IgG molecule is important for stability and optimal half-life of infused immunoglobulin in vivo.

III. EXPERIMENTAL AUTOIMMUNE DISEASE

Prevention or attenuation of experimental autoimmune disease with human IVIg or with normal homologous immunoglobulin provides a useful approach to the study of the immunomodulatory effects of IVIg. IVIg has been shown to prevent renal disease and to suppress hyperproduction of IgE in $HgCl_2$-induced autoimmune disease of Brown-Norway rats (Rossi et al., 1991a); prevent S retinal antigen-induced experimental autoimmune uveoretinitis (EAU) in genetically susceptible rats and induce antigen-specific T cell anergy in tolerant animals (Saoudi et al.,

1993); suppress the occurrence of experimental allergic encephalomyelitis, an effect mediated, at least in part, by inhibition of the overproduction of TNFα (Achiron et al., 1994); inhibit or delay the occurrence of experimental autoimmune arthritis induced in Lewis rats by *Mycobacterium tuberculosis* in Freund's adjuvant (Achiron et al., 1994); diminish the frequency of fetal resorptions in mice with passively transferred anti-cardiolipin antibodies (Bakimer et al., 1993). Infusion of IVIg has lead to a decrease in circulating titers of anti-microsomal autoantibodies in SCID mice humanized with cells of patients with primary biliary cirrhosis (Hammarström et al., 1993). In addition, normal mouse immunoglobulin has been shown to prevent or delay autoimmune manifestations in several models of spontaneously occurring autoimmune diseases in mice, e.g., diabetes in NOD mice when injected neonatally with immunoglobulin (Forsgren et al., 1991), and that of lupus-like disease in (NZB × NZW) F1 mice having received immunoglobulins from polyclonally stimulated BALB/c mice (Hentati et al., 1994). Repeated administration of normal polyclonal mouse immunoglobulin at doses equivalent to those used for human IVIg therapy to NOD mice at birth, reduced the prevalence of insulitis at 15 weeks and the development of diabetes as compared with untreated mice (Andersson et al., 1991). Administration of high doses of a mixture of natural monoclonal antibodies or of a single natural monoclonal antibody at the same age also efficiently prevented the development of diabetes in NOD mice. The effects of natural antibodies were based on variable region specificity since some but not all monoclonal antibodies tested inhibited the development of the disease (Andersson et al., 1991). The monoclonal antibodies that were the most efficient in inhibiting diabetes had previously shown to be polyreactive and idiotypically "connected." The development of the Vh gene repertoire in NOD mice differs from that of other mouse strains in that adult NOD animals retain an overrepresentation of D-proximal Vh genes and utilize the VH7183.1 gene segment whereas rearrangements utilizing this gene are nonfunctional in normal adult Balb/c and C57Bl/6 mice. Prevention of disease by the administration of natural monoclonal antibody was associated with the absence of functional 7183.1 rearrangements in splenic B cells and with a decrease in the frequency of Vh7183 rearrangements utilizing the 7183.1 gene. The data suggest that the presence of functional Vh7183.1 rearrangements in the adult NOD mouse reflects an aberrant development in the immune repertoire in the animal that is related to the emergence of the autoimmune disease. The data also suggest that natural antibodies may be effective in preventing autoimmunity by interfering with the selective processes of the B cell repertoire and that B cells influence the development of T cell-mediated autoimmune disorders.

IV. INTERACTIONS OF INTRAVENOUS IMMUNOGLOBULIN WITH MOLECULES AND CELLS OF THE IMMUNE SYSTEM

The spectrum of antibody reactivities of variable regions expressed in IVIg provides the basis for the immunomodulatory effects of immunoglobulin. Some of the target molecules for natural IgG antibodies present in IVIg are molecules which contribute to the initiation and control of immune responses and/or molecules, for which targeted immunomanipulation may be effective in preventing human or experimental autoimmune disease. Table 3 lists such molecules of the immune system to which antibody reactivities have been identified in IVIg preparations.

Table 3. Reported Antibody Reactivities Present in IVIg Against
Molecules and Cells of the Immune System

Variable regions (idiotypes) of immunoglobulins and B cell antigen receptors

Variable and framework determinants of αβ T cell receptors

Other surface molecules of B cells, T cells and monocytes, including:
    CD5
    CD4
    MHC class I
    RGD-expressing adhesion molecules

Cytokines, cytokine receptors

Fc Receptors

There is compelling evidence for a direct interaction of IVIg with Fcγ receptors
(FcγR), leading to functional blockade of the receptors on phagocytic cells in vivo.
This interaction accounts for the rapid and transient reversal of peripheral autoimmune cytopenias, e.g., for the increase in platelet numbers in patients with ITP
treated with IVIg. Thus: i) intravenous infusion of Fcγ fragments prepared from
IVIg corrects acute autoimmune thrombocytopenia with kinetics and efficacy similar to those of treatment with intact IVIg (Debré et al., 1993); ii) infusion of monoclonal anti-FcγRIII antibody results in reversal of thrombocytopenia in ITP (Clarkson et al., 1986); iii) administration of IVIg is followed by a decrease in the clearance
of autologous erythrocytes coated with anti-D IgG antibodies (Fehr et al., 1982;
Salama et al., 1983); iv) peripheral blood monocytes from IVIg-treated patients
with ITP exhibit a decreased ability to form FcγR-dependent rosettes with IgG-
coated erythrocytes (Kimberly et al., 1984). In addition to blockade of receptors on
phagocytes, the binding of Fc of IgG to FcγR is likely to affect the function of B cells
and monocytes through the ability of Fc to trigger intracellular signalling upon
binding to Fc receptors on these cells (Fridman, 1993; Unkeless et al., 1988). Thus,
IVIg downregulates immunoglobulin synthesis by B cells and alters patterns of
secretion of monocytic cytokines in vitro through Fc-dependent mechanisms. The
binding of IgG to FcγR on normal peripheral blood mononuclear cells induces the
release of soluble FcγR in vitro, and intravenous infusion of Fcγ fragments was
shown to be followed by an increase in the serum concentration of sCD16 in vivo
(Debré et al., 1993; Lowy et al., 1983) (Figure 3). Although soluble forms of FcγR are
known to participate in the isotypic control of immunoglobulin production (Galon
et al., 1995), the clinical relevance of these effects in relation to IVIg therapy remains
as yet unclear.

Complement and Immune Complexes

The ability of IVIg to interfere with complement activation was first demonstrated
in two in vivo models, one of complement-dependent hepatic clearance of IgM-
sensitized guinea pig erythrocytes (Basta et al., 1989b) and the other of Forsmann
shock in guinea pigs, in which rabbit IgG antibodies to endothelial cells induce

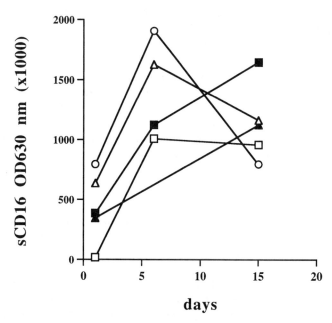

days

Figure 3. Changes in the serum concentration of sCD16 following administration of Fcγ fragments to patients with acute immune thrombocytopenic purpura. Soluble CD16 was quantitated using a dot-blot assay with ^{125}I-radiolabeled 3G8 anti-CD16 mAb. Concentrations of sCD16 are expressed as units of optical density at 630 nm. Fcγ fragments were infused on day 0. Each curve depicts one patient. Adapted from Debré et al., 1993.

acute complement-mediated tissue damage (Basta et al., 1989a). In the latter model, guinea pigs were treated with IVIg 3 h before they were subjected to otherwise lethal doses of anti-Forsmann antiserum. The median duration of survival was increased five times and mortality prevented in 38% of the animals. The mechanism involved in the protective effect of IVIg was shown to be an ability of normal immunoglobulin G to prevent C3 and C4 uptake on IgG- and IgM-coated targets (Basta et al., 1989a). The effect was not dependent on an inhibition of C1 uptake and the interference of IVIg with early steps of classical complement pathway activation, but rather on the ability of IVIg to bind the activated fragments C3b and C4b and subsequently prevent their binding to targets of complement activation. Inhibition by IVIg of the binding of C3 and C4 to target cells is one explanation for the beneficial effects of IVIg therapy in conditions where complement-mediated tissue injury plays a major role, e.g., in acute dermatomyositis, where a destruction of the endomyosial capillaries by the membrane attack complex of complement is the major pathogenic event (Basta and Dalakas, 1994). Thus, treatment with IVIg of patients with steroid-resistant dermatomyositis prevented the deposition of C3b and formation of membrane attack complexes on target cells in situ, as shown by semi-quantitative immunohistochemistry of patients' biopsy samples (Basta and Dalakas, 1994). Recent data indicate that the capacity of normal immunoglobulin to inhibit C3 and C4 uptake by immune complexes is not restricted to IgG but that, on a molar basis, monomeric serum IgA and IgM are more active than IgG in inhibiting complement activation (Miletic et al., 1996).

IVIg alters the amount of C3 and C4 in immune complexes and may further alter immune complex size and composition by bringing in rheumatoid factor activity and anti-idiotypic antibodies to some of the idiotypes expressed by complexed immunoglobulins. IVIg is thus likely to modify the structure, molecular weight, solubility and phlogistic potential of complexes in immune complex-mediated conditions. Hence, the addition of IVIg in vitro to renal biopsy material from patients with immune complex-mediated glomerulonephritis, resulted in a sharp decrease in the amount of immunoglobulin deposits in glomeruli (Sato et al., 1986).

Cytokines and Cytokine Receptors

There are multiple ways by which IVIg may modulate cytokine production and cytokine-mediated functions: i) IVIg selectively induces or downregulates the production of monocytic and T cell cytokines; ii) IVIg contains natural antibodies to cytokines, some of which exhibit neutralizing properties; and iii) IVIg alters expression of cytokine receptors and cytokine receptor-mediated functions.

The ability of IVIg to modulate the production and release of proinflammatory monocytic cytokines provides the basis for the rapid anti-inflammatory effects of IVIg that are observed in acute inflammatory conditions, e.g., in Kawasaki's syndrome and juvenile rheumatoid arthritis. In the latter conditions, infusion of IVIg is followed by a decrease in body temperature within two hours and improvement in inflammatory markers such as ESR and serum levels of C-reactive protein within one or two days. Culture of normal human peripheral blood monocytes with normal IgG was shown to result in the production and release of IL-1ra (Poutsiaka et al., 1991; Ruiz de Souza et al., 1995). The effect of IVIg is selective in that IVIg triggers gene transcription and secretion of IL-1ra and IL-8, without inducing the production of IL-1α, IL-1β, TNFα nor IL-6 by monocytes (Ruiz de Souza et al., 1995) (Figure 4). The effect of IVIg is dose-dependent and requires both the Fc and F(ab')$_2$ portions of IgG. The enhancing effect of IVIg on the synthesis of IL-1ra and IL-8 by monocytes is increased in the presence of autologous lymphocytes in cultures (Ruiz de Souza et al., 1995). Conflicting results have been reported regarding the production of IL-1 and TNFα in LPS-stimulated monocyte cultures in the presence of IVIg (Iwata et al., 1987; Kuhnert et al., 1990; Shimozato et al., 1991). Only scant information is available on changes in patterns of cytokine production in patients following administration of IVIg, due to our present limitations in methods to assess cytokine production in vivo. These limitations extend to T cell cytokines which often require, in order to be measured, that patients' cells are stimulated in vitro prior to quantitating cytokine production in cell cultures. IVIg has been shown to cause a significant suppression of the production of several T cell lymphokines upon activation of mononuclear cells with PMA/ionomycin in vitro (Andersson et al., 1993). Thus, using a technology based on immunocytochemistry with primary cytokine-specific antibodies, which enables the study of the production of cytokines at a single cell level, Andersson et al. have observed that the synthesis of IL-2, TNFβ, GM-CSF, IL-3, IL-4, IL-5 and IL-10 was reduced for up to 48 h of stimulation with IVIg (Andersson et al., 1993). The same group further demonstrated that IVIg downregulates the production of TNFβ and IFNγ in mono-

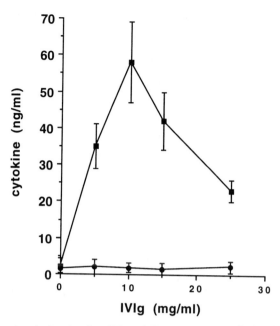

Figure 4. Selective induction by IVIg of IL-1ra in serum-free cultures of normal peripheral blood mononuclear cells (PBMC). Purified PBMC (1×10^6 NSE$^+$ cells/ml) from healthy donors were cultured in the presence of IVIg at indicated concentrations for 24 h at 37°CC. The concentration of IL-1 ra (squares), and IL-1β (circles) was determined in culture supernatants by ELISA. The figure depicts mean values ± SEM obtained in 5 individuals. Adapted from Ruiz-de-Souza et al., 1995.

nuclear cells stimulated with anti-CD3 mAb or with streptococcal pyrogenic exo-toxin A as a source of superantigen for T cells (Skansén-Saphir et al., 1994). Evidence is still lacking on the mechanisms by which IVIg affects the production of cytokines and on how it may alter the balance between Th1 and Th2-type CD4$^+$ T helper lymphocytes in vivo.

Normal IgG was shown to contain natural antibodies against IL-1α, TNFα and IL-6 (Abe et al., 1994; Bendtzen et al., 1990; Svenson et al., 1990). Natural anti-cytokine antibodies could inhibit cytokine-mediated effects when produced in excess in systemic inflammatory disorders. Unpublished evidence from our laboratory suggests that normal IgG also contains antibodies to certain cytokine receptors and that it may modulate cytokine production by interfering with induction of transcription of cytokine genes, either directly through "transcription factor-like" effects of IgG or indirectly by stimulating membrane molecules which would in turn trigger intracellular pathways regulating cytokine gene transcription.

Idiotypes of Immunoglobulins

Interactions between IVIg and variable regions of autoantibodies provide the basis for the ability of IVIg to regulate autoreactive B cell clones in vivo. Lines of evidence that we have accumulated demonstrating that IVIg contains antibodies

Table 4. Evidence for the Presence in IVIg of Complementary
Antibodies to Idiotypes of Autoantibodies

F(ab')2 fragments of IVIg inhibit autoantibody activity of F(ab')2 fragments of Ig
from patients with autoimmune disease

Autoantibodies are selectively retained on affinity columns of F(ab')2 fragment
of IVIg coupled to Sepharose

F(ab')2 fragments of IVIg compete with heterologous anti-idiotypic antibodies for
the binding to idiotypes of autoantibodies

Infusion of IVIg into patients with autoimmune disease results in the selective
downregulation or upregulation of B cell clones that are complementary to
variable regions of IVIg

---

that recognize idiotypes of disease-associated and of natural autoantibodies and
antigen receptors on B lymphocytes, are summarized in Table 4.

We have shown that intact IVIg and F(ab')$_2$ fragments of IVIg neutralize the
functional activity of various autoantibodies and/or inhibit the binding of the
autoantibodies to their respective autoantigens in vitro. Inhibition of autoantibody
activity by IVIg has been observed in the case of autoantibodies to factor VIII
(Sultan et al., 1984), thyroglobulin, DNA, intrinsic factor (Rossi and Kazatchkine,
1989), peripheral nerve (van Doorn et al., 1990), neutrophil cytoplasmic antigens
(Rossi et al., 1991b), platelet gpIIb IIIa (Berchtold et al., 1989), the acetylcholine
receptor (Liblau et al., 1991), endothelial cells (Ronda et al., 1994b), phospholipids
(Caccavo et al., 1994), nephritic factor (Fremeaux-Bacchi et al., 1992) and retinal
autoantigens (Kazatchkine et al., 1994) (Figure 5). Recently, it was shown that IVIg
contains antibodies directed to the cross-reactive 4B4 idiotype that is strongly
associated with Sjögren's syndrome (Dekeyser et al., 1996). In most cases, inhibition of autoantibody activity by IVIg was found to be dose-dependent with a
bell-shaped pattern of inhibition curves; maximal inhibition was reached at specific molar ratios between patient's IgG and IVIg that differed depending on the
autoantibodies and the patients (Rossi et al., 1989). The neutralizing capacity of
IVIg toward autoantibodies likely explains the rapid fall in the plasma titer of
anti-factor VIII and ANCA autoantibodies that has been seen in patients with
anti-factor VIII autoimmune disease and with ANCA-positive vasculitis following
treatment with IVIg (Figure 2) (Jayne et al., 1991, Sultan et al., 1984). In patients
with these diseases, a direct relationship has been found between the ability of IVIg
to neutralize autoantibody activity in vitro and that of IVIg to decrease autoantibody titers in treated patients in vivo (Jayne et al., 1991; Rossi et al., 1988).

Evidence that the inhibitory capacity of IVIg is related to the presence in IVIg of
antibodies directed to idiotypes of autoantibodies came from affinity chromatography experiments using columns of F(ab')$_2$ fragments of IVIg coupled to Sepharose.
IgG or F(ab')$_2$ fragments of IgG with autoantibody activity purified from patients'
serum, were loaded on the columns before the columns were washed and then
eluted at acid pH. Specific autoantibody activity, expressed as arbitrary units per
mg of protein, was measured in the acid eluate and compared with that of the
material that had been applied on the columns. A 1.3- to 50-fold increase in specific

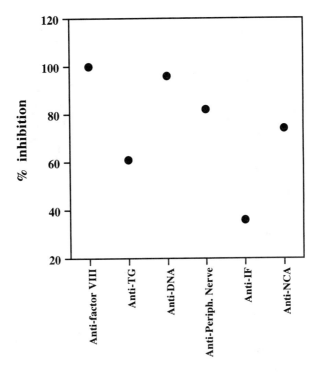

Figure 5. Inhibition of autoantibody by F(ab')$_2$ fragments of IVIg in vitro. F(ab')$_2$ fragments of IgG purified from patient serum were incubated with increasing amounts of F(ab')$_2$ fragments of IVIg. The figure represents maximal inhibition of autoantibody activity achieved at specific mole to mole ratios of F(ab')$_2$ fragments of IVIg and F(ab')$_2$ fragments of autoantibodies.

anti-factor VIII, anti-DNA, anti-thyroglobulin, anti-peripheral nerve, anti-neutrophil cytoplasmic antigen (ANCA), anti-intrinsic factor and anti-retinal antigen autoantibody activity was observed in the eluates, demonstrating that F(ab')$_2$ fragments of IVIg specifically bind idiotypic determinants located in or close to the antigen-binding site of the autoantibodies, with high affinity (Figure 6). Furthermore, the analysis of densitometric patterns of immunoblots on endothelial cell protein extracts of IgG purified from serum of patients with SLE prior to and after affinity chromatography on Sepharose-bound F(ab')$_2$ fragments of IVIg, demonstrated that IVIg reacts selectively with certain antibody species within the polyclonal population of anti-endothelial cell autoantibodies (Ronda et al., 1994a).

We have further shown that IVIg share anti-idiotypic reactivity toward idiotypes of autoantibodies with heterologous anti-idiotypic reagents, as additional evidence that IVIg contains anti-idiotypes to autoantibodies. Thus, IVIg was shown to compete with monoclonal and polyclonal anti-idiotypic antibodies for the binding to idiotypes expressed by anti-factor VIII (Dietrich et al., 1990) and anti-thyroglobulin (TG) autoantibodies (Dietrich and Kazatchkine, 1990). A paratope-related idiotype defined by a mouse monoclonal antibody termed 20F2, expressed by anti-factor VIII autoantibodies of a patient with anti-factor VIII autoimmune dis-

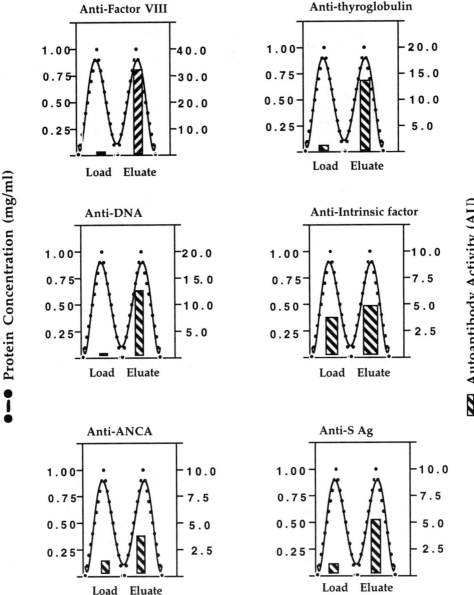

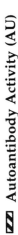

Figure 6. Selective retention of autoantibody activity on affinity columns of F(ab')$_2$ fragments of IVIg coupled to Sepharose. IgG or F(ab')$_2$ fragments containing autoantibody activity were chromatographed on Sepharose-bound F(ab')$_2$ fragments of IVIg. The affinity matrix was washed until no protein was detected in the effluent and bound protein was then eluted at pH 2.8. Autoantibody activity was measured in the loaded material and in the acid-eluted fraction. Peaks represent total protein content in the fractions. Hatched bars depict specific autoantibody activity in the fractions, as measured by ELISA. Adapted from Rossi et al., 1989; Rossi et al., 1991b.

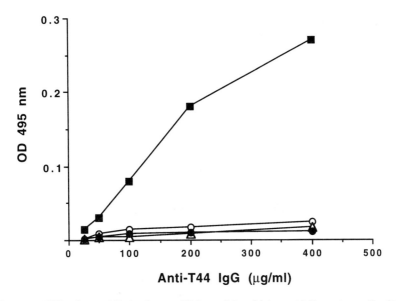

Figure 7. IVIg shares idiotypic specificity with rabbit anti-idiotypic antibodies to anti-thyroglobulin autoantibodies. The figure depicts the binding of rabbit anti-idiotypic anti-T44 antibody to F(ab')$_2$ fragments of IgG of a patient with autoimmune thyroiditis, that had been eluted from Sepharose-bound F(ab')$_2$ fragments of IVIg (closed squares), F(ab')$_2$ fragments in the effluent of the affinity column (open circles), unchromatographed F(ab')$_2$ fragments of patient IgG (closed diamonds), and F(ab')$_2$ fragments of IVIg (open triangles). Binding was measured by using an ELISA with plates coated with 40 µg/ml of F(ab')$_2$ fragments of patient IgG. Adapted from Dietrich and Kazatchkine, 1990.

ease, was also recognized by IVIg. IVIg was capable of neutralizing anti-factor VIII activity of patient's anti-factor VIII autoantibodies that had been affinity purified on a 20F2 mAb affinity column (Dietrich et al., 1990). Similar results to those observed with anti-factor VIII autoantibodies, were obtained with anti-TG autoantibodies (Dietrich and Kazatchkine, 1990; Kaveri et al., 1993), demonstrating that IVIg contains anti-idiotypes directed against cross-reactive idiotypes expressed by disease-associated autoantibodies (Figure 7). Additional evidence for reactivity between IVIg and idiotypic determinants of an antibody molecule comes from the demonstration of the binding of IVIg to a synthetic peptide derived from the CDR2/FR3 region of the V1 S107 heavy chain (Kaveri et al., 1990). This peptide termed T15H(50-73) originates from the V region of the T15 idiotype of mouse and human anti-phosphorylcholine antibodies (Halpern et al.; 1991, Kang et al., 1988). IVIg bound to the immobilized T15 peptide and specific anti-T15 peptide antibodies were isolated from IVIg through peptide-Sepharose affinity chromatography. The isolated anti-peptide antibodies were further shown to exhibit self-binding properties. These studies raise the issue of the significance of antibodies in IVIg that recognize an evolutionarily conserved hypervariable antibody structure that may express regulatory functions within the idiotypic network, in addition to demonstrating the binding of IVIg to an idiotype.

Table 5. V Region-Dependent Connectivity Within the IgG Fraction of the
Serum of a Single Donor and Within Pooled IgG Originating from a
Large Number of Donors*

	Coupled (mg)	Loaded (mg)	Loaded/ coupled	Eluted (mg)	Loaded/ eluted
F(ab')$_2$ IVIg/ F(ab')$_2$ IVIg	302	540	1.78	4	135 (0.74%)
F(ab')$_2$ IgG/ F(ab')$_2$ IgG/	88	198	2.27	0.3	660 (0.15 %)

*F(ab')$_2$ fragments of IVIg and F(ab')$_2$ fragments of IgG from a single donor were chromatographed on Sepharose-bound F(ab')$_2$ fragments of IVIg and on Sepharose-bound F(ab')$_2$ fragments of the same individual's IgG, respectively. The amounts of F(ab')$_2$ fragments of that had been coupled to Sepharose, of F(ab')$_2$ fragments loaded on the columns and of F(ab')$_2$ fragments recovered in acid eluates from the columns.

Since IVIg contain both natural autoantibodies and anti-idiotypes to autoanti-bodies, it may be expected that F(ab')$_2$–F(ab')$_2$ dimers form in IVIg pools. Such dimers have been shown to occur and to involve up to 30% of IgG molecules in therapeutic preparations of IVIg (Tankersley, 1994). Dimers of complementary variable regions within IVIg pools were directly demonstrated by electron micros-copy (Roux and Tankersley, 1990). The relative amount of dimers in preparations of IVIg increases with the number of donors contributing to the plasma pool (Tankersley et al., 1988). Dimers in IVIg preferentially form between autoanti-bodies and anti-autoantibodies rather than between antibodies to non-self antigens (e.g., vaccinal antigens) and anti-idiotypes to these antibodies. Thus, IgG involved in dimer formation in IVIg contains higher levels of specific autoreactivity than IVIg molecules not engaged in dimer formation (Dietrich et al., 1992b; Vassilev et al., 1995). Variable region-connected IgG molecules may be demonstrated in pools of IVIg by affinity chromatography. Although present in smaller amounts, dimers of complementary IgG molecules may also be evidenced in the IgG fraction of the serum of an individual donor (Table 5). Interactions between complementary vari-able regions in IVIg may also be analyzed by using quantitative immunoblotting, where "anti-idiotypic IgG" is blotted onto F(ab')$_2$ fragments of IVIg that have been separated by isoelectric focusing prior to transfer on nitrocellulose membranes (Ayouba et al., 1996). Average affinities of F(ab')$_2$ fragments of IVIg with comple-mentary molecules in the same IVIg preparation were found to be in the micromo-lar range.

In addition to recognizing idiotypic determinants on autoantibodies of the IgG isotype, IVIg reacts with idiotypes expressed by IgM autoantibodies of healthy individuals and autoantibodies of the IgM isotype in patient serum (Rossi et al., 1990; van Doorn et al., 1990). Thus, we have demonstrated that F(ab')$_2$ fragments of IVIg bind to natural polyreactive IgM antibodies secreted by EBV-transformed normal B lymphocytes. No correlation was observed between the degree of polyre-activity of IgM autoantibodies and their relative reactivity with IVIg. The presence of antibodies in IVIg that are idiotypically connected with natural IgG and IgM antibodies reflects the physiological situation in which IgG molecules, as well as IgG and IgM molecules, express idiotypic complementarity in autologous serum. In other words and as discussed later, autoreactivity of IgG in whole serum is controlled in part by autologous anti-idiotypic IgG and autologous anti-idiotypic IgM (Adib et al., 1990; Hurez et al., 1993).

Interactions between complementary immunoglobulins within pools of IgG in IVIg preparations may result in additive or synergistic enhancement or else in inhibition of specific antibody activities in the pool (Dietrich et al., 1992a). One particular source of anti-idiotypic activity against autoantibodies in IVIg is the plasma of patients who recovered from autoimmune disease and in whom recovery has been associated with the generation of anti-idiotypes against acute phase autoantibodies. The occurrence of anti-idiotypes in post-recovery sera has been documented in several autoimmune conditions including anti-factor VIII autoimmune disease, ANCA-positive vasculitis, Guillain-Barré syndrome, anti-fibrinogen antibodies, SLE and in the serum of non-affected children born to myasthenic mothers (Lefvert, 1994; Lefvert and Osterman, 1983; Lundkvist et al., 1993; Rossi et al., 1991b; Ruiz-Arguelles, 1988; Sultan et al., 1987; Zouali and Eyquem, 1983). We have also gathered evidence that the plasma of healthy donors over the age of 65 years and pooled IgG from multiparous women contain higher amounts of anti-idiotypic activity against, e.g., autoantibodies to factor VIII than plasma of healthy young adult males (Dietrich et al., 1992a). It may be speculated that plasmas containing high anti-idiotypic activity to autoantibodies could represent a privileged source to prepare IVIg for immunomodulation of autoimmune disease.

Membrane Molecules of Lymphocytes

In addition to binding to idiotypes of immunoglobulins, IVIg reacts with a number of membrane molecules of T cells, B cells and monocytes that are relevant for the control of autoreactivity and induction of tolerance to self. Thus, IVIg has been shown to contain antibodies to variable and constant regions of the human $\alpha\beta$ T cell receptor, cytokines and cytokine receptors, CD5, CD4 and HLA class I molecules. We believe that antibodies directed to such functional molecules of lymphocytes are important for the immunomodulatory effects of normal immunoglobulin.

The binding of IVIg to variable and constant regions of the human $\alpha\beta$ TCR has been documented in two studies using synthetic peptides derived from the TCR. Overlapping synthetic hexadecapeptides of human TCRβ YT35 were used to assess the binding of IVIg by ELISA in one study (Marchalonis et al., 1992); overlapping TCR peptides attached to polyethylene pins ("Pepscan" technology) mapped using anti-TCR mAbs have been used in the second study (Kruger et al., 1993). Both studies demonstrated the binding of IVIg to determinants of the constant region of the β chain of the TCR as well as to framework and clonotypic determinants of the variable region of the receptor (Marchalonis et al., 1992). By using affinity purification, an anti-Vβ8-enriched fraction was purified from IVIg that displayed high levels of binding to specific Vβ8 TCR peptides (Marchalonis et al., 1992). The presence of autoantibodies to defined human TCR peptides in IVIg provides the therapeutic preparations with a potential for modulation of specific T cell immune responses. The ability of IVIg to inhibit superantigen-elicited T cell activation has recently been documented (Takei et al., 1993). The mechanism by

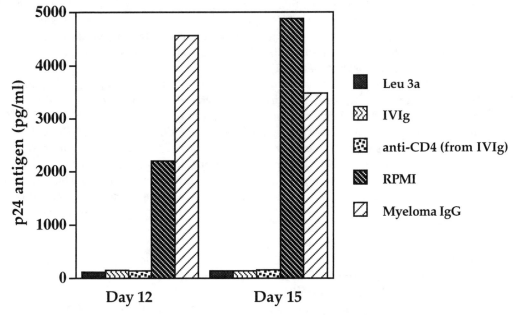

Figure 8. Anti-CD4 antibodies in IVIg. The figure depicts the inhibition by affinity-purified anti-CD4 antibodies from IVIg of infection of the human CD4[+] T cell line H9 with HIV. H9 cells (3×10^5) were preincubated with Leu3a (0.25 µg), affinity-purified anti-CD4 antibodies from IVIg (2 µg), IVIg (10 µg) or myeloma IgG (10 µg) before infection with HIV (8×10^{-3} infectious units/cell). The cells were then cultured for 15 days. The concentration of p24 antigen in culture supernatants was determined by ELISA at days 12 and 15. Adapted from Hurez et al., 1994.

which IVIg was inhibitory did not depend however on binding to TCR, but rather on direct neutralization of staphylococcal toxin superantigens by specific antibodies in IVIg (Takei et al., 1993). We have recently addressed this question and observed that the addition of IVIg to normal PBMC stimulated with staphylococcal enterotoxin B (SEB) superantigen resulted in an increase in the proportion of CD3 blast cells expressing the Vβ markers of the subfamilies of T cells which expand in presence of SEB. These observations indicated that SEB-activated T cells are rescued from the inhibition of proliferation which is induced by IVIg in stimulated T cell cultures (Baudet et al., 1995).

Antibodies to CD5 in IVIg were identified by the ability of IVIg and F(ab')$_2$ fragments of IVIg to inhibit the binding of labeled CD5 mAb to a CD5-expressing human T cell line and to bind to mouse L cells that expressed human CD5 following stable transfection with CD5 cDNA (Vassilev et al., 1993). Antibodies to CD4 have been characterized in IVIg using both immunochemical and functional approaches (Hurez et al., 1994). IVIg and F(ab')$_2$ fragments of IVIg bound to a recombinant soluble form of human CD4, as assessed by ELISA, immunoblotting and real time analysis of complex formation in the fluid phase using the BIAcore setup. Anti-CD4 antibodies were isolated from IVIg by affinity chromatography on rCD4-Sepharose and shown to bind to human CD4[+] T cells. The affinity-purified anti-CD4 fraction of IVIg inhibited the proliferative responses in MLR and in vitro

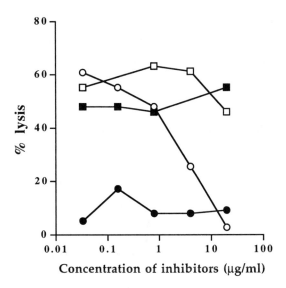

Figure 9. Anti-MHC class I antibodies in IVIg. The figure depicts the inhibition of class I-restricted T cell-mediated cytotoxicity by affinity-purified anti-class I B07.75-84 peptide antibodies from IVIg. A CD8+ human T cell line specific for the M.58-66 influenza virus peptide used as a source of effector cells was incubated with affinity-purified anti-B07.75-84 peptide antibodies from IVIg (open circles), human myeloma IgG (open squares), mouse monoclonal anti-class I antibody W6/32HL (closed circles) or medium alone (closed squares). ^{51}Cr-labeled target cells sensitized with the viral peptide were incubated with effector cells at a 10:1 E/T ratio. ^{51}Cr release was measured in supernatants. Adapted from Kaveri et al., 1996.

infection of CD4+ T cells with HIV (Hurez et al., 1994) (Figure 8). Recent observations from our laboratory (Vassilev, T et al., unpublished) indicate that IVIg also contains antibodies to the RGD sequence that is essential to the interaction between several integrins and their respective ligands.

Another target molecule for IVIg on immunocompetent cells is HLA class I. We have shown that IVIg contains antibodies to the B07.75-84 peptide which corresponds to a conserved region of the α1 helix of the first domain of HLA-B7 01, a non-polymorphic determinant of HLA class I molecules (Kaveri et al., 1996). Intact IVIg and F(ab')$_2$ fragments of IVIg bound to the peptide as well as to purified soluble HLA and to HLA on human T cells. The binding of anti-peptide antibodies to HLA was inhibited by free peptide. Anti-peptide antibodies isolated from IVIg by affinity chromatography inhibited CD8-mediated class I-restricted cytotoxicity of an influenza virus-specific human T cell line toward an influenza peptide-primed target cell (Figure 9). The presence in IVIg of antibodies to critical regions of HLA class I suggests a role for IVIg in modulation of class I-restricted cellular interactions in the immune response. Of relevance are recent observations that administration of IVIg to hyperimmunized dialyzed patients decreases the plasma titer of cytotoxic anti-class I antibodies allowing, in certain cases, to perform an allotransplantation in patients with otherwise positive cross-match (Glotz et al., 1995).

V. IMMUNOMODULATORY EFFECTS OF INTRAVENOUS IMMUNOGLOBULIN IN AUTOIMMUNE DISEASES

Clinical observations in autoimmune patients treated with IVIg together with experimental data obtained in animals infused with normal homologous immuno-globulin have provided several lines of evidence documenting that normal immu-noglobulin participates in the selection of B and T cell repertoires (Table 6). Selec-tion of immune repertoires, e.g., of autoreactive antibody repertoires, is thus one physiological function of natural antibodies in healthy individuals.

Homologous Immunoglobulin Selects T and B Cell Repertoires in Mice

A striking effect of the administration of normal mouse immunoglobulin into normal adult mice is thymocyte depletion, with double positive immature thymo-cytes being more susceptible to homologous immunoglobulin than single positive mature T cells (Sundblad et al., 1994). Depletion in immature T cells contrasts with activation of CD4+ T cells in the periphery (spleen) (Sundblad et al., 1991). In line with the above evidence, recent experiments from our laboratory (Vassilev, T et al., unpublished) indicate that infusion of IVIg into SCID mice humanized with PBMCs from healthy donors induce expression of activation markers on T cells. There is evidence in the mouse that normal immunoglobulins participate in the selection of TCR repertoires (Martinez et al., 1986) suggesting that dysfunctional antibody repertoires could participate in the generation of T cell-mediated diseases and providing a putative mechanism of action of IVIg in T cell-dependent autoim-mune disease. Of relevance to the latter concept is the observation that immuno-globulin-mediated selection of T cell repertoires specifically applies to T cells that are naturally activated (autoreactive) (Coutinho et al., 1987) and the observations of therapeutic effects of normal immunoglobulin in NOD mice and rats with EAE and adjuvant arthritis (Andersson et al., 1991; Forsgren et al., 1991; Achiron et al., 1994).

Infusion of normal homologous immunoglobulin into adult mice also results in depletion of immature bone marrow B cells and in the selective activation of certain peripheral B cells. Thus, administration to normal Balb/c mice for five days intra-venously of pooled IgG from healthy Balb/c or C57BL/6 mice resulted in a dose-dependent depletion in small sIgM-B220+ B cells, both in frequencies and in abso-lute numbers (Sundblad et al., 1991). The effect was seen with polyclonal homologous IgG but not with equivalent doses of monoclonal IgG nor with human IgG, suggesting that pre B/B cell depletion is dependent on specific variable regions present in the homologous immunoglobulin pool. Bone marrow B cell depletion was independent of T cells as shown in experiments using athymic mice. Direct evidence for the ability of IgG to interact with target pre B/B cells has been obtained by adding IgG to bone marrow cell cultures (Sundblad et al., 1994). Variable region specificity of the selection of emergent bone marrow B cell reper-toires by normal immunoglobulin was obtained by analyzing the Vh gene reper-toires of bone marrow cells of immunoglobulin-treated mice. Vh gene family expression was compared in the bone marrow and peripheral B cells in germ-free and in conventionally raised Balb/c mice (Freitas et al., 1991). Adult germ-free animals showed the same Vh gene family usage in peripheral tissues as in the bone marrow whereas peripheral B cell repertoires of conventional Balb/c mice differed

Table 6. Evidence for Selection of Immune Repertoires in
Recipients of Normal Immunoglobulin

Depletion of immature thymocytes and selection of pre-immune B cell repertoires in the
    bone marrow and peripheral lymphoid tissues, follow infusion of homologous Ig in mice.

Subsets of splenic lymphocytes are selectively activated in mice following administration
    of normal homologous Ig.

Disease-related autoantibodies may be suppressed for prolonged periods of time following
    treatment of autoimmune patients with IVIg.

IVIg therapy results in increased serum concentrations of IgM; B cell clones that are
    complementary (anti-idiotypic) to variable regions of IVIg are selectively downregulated
    or upregulated in patients receiving IVIg.

Normal patterns of spontaneous fluctuations of autoantibodies in serum are restored
    following infusion of IVIg into autoimmune patients.

from those in bone marrow with decreased utilization of the Vh7183 family and
increased frequency of the VhX24 family. Administration of normal homologous
IgG selectively decreased the usage of the Vh7183 family in germ-free mice. These
data indicated that bone marrow B cells are not eliminated randomly by immunoglobulin but in a fashion dependent on the Vh genes they express and thus that
polyclonal serum immunoglobulin affects the selection of antibody repertoires.
Further studies by Sundblad et al., demonstrated that the administration of normal
mouse IgG into adult Balb/c mice resulted in an increase in blast B cells in the
spleen of treated animals, associated with an increase in the number of splenic
immunoglobulin-secreting cells (Sundblad et al., 1991). By assaying plasma cells
and serum IgG for reactivities with a panel of antigens, it was shown that certain
autoantibodies (e.g., anti-thyroglobulin and rheumatoid factor) were more frequently produced by plasma cells of immunoglobulin-treated than untreated animals.

VI. SUPPRESSION OF AUTOANTIBODIES BY INTRAVENOUS
IMMUNOGLOBULIN

The suppressive effects of IVIg on disease-associated autoantibodies in patients
with autoimmune disease are short-term and long-term. In the short-term, i.e.,
within hours following infusion of IVIg, the serum titer of autoantibodies may
rapidly decrease (Figure 2), due to complementary (idiotypic) neutralizing interactions between patient autoantibodies and anti-idiotypes to autoantibodies present
in IVIg. Neutralization of circulating autoantibodies by passively transferred anti-
idiotypes is somewhat analogous to the neutralization of autoantibodies by autologous anti-idiotypes generated in patients who recover spontaneously from autoimmune disease (Abdou et al., 1981; Ruiz-Arguelles, 1988; Sultan et al., 1987).

As first observed in patients with anti-factor VIII autoimmune disease (Sultan et
al., 1984), the suppressive effect of IVIg infusion on circulating autoantibodies may
be long lasting, far beyond the half-life of infused immunoglobulin. As discussed
below, these long-term suppressive effects are dependent on the selection of B cell

repertoires in IVIg recipients. There is also in vitro evidence for a direct inhibitory capacity of IVIg on immunoglobulin production by B cells. In an early study, a decrease in non-specific immunoglobulin production has been observed in poke-weed mitogen-stimulated lymphocyte cultures of cells of patients with ITP follow-ing IVIg therapy (Tsubakio et al., 1983). IVIg was shown to modulate antibody responses, possibly by enhancing suppressor T cell functions. Thus, the ability of Con A-activated cells to suppress autologous antibody responses in cultures of PBMCs was enhanced in patients with ITP that responded positively to IVIg (Delfraissy et al., 1985). IVIg has also been shown to dose-dependently suppress the production of IgM by EBV-transformed B lymphoblastoid cells (Kondo et al., 1994). The effect of IVIg was blocked by pretreatment of the B cells with anti-FcγRIII receptor antibody or anti-Fcγ antibody, indicating that the effect was at least in part dependent on the Fc portion of IVIg. Intact IVIg inhibited pokeweed mitogen-stimulated antibody production by B cells (Hashimoto et al., 1986; Kondo et al., 1991; Stohl, 1986), an effect also shown to be dependent on the constant region of IgG (Kondo et al., 1991). Thus, autoantibody production by B cells may be non-specifically reduced by Fc-dependent mechanisms; it may also be specifically downmodulated by anti-idiotypes present in IVIg and directed against B cell antigen receptor on autoantibody-producing cells, an effect that is likely to require the cooperation of the Fc portion of IVIg with the variable region targeting the idiotype-expressing B cell (Kohler et al., 1988).

IVIg inhibits proliferation of in vitro-activated B and T lymphocytes by as yet poorly understood mechanisms (Kawada and Terasaki, 1987; Leung et al., 1995; Van Schaik et al., 1992). In addition to in vitro-activated lymphocytes, IVIg was shown to inhibit the proliferation of autonomously growing cell lines of different origins. These observations suggest that IVIg may interfere with the expression of genes involved in cell cycle and that IgG could exert through these mechanisms some of its homeostatic functions. Mitogenic responses of normal human periph-eral blood mononuclear cells to PHA, Con A and pokeweed mitogen were shown to be suppressed in IVIg-supplemented cultures in a dose-dependent fashion (Van Schaik et al., 1992). The effect was due to IVIg since it was reversible following removal of IVIg by washing. IgG levels required for this anti-proliferative effect were "supraphysiological" but within those that are achieved upon treatment with IVIg (Van Schaik et al., 1992).

B Cell Clones that Are Anti-Idiotypic to IVIg Are Selectively Downregulated or Upregulated in Patients Receiving IVIg

We have analyzed the changes in antibody repertoires that followed the infusion of IVIg in a patient with autoimmune thyroiditis, taking advantage of the presence in this particular patient of anti-thyroglobulin IgG autoantibodies that bear a disease-specific idiotype termed T44 (Dietrich et al., 1993). Within 24 h after infusion of IVIg, serum IgG levels sharply increased to 1.5 times pre-infusion levels and then decreased to return to baseline levels after four weeks, as expected from the known half-life of IgG. Following the second infusion of the same dose of the same IVIg preparation, the concentration of serum IgG increased to 2.2 times pre-infusion levels that is higher than would have been expected from the amount of transfused immunoglobulin. We interpret this increase as reflecting a secondary immune

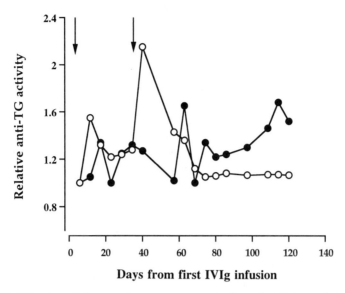

Figure 10. Kinetics of changes in serum concentration of anti-thyroglobulin (TG) antibodies in a patient with autoimmune thyroiditis following infusions of IVIg. Open circles depict total IgG anti-TG activity in serum. Closed circles depict anti-TG activity in the IVIg-reactive fraction of patient IgG purified by affinity chromatography on IVIg-Sepaharose. Anti-TG activity was measured by ELISA. Arrows denote infusions of IVIg. Adapted from Dietrich et al., 1993.

response triggered by variable regions (idiotypes) of IVIg. Interestingly, serum levels of IgM decreased within the first 24 h following infusion of IVIg, which may be the consequence of complementary variable region-dependent interactions between infused IgG and circulating IgM (see below). IgM levels then increased, the second infusion having resulted in a cumulative increase in the production of IgM and the persistence of elevated levels of IgM in serum for more than 14 weeks. These observations provide direct evidence that IVIg triggers subsets of B cells in the recipient to produce antibodies.

Analysis of the changes in antibody repertoires in patient's serum indicated that the antibody activities did not vary as would have been expected from just the passive transfer of antibody specificities contained in IVIg. Thus, although IVIg contain high amounts of anti-phosphorylcholine and anti-gliadin antibodies, no changes were observed in the serum titers of anti-phosphorylcholine IgG whereas the titer of anti-gliadin antibodies increased sharply in serum 24 h after infusion of IVIg. We further analyzed the kinetics of changes in serum levels of anti-IVIg activity of IgG in patient's serum by measuring sequentially the amount of patient's IgG that was retained on an affinity column of IVIg-Sepharose. As shown in Figure 10, the relative changes in the concentration of IVIg-reactive IgG in serum did not follow the changes in the concentration of total serum anti-thyroglobulin IgG. The concentration of the subpopulation of the patient's serum anti-thyroglobulin antibodies reactive with (anti-idiotypic to) IVIg increased from the third week onward following IVIg infusion, whereas total anti-thyroglobulin activity in serum remained stable. The data indicate that a distinct subpopulation of anti-thyroglobulin B cells reactive with variable regions of normal IgG antibodies present in IVIg has been stimulated in vivo following infusion of IVIg. Whereas certain clones of B cells expressing complementary idiotypes to antibodies in IVIg are stimulated following infusion of IVIg, other clones may be selectively downregulated. Thus, we have observed that within the population of IVIg-reactive patient's anti-thyroglobulin IgG, clones expressing the T44 idiotype were downregulated for eight weeks from the fourth week following the infusion of IVIg. We had previously shown that IVIg contains antibodies reactive with T44 Id$^+$ anti-thyroglobulin IgG (Dietrich and Kazatchkine, 1990). Our observations suggest that the infusion of IVIg may induce subtle changes in the concentration of circulating autoantibodies that may not be apparent from the analysis of the total polyclonal population of antibodies of a given specificity.

Further evidence for variable region-mediated changes in idiotypic network function in individuals receiving IVIg came from the analysis of the kinetics of spontaneous fluctuations of autoantibody levels in the serum of patients before and after treatment with IVIg. We had previously demonstrated that changes in serum levels of natural autoantibodies in healthy individuals are not random but exhibit "highly organized" reproducible oscillatory patterns (Varela et al., 1991). These patterns were not found upon analysis of the kinetics of the fluctuations of disease-related autoantibodies in the serum of patients with autoimmune thyroiditis. The observation that perturbed oscillatory patterns were observed in the case of both anti-thyroglobulin and anti-DNA autoantibodies suggest the presence of an altered network rather than a restricted clonal defect in autoimmune thyroiditis. Interestingly, the analysis of serum fluctuations of anti-DNA and anti-thyroglobulin autoantibodies in a patient in the weeks that followed infusion of IVIg, demonstrated the restoration of a normal pattern of fluctuations of autoantibodies in serum (Dietrich et al., 1993).

A Role for IVIgM?

Variable region-dependent interactions control the expression of IgG autoreactivity in serum. Thus, low or undetectable levels of autoreactive IgG are maintained in whole serum under physiological conditions, whereas high levels of autoreactivity are present in IgG isolated from normal serum (Adib et al., 1990; Berneman et al., 1993; Hurez et al., 1993; Mouthon et al., 1995b; Ronda et al., 1994b) (Figure 11). Evidence for the role of idiotypic regulation of IgG reactivity by IgM is derived from the following observations: i) purified serum IgM dose-dependently inhibits the binding of purified autologous IgG of healthy individuals and purified IgG from the serum of patients with autoimmune diseases, to panels of self antigens; ii) purified serum IgM binds to F(ab')$_2$ fragments of autologous IgG in a dose-dependent manner; iii) binding to autoantigens of IgG in the serum of SCID mice reconstituted with normal human PBMCs (huSCID) is higher than that of the purified IgG fraction of the serum. Lack of control of IgG autoreactivity in the serum of huSCID may be related to the low amount of human IgM in these mice (Hurez et al., 1993). The latter observations are relevant to autoimmune disease since, for example, the loss of IgG ANCA autoantibody activity in the serum of patients in clinical remission of ANCA-positive vasculitis is associated with the presence in serum of anti-idiotypic antibodies of the IgM isotype directed against

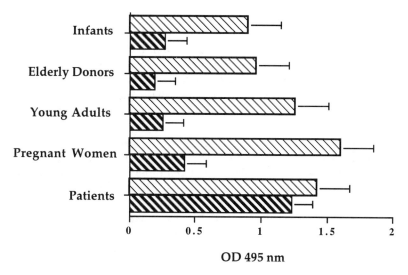

Figure 11. Autologous IgM controls autoreactivity of IgG in normal serum. The figure depicts the reactivity toward self antigens of IgG in whole serum (dark hatched columns) as compared with IgG purified from serum (light hatched columns). The experiments were performed using IgG from infants, elderly donors, young adults, pregnant women and patients with autoimmune thyroiditis, as indicated. Each column represents mean OD ± SD of binding of IgG of 20 individuals.

patient's acute phase IgG ANCA autoantibodies (Jayne et al., 1993; Rossi et al., 1991b). There is in vitro evidence that IgM-dependent regulation of IgG autoreactivity in serum may be defective in autoimmune conditions (Hurez et al., 1993; Ronda et al., 1994b). Thus, in the serum of patients with SLE and in patients with autoimmune thyroiditis, IgG autoreactivity to protein antigens in endothelial cells (SLE) and to thyroglobulin (autoimmune thyroiditis), is similar when tested in whole serum and in the purified IgG fraction of serum, suggesting a lack of IgM-dependent control in these pathological sera. IgM has an essential if not exclusive role in controlling levels of IgG autoreactivity in serum, as indicated by the lack of regulatory capacity of mouse serum from μ knockout animals as compared with serum of μ sufficient animals (A. Coutinho, personal communication). Taken together, these results argue in support of a future use of therapeutic preparations of pooled normal IgM alone or as complementary therapy with IVIg, for immunomodulation of human autoimmune disease (Hurez et al., 1996).

ACKNOWLEDGMENTS

These studies were supported by Institut National de la Santé et de la Recherche Médicale (INSERM), Centre National de la Recherche Scientifique (CNRS), France, The Central Laboratory of the Swiss Red Cross, Bern, Switzerland, the Laboratoire Français des Biotechnologies, les Ulis, France and Sandoz France. The authors are grateful to A. Coutinho, B. Bellon, G. Dietrich, V. Hurez, S. Lacroix-Desmazes, L. Mouthon, A. Pashov, N. Ronda, F. Rossi, V. Ruiz de Souza, S. Spalter, Y. Sultan, and T. Vassilev for their contributions.

REFERENCES

Abdou, N.I., H. Wall, H.B. Lindsley, J.F. Halsey, and T. Susuki. 1981. Network theory in autoimmunity: in vitro suppression of serum anti-DNA antibody binding to DNA by anti-idiotypic antibody in systemic lupus erythematosus. *J. Clin. Invest.* **67**, 1297–1304.

Abe, Y., A. Horiuchi, M. Miyake, and S. Kimura. 1994. Anti-cytokine nature of human immunoglobulin: one possible mechanism of the clinical effect of intravenous therapy. *Immunol. Rev.* **139**, 5–19.

Achiron, A., R. Margalit, R. Hershkoviz, D. Markovits, T. Reshef, E. Melamed, I.R. Cohen, and O. Lider. 1994. Intravenous immunoglobulin treatment of experimental T cell-mediated autoimmune disease. Upregulation of T cell proliferation and downregulation of tumor necrosis factor alpha secretion. *J. Clin. Invest.* **93**, 600–605.

Adib, M., J. Ragimbeau, S. Avrameas, and T. Ternynck. 1990. IgG autoantibody activity in normal mouse serum is controlled by IgM. *J. Immunol.* **145**, 3807–3813.

Andersson, A., S. Forsgren, A. Soderstrom, and D. Holmberg. 1991. Monoclonal natural antibodies prevent development of diabetes in the non-obese diabetic (NOD) mouse. *J. Autoimmunity* **4**, 733–742.

Andersson, U.G., L. Bjork, U. Skansén-Saphir, and J.P. Andersson. 1993. Down-regulation of cytokine production and IL-2 receptor expression by pooled human IgG. *Immunology* **79**, 211–216.

Ayouba, A., G. Peltre, and A. Coutinho. 1996. Quantitative analysis of multiple V region interactions among normal human IgG. *Eur. J. Immunol.* **26**, 710–716.

Bakimer, R., B. Guilburd, N. Zurgil, and Y. Shoenfeld. 1993. The effect of intravenous γ-globulin on the induction of experimental antiphospholipid syndrome. *Clin. Immunol. Immunopathol.* **69**, 97–102.

Basta, M., and M.C. Dalakas. 1994. High-dose intravenous immunoglobulin exerts its beneficial effect in patients with dermatomyositis by blocking endomysial deposition of activated complements fragments. *J. Clin. Inv.* **94**, 1729–1735.

Basta, M., P. Kirshbom, M.M. Frank, and L.F. Fries. 1989a. Mechanism of therapeutic effect of high-dose intravenous immunoglobulin. Attenuation of acute, complement-dependent immune damage in a guinea pig model. *J. Clin. Invest.* **84**, 1974–1981.

Basta, M., P.F. Langlois, M. Marques, M.M. Frank, and L.F. Fries. 1989b. High-dose intravenous immunoglobulin modifies complement-mediated in vivo clearance. *Blood* **74**, 326–333.

Baudet, V., V. Hurez, C. Lapeyre, S.V. Kaveri, and M.D. Kazatchkine. 1995. Intravenous immunoglobulin (IVIg) enhances the selective expansion of Vβ3+ and Vβ17+ ab T cells induced by superantigen. *Scand. J. Immunol.*, in press.

Bendtzen, K., M. Svenson, V. Jonsson, and E. Hippe. 1990. Autoantibodies to cytokines — friends or foes? *Immunol. Today* **11**, 167–169.

Berchtold, P., G.L. Dale, P. Tani, and R. McMillan. 1989. Inhibition of autoantibody binding to platelet glycoprotein IIb/IIIa by anti-idiotypic antibodies in intravenous immunoglobulins. *Blood* **74**, 2414–2417.

Berneman, A., B. Guilbert, S. Eschrich, and S. Avrameas. 1993. IgG auto- and polyreactivities of normal human sera. *Mol. Immunol.* **30**, 1499–1510.

Blanchette, V.S., P. Imbach, and M. Andrew. 1994. A prospective randomized trial of intravenous immunoglobulin G, oral prednisolone and intravenous anti-D in childhood acute idiopathic thrombocytopenic purpura. *Lancet* **344**, 703–707.

Blasczyk, R., U. Westhoff, and H. Grossewilde. 1993. Soluble CD4, CD8, and HLA molecules in commercial immunoglobulin preparations. *Lancet* **341**, 789–790.

Caccavo, D., F. Vaccaro, G.M. Ferri, A. Amoroso, and L. Bonomo. 1994. Antiidiotypes against antiphospholipid antibodies are present in normal polyspecific immunoglobulins for therapeutic use. *J. Autoimmunity* **7**, 537–548.

Clarkson, S.B., J.B. Bussel, R.P. Kimberly, J.E. Valinsky, R.L. Nachman, and J.C. Unkeless. 1986. Treatment of refractory immune thrombocytopenic purpura with an anti-Fc gamma-receptor antibody. *N. Engl. J. Med.* **314**, 1236–1239.

Coutinho, A., and M.D. Kazatchkine. 1994. *Autoimmunity. Physiology and Disease.* John Wiley & Sons Inc., New York.

Coutinho, A., C. Marquez, P.M.F. Araujo, P. Pereira, M. Toribio, M.A. Marcos, and A.C. Martinez. 1987. A functional idiotypic network of T helper cells and antibodies limited to the compartment of "naturally" activated lymphocytes in normal mice. *Eur. J. Immunol.* **17**, 821–825.

Coutinho, A., M.D. Kazatchkine, and S. Avrameas. 1996. Natural autoantibodies. *Curr. Opin. Immunol.* 812–818.

Dalakas, M., I. Illa, J. Dambrosia, S. Soueidan, D. Stein, C. Otero, S. Dinsmore, and S. McCrosky. 1993. A controlled trial of high-dose intravenous immune globulin infusions as treatment for dermatomyositis. *N. Engl. J. Med.* **329**, 1993–2000.

Debré, M., M.C. Bonnet, W.H. Fridman, E. Carosella, N. Philippe, P. Reinert, E. Vilmer, C. Caplan, J.L. Teillaud, and C. Griscelli. 1993. Infusion of Fcγ fragments for the treatment of children with acute immune thrombocytopenic purpura. *Lancet* **342**, 945–949.

Dekeyser, F., M.D. Kazatchkine, F. Rossi, H. Dang, and N. Talal. 1996. Pooled human immunoglobulins contain anti-idiotypes with reactivity against the 4B4/P36 cross-reactive idiotype. *Clin. Exp. Rheumatol.*, in press.

Delfraissy, J.F., G. Tchernia, Y. Laurian, C. Wallon, and P. Galanaud. 1985. Suppressor cell function after intravenous gammaglobulin treatment in adult chronic idiopathic thrombocytopenic purpura. *Br. J. Haematol.* **60**, 315–322.

Dietrich, G., and M.D. Kazatchkine. 1990. Normal immunoglobulin G (IgG) for therapeutic use (intravenous Ig) contain antiidiotypic specificities against an immunodominant, disease-associated, cross-reactive idiotype of human anti-thyroglobulin autoantibodies. *J. Clin. Invest.* **85**, 620–625.

Dietrich, G., M. Algiman, Y. Sultan, U.E. Nydegger, and M.D. Kazatchkine. 1992a. Origin of anti-idiotypic activity against anti-factor VIII autoantibodies in pools of normal human immunoglobulin G (IVIg). *Blood* **79**, 2946–2951.

Dietrich, G., S.V. Kaveri, and M.D. Kazatchkine. 1992b. A V region-connected autoreactive subfraction of normal human serum immunoglobulin G. *Eur. J. Immunol.* **22**, 1701–1706.

Dietrich, G., P. Pereira, M. Algiman, Y. Sultan, and M.D. Kazatchkine. 1990. A monoclonal anti-idiotypic antibody against the antigen-combining site of anti-factor VIII autoantibodies defines an idiotope that is recognized by normal human polyspecific immunoglobulins for therapeutic use (IVIg). *J. Autoimmunity* **3**, 547–557.

Dietrich, G., F. Varela, V. Hurez, M. Bouanani, and M.D. Kazatchkine. 1993. Selection of the expressed B cell repertoire by infusion of normal immunoglobulin G in a patient with autoimmune thyroiditis. *Eur. J. Immunol.* **23**, 2945–2950.

Eibl, M.M., and R.J. Wedgwood. 1993. Intravenous immunoglobulin: a review. *Immunodeficiencies* 659–688.

Fehr, J., V. Hofmann, and U. Kappeler. 1982. Transient reversal of thrombocytopenia in idiopathic thrombocytopenic purpura by high-dose intravenous gammaglobulin. *N. Engl. J. Med.* **306**, 1254–1258.

Forsgren, S., A. Andersson, V. Hillorn, A. Soderstrom, and D. Holmberg. 1991. Immunoglobulin-mediated prevention of autoimmune diabetes in the non-obese diabetic (NOD) mouse. *Scand. J. Immunol.* **34**, 445–451.

Freitas, A.A., A.C. Viale, A. Sundblad, C. Heusser, and A. Coutinho. 1991. Normal serum immunoglobulins participate in the selection of peripheral B-cell repertoires. *Proc. Natl. Acad. Sci. USA* **88**, 5640–5644.

Fremeaux-Bacchi, V., F. Maillet, L. Berlan, and M.D. Kazatchkine. 1992. Neutralizing antibodies against C3Nef in intravenous immunoglobulin. *Lancet* **340**, 63–64.

Fridman, W. 1993. Regulation of B-cell activation and antigen presentation by Fc receptors. *Curr. Opin. Immunol.* **5**, 355–360.

Gajdos, P., H. Outin, D. Elkharrat, D. Brunel, P.D. Rohan-Chabot, J.C. Raphael, M. Goulon, C. Goulon-Goeau, and E. Morel. 1984. High-dose intravenous gammaglobulin for myasthenia gravis. *Lancet* **i**, 406–407.

Galon, J., C. Bouchard, W.H. Fridman, and C. Sautes. 1995. Ligands and biological activities of soluble Fc gamma receptors. *Immunol. Lett.* **44**, 175–181.

Gelfand, E.W., B. Esterl, and B.D. Mazer. 1994. Benefit of 12% solution of intravenous immunoglobulin in the treatment of steroid-dependent asthma. *Immunoglobulins: Extending the Horizon*, 49–62.

Glotz, D., J.P. Haymann, P. Niaudet, P. Lang, P. Druet, and J. Bariety. 1995. Successful kidney transplantation of immunized patients after desimmunization with normal human polyclonal immunoglobulins for intravenous use (IVIg). *Transplant. Proc.*, in press.

Halpern, R., S.V. Kaveri, and H. Kohler. 1991. Human anti-phosphorylcholine antibodies share idiotopes and are self-binding. *J. Clin. Invest.* **88**, 476–482.

Hammarström, L., M.R. Abedi, M.S. Hassan, and C.I. Edward-Smith. 1993. The SCID mouse as a model for autoimmunity. *J. Autoimmunity* **6**, 667–674.

Hashimoto, F., Y. Sakiyama, and S. Matsumoto. 1986. The suppressive effect of gammaglobulin preparations on in vitro pokeweed mitogen-induced immunoglobulin production. *Clin. Exp. Immunol.* **65**, 409–415.

Hentati, B., M.N. Sato, B. Payelle-Brogard, S. Avrameas, and T. Ternynck. 1994. Beneficial effect of polyclonal immunoglobulins from malaria-infected Balb/c mice on lupus-like syndrome of (NZB × NZW)F1 mice. *Eur. J. Immunol.* **24**, 8–15.

Hughes, R. 1996. Plasma exchange versus intravenous immunoglobulin for Guillain-Barré syndrome. *Japan J. Apheresis* **15**, S12.

Hurez, V., S.V. Kaveri, and M.D. Kazatchkine. 1993. Expression and control of the natural autoreactive IgG repertoire in normal human serum. *Eur. J. Immunol.* **23**, 783–789.

Hurez, V., S.V. Kaveri, A. Mouhoub, G. Dietrich, J.C. Mani, D. Klatzmann, and M.D. Kazatchkine. 1994. Anti-CD4 activity of normal human immunoglobulins G for therapeutic use (Intravenous immunoglobulin, IVIg). *Therap. Immunol.* **1**, 269–278.

Hurez, V., M.D. Kazatchkine, S. Ramanathan, B. Basuyaux, A. Pashov, T. Vassilev, Y. De-Kozak, B. Bellon, and S.V. Kaveri. 1996. Inhibition of autoantibody activity by pooled normal human polyspecific IgM: potential implications for immunoglobulin therapy of autoimmune diseases, in preparation.

Imbach, P., S. Barandun, V. d'Apuzzo, C. Baumgartner, A. Hirt, A. Morell, E. Rossi, M. Schoni, M. Vest, and H. P. Wagner. 1981. High-dose intravenous gammaglobulin for idiopathic thrombocytopenic purpura in childhood. *Lancet* **i**, 1228–1230.

Iwata, M., T. Shimozato, H. Tokiwa, and E. Tsubura. 1987. Antipyretic activity of a human immunoglobulin preparation for intravenous use in a experimental model of fever in rabbits. *Infect. Immun.* **55**, 547–552.

Jayne, D.R.W., M. Davies, C. Fox, and C.M. Lockwood. 1991. Treatment of systemic vasculitis with pooled intravenous immunoglobulin. *Lancet* **ii**, 1137–1139.

Jayne, D.R.W., V.L.M. Esnault, and C.M. Lockwood. 1993. ANCA anti-idiotype antibodies and the treatment of systemic vasculitis with intravenous immunoglobulin. *J. Autoimmunity* **6**, 207–219.

Kang, C.-Y., T.K. Brunck, T. Kieber-Emmons, J.E. Blalock, and H. Kohler. 1988. Inhibition of self-binding antibodies (autobodies) by a Vh-derived peptide. *Science* **240**, 1034–1036.

Kaveri, S., T. Vassilev, V. Hurez, R. Lengagne, C. Lefranc, S. Cot, P. Pouletty, D. Glotz, and M. Kazatchkine. 1996. Antibodies to a conserved region of HLA class I molecules, capable of modulating CD8 T cell-mediated function, are present in pooled normal immunoglobulin for therapeutic use (IVIg). *J. Clin. Invest.* **97**, 865–869.

Kaveri, S.V., C.Y. Kang, and H. Kohler. 1990. Natural mouse and human antibodies bind to a peptide derived from a germline variable heavy chain: Evidence for evolutionary conserved self-binding locus. *J. Immunol.* **145**, 4207–4213.

Kaveri, S.V., H.T. Wang, D. Rowen, M.D. Kazatchkine, and H. Kohler. 1993. Monoclonal anti-idiotypic antibodies against human anti-thyroglobulin autoantibodies recognize idiotopes shared by disease-associated and natural anti-thyroglobulin autoantibodies. *Clin. Immunol. Immunopathol.* **69**, 333–340.

Kawada, K., and P.I. Terasaki. 1987. Evidence for immunosuppression by high-dose gammaglobulin. *Exp. Hematol.* **15**, 133–136.

Kazatchkine, M.D., G. Dietrich, V. Hurez, N. Ronda, B. Bellon, F. Rossi, and S.V. Kaveri. 1994. V region-mediated selection of autoreactive repertoires by intravenous immunoglobulin (IVIg). *Immunol. Rev.* **139**, 79–107.

Kimberly, R.P., J.E. Salmon, J.B. Bussel, M. Kuntz-Crow, and M.W. Hilgartner. 1984. Modulation of mononuclear phagocyte function by intravenous gamma globulin. *J. Immunol.* **132**, 745–750.

Kohler, H., T. Kieber-Emmons, S. Srinivasan, S. Kaveri, W. J.W. Morrow, S. Muller, C.-Y. Kang, and S. Raychaudhuri. 1988. Revised immune network concepts. *Clin. Immunol. Immunopathol.* **52**, 104–116.

Kondo, N., T. Ozawa, K. Mushiake, F. Motoyoshi, T. Kameyama, K. Kasahara, H. Kaneko, M. Yamashina, Y. Kato, and T. Orii. 1991. Suppression of immunoglobulin production of lymphocytes by intravenous immunoglobulin. *J. Clin. Immunol.* **11**, 152–158.

Kondo, N., K. Kasahara, T. Kameyama, Y. Suzuki, N. Shimozawa, S. Tomatsu, Y. Nakashima, T. Hori, A. Yamagishi, T. Ogawa, H. Iwata, Y. Takahashi, R. Takenaka, M. Haga, and T. Orii. 1994. Intravenous immunoglobulins suppress immunoglobulin production by suppressing Ca^{2+}-dependent signal transduction through Fcγ receptors in B lymphocytes. *Scand. J. Immunol.* **40**, 37–42.

Kruger, M., E. Rodriguez, C. Killion, E. McLaughlin-Taylor, and R. Goodenow. 1993. Identification and isolation of anti-T cell receptor antibodies in gammagard. In *Intravenous IgIV: Current status of clinical applications and research topics*, in press.

Kuhnert, P., L. Schalch, and T.W. Jungi. 1990. Cytokine induction in human mononuclear cells stimulated by IgG-coated culture surfaces and by IgG for infusion. *Clin. Immunol. Immunopathol.* **57**, 218–222.

Lacroix-Desmazes, S., L. Mouthon, A. Coutinho, and M.D. Kazatchkine. 1995. Analysis of the natural human IgG antibody repertoire: life-long stability of reactivities towards self-antigens contrasts with age-dependent diversification of reactivities against bacterial antigens. *Eur. J. Immunol.* **25**, 2598–2604.

Lalezari, P., M. Korshidi, and M. Petrosova. 1986. Autoimmune neutropenia of infancy. *J. Pediatr.* **109**, 764–769.

Lefvert, A.K. 1994. Human and experimental myasthenia gravis. *Autoimmunity: Physiology and Disease*, 267–305.

Lefvert, A.K., and P.O. Osterman. 1983. Neonates to myasthenic mothers: a clinical study and an investigation of kinetic and biochemical properties of the acetylcholine receptor antibodies. *Neurology* **33**, 133–138.

LeHoang, P., D. Jobin, and M.D. Kazatchkine. 1996. Treatment of birdshot retinochoroidopathy with intravenous immunoglobulins. *Am. J. Ophthalmol.*, submitted.

Leung, D.Y.M., M. Gately, A. Trumble, B. Ferguson-Darnell, P.M. Schlievert, and L.J. Picker. 1995. Bacterial superantigens induce T cell expression of the skin-selective homing receptor, the cutaneous lymphocyte-associated antigen, via stimulation of interleukin 12 production. *J. Exp. Med.* **181**, 747–753.

Liblau, R., P. Gajdos, F.A. Bustarret, R.E. Habib, J.F. Bach, and E. Morel. 1991. Intravenous gammaglobulin in myasthenia gravis: Interaction with anti-acetylcholine receptor autoantibodies. *J. Clin. Immunol.* **11**, 128–131.

Lowy, I., C. Brezin, C. Neauport-Sautès, J. Thèze, and W.H. Fridman. 1983. Isotype regulation of antibody production: T cell hybrids can be selectively induced to produce IgG and IgG2 subclass-specific suppressive immunoglobulin-binding factors. *Proc. Natl. Aced. Sci. USA* **80**.

Lundkvist, I., P.A. Van-Doorn, M. Vermeulen, and A. Brand. 1993. Spontaneous recovery from Guillain-Barré syndrome is associated with anti-idiotypic antibodies recognizing a cross-reactive on anti-neuroblastoma cell line antibodies. *Clin. Immunol. Immunopathol.* **67**, 192–198.

Marchalonis, J.J., H. Kaymaz, F. Dedeoglu, S.F. Schlutter, D.E. Yocum, and A.B. Edmundson. 1992. Human autoantibodies reactive with synthetic autoantigens from T-cell receptor β chain. *Proc. Natl. Acad. Sci. USA* **89**, 3325–3329.

Martinez, A.C., M.L. Toribio, P. Pereira, A. De la Hera, P.-A. Cazenave, and A. Coutinho. 1986. Maternal transmission of idiotypic network interactions selecting available T cell repertoires. *Eur. J. Immunol.* **16**, 1445–1451.

McGuire, W.A., H.H. Yang, E. Bruno, J. Brandt, R. Briddell, T.D. Coates, and R. Hoffman. 1987. Treatment of antibody-mediated pure red-cell aplasia with high-dose intravenous gammaglobulin. *N. Engl. J. Med.* **317**, 1004–1008.

McIntyre, E.A., D.C. Linch, M.G. Macey, and A.C. Newland. 1985. Successful response to intravenous immunoglobulin in autoimmune hemolytic anemia. *Br. J. Haematol.* **60**, 387–388.

Miletic, V.D., C.G. Hester, and M.M. Frank. 1996. Regulation of complement activity by Immunoglobulin. *J. Immunol.* **156**, 749–757.

Mouthon, L., M. Haury, S. Lacroix-Desmazes, C. Barreau, A. Coutinho, and M.D. Kazatchkine. 1995a. Analysis of the normal human IgG antibody repertoire. Evidence that IgG autoantibodies of healthy adults recognize a limited and conserved set of protein antigens in homologous tissues. *J. Immunol.* **154**, 5769–5778.

Mouthon, L., A. Nobrega, N. Nicolas, S. Kaveri, C. Barreau, A. Coutinho, and M. Kazatchkine. 1995b. Invariance and restriction towards a limited set of self-antigens characterize neonatal IgM antibody repertoires and prevail in autoreactive repertoires of healthy adults. *Proc. Natl. Acad. Sc. USA* **92**, 3839–3844.

Nobrega, A., M. Haury, A. Grandien, E. Malanchere, A. Sundblad, and A. Coutinho. 1993. Global analysis of antibody repertoires. II. Evidence for specificity, self-selection and the immunological "homunculus" of antibodies in normal serum. *Eur. J. Immunol.* **23**, 2851–2859.

Oda, H., A. Honda, and K. Sugita. 1985. High dose intact IgG infusion in refractory autoimmune hemolytic anemia (Evans syndrome). *J. Pediatr.* **107**, 744–746.

Poutsiaka, D.D., B.D. Clark, E. Vannier, and C.A. Dinarello. 1991. Production of IL-receptor antagonist and IL-1β by peripheral blood mononuclear cells is differentially regulated. *Blood* **78**, 1275–1279.

Ronda, N., M. Haury, A. Nobrega, A. Coutinho, and M.D. Kazatchkine. 1994a. Selectivity of recognition of variable (V) regions of autoantibodies by intravenous immunoglobulin (IVIg). *Clin. Immunol. Immunopathol.* **70**, 124–128.

Ronda, N., M. Haury, A. Nobrega, S.V. Kaveri, A. Coutinho, and M.D. Kazatchkine. 1994b. Analysis of natural and disease-associated autoantibody repertoires: anti-endothelial cell IgG autoantibody activity in the serum of healthy individuals and patients with systemic lupus erythematosus. *Int Immunol.* **6**, 1651–1660.

Rossi, F., and M.D. Kazatchkine. 1989. Antiidiotypes against autoantibodies in pooled normal human polyspecific Ig. *J. Immunol.* **143**, 4104–4109.

Rossi, F., Y. Sultan, and M.D. Kazatchkine. 1988. Anti-idiotypes against autoantibodies and alloantibodies to Factor VIII:C (anti-haemophilic factor) are present in therapeutic polyspecific normal immunoglobulins. *Clin. Exp. Immunol.* **74**, 311–316.

Rossi, F., G. Dietrich, and M.D. Kazatchkine. 1989. Anti-idiotypes against autoantibodies in normal immunoglobulins: Evidence for network regulation of human autoimmune responses. *Immunol. Rev.* **110**, 135–149.

Rossi, F., B. Guilbert, C. Tonnelle, T. Ternynck, F. Fumoux, S. Avrameas, and M.D. Kazatchkine. 1990. Idiotypic interactions between normal human polyspecific IgG and natural IgM antibodies. *Eur. J. Immunol.* **20**, 2089–2094.

Rossi, F., B. Bellon, M.C. Vial, P. Druet, and M.D. Kazatchkine. 1991a. Beneficial effect of human therapeutic intravenous immunoglobulins (IVIg) in mercuric-chloride-induced autoimmune disease of Brown-Norway rats. *Clin. Exp. Immunol.* **84**, 129–133.

Rossi, F., D.R.W. Jayne, C.M. Lockwood, and M.D. Kazatchkine. 1991b. Anti-idiotypes against anti-neutrophil cytoplasmic antigen autoantibodies in normal human polyspecific IgG for therapeutic use and in the remission sera of patients with systemic vasculitis. *Clin. Exp. Immunol.* **83**, 298–303.

Roux, K.H., and D.L. Tankersley. 1990. A view of the human idiotypic repertoire: Electron microscopic and immunologic analyses of spontaneous idiotype-anti-idiotype dimers in pooled human IgG. *J. Immunol.* **144**, 1387–1395.

Ruiz-Arguelles, A. 1988. Spontaneous reversal of acquired autoimmune dysfibrinogenemia probably due to an anti-idiotypic antibody directed to an interspecies cross-reactive idiotype expressed on anti-fibrinogen antibodies. *J. Clin. Invest.* **82**, 958–963.

Ruiz de Souza, V., M.P. Carreno, S.V. Kaveri, J.M. Cavaillon, M.D. Kazatchkine, and N. Haeffner-Cavaillon. 1995. Selective induction of IL-1ra and IL-8 in human monocytes by normal polyspecific immunoglobulin G for therapeutic use (IVIg). *Eur. J. Immunol.* **25**, 1267–1273.

Salama, A., C. Mueller-Eckhardt, and V. Kiefel. 1983. Effect of intravenous immunoglobulin in immune thrombocytopenia. Competitive inhibition of reticuloendothelial system function by sequestration of autologous red blood cells? *Lancet* **ii**, 193–195.

Saoudi, A., V. Hurez, Y. de Kozak, J. Kuhn, S.V. Kaveri, M.D. Kazatchkine, P. Druet, and B. Bellon. 1993. Human immunoglobulin preparations for intravenous use prevent experimental autoimmune uveoretinitis. *Int. Immunol.* **5**, 1559–1567.

Sato, M., H. Kojima, and S.J. Koshikawa. 1986. Modification of immune complexes deposited in glomeruli in tissue sections treated with sulfonized gamma-globulin. *Clin. Exp. Immunol.* **64**, 623–628.

Shimozato, T., M. Iwata, H. Kawada, and N. Tamura. 1991. Human immunoglobulin preparation for intravenous use induces elevation of cellular cyclic adenosine 3′:5′-monophosphate levels, resulting in suppression of tumor necrosis factor alpha and interleukin-1 production. *Immunology* **72**, 497–501.

Skansén-Saphir, U., J. Andersson, L. Bjork, and U. Andersson. 1994. Lymphokine production induced by streptococcal pyrogenic exotoxin-A is selectively down-regulated by pooled human IgG. *Eur. J. Immunol.* **24**, 916–922.

Stohl, W. 1986. Cellular mechanisms in the in vitro inhibition of pokeweed mitogen-induced B cell differentiation by immunoglobulin for intravenous use. *J. Immunol.* **136**, 4407–4413.

Sultan, Y., M.D. Kazatchkine, P. Maisonneuve, and U.E. Nydegger. 1984. Anti-idiotypic suppression of autoantibodies to Factor VIII (antihaemophilic factor) by high-dose intravenous gammaglobulin. *Lancet* **ii**, 765–768.

Sultan, Y., F. Rossi, and M.D. Kazatchkine. 1987. Recovery from anti-VIII:C (antihemophilic factor) autoimmune disease is dependent on generation of antiidiotypes against anti-VIII:C autoantibodies. *Proc. Natl. Acad. Sci. USA* **84**, 828–831.

Sundblad, A., F. Huetz, D. Portnoi, and A. Coutinho. 1991. Stimulation of B and T cells by in vivo high dose immunoglobulin administration in normal mice. *J. Autoimmunity* **4**, 325–339.

Sundblad, A., M. Marcos, E. Malenchere, A. Castro, M. Haury, F. Huetz, A. Nobrega, and A. Coutinho. 1994. Observations on the mode of action of normal immunoglobulin at high-doses. *Immunol. Rev.* **139**, 125–158.

Svenson, M., M.B. Hansen, and K. Bendtzen. 1990. Distribution and characterization of autoantibodies to interleukin 1α in normal human sera. *Scand. J. Immunol.* **32**, 695–701.

Takei, S., Y. Arora, and S.M. Walker. 1993. Intravenous immunoglobulin contains specific antibodies inhibitory to activation of T cells by staphylococcal toxin superantigens. *J. Clin. Invest.* **91**, 602–607.

Tankersley, D.L., M.S. Preston, and J.S. Finlayson. 1988. Immunoglobulin G dimer: an idiotype-anti-idiotype complex. *Mol. Immunol.* **25**, 41–48.

Tankersley, D.L. 1994. Dimer formation in immunoglobulin preparations and speculations on the mechanisms of action of intravenous immunoglobulin in autoimmune diseases. *Immunol. Rev.* **139**, 159–172.

Tsubakio, T., Y. Kurata, S. Katagiri, Y. Kanakura, T. Tamakai, J. Kuyama, Y. Kanayama, T. Yoonezawa, and S. Taurui. 1983. Alteration of T cell subsets and immunoglobulin synthesis in vitro during high-dose gammaglobulin therapy in patients with idiopathic thrombocytopenic purpura. *Clin. Exp. Immunol.* **53**, 697–702.

Unkeless, J.C., E. Scigliano, and V.H. Freedman. 1988. Structure and function of human receptors for IgG. *Ann. Rev. Immunol.* **6**, 251–281.

van der Meché, F.G.A., P.I.M. Smith, and Dutch Guillain-Barré Study Group. 1992. A randomized trial comparing intravenous immune globulin and plasma exchange in Guillain-Barré syndrome. *N. Engl. J. Med.* **326**, 1123–1129.

van Doorn, P.A., F. Rossi, A. Brand, M. van Lint, M. Vermeulen, and M.D. Kazatchkine. 1990. On the mechanism of high dose intravenous immunoglobulin treatment of patients with chronic inflammatory demyelinating polyneuropathy. *J. Neuroimmunol.* **29**, 57–64.

Van Schaik, I.N., I. Lundkvist, M. Vermeulen, and A. Brand. 1992. Polyvalent Immunoglobulin for Intravenous Use Interferes with cell proliferation in vitro. *J. Clin. Immunol.* **12**, 325–334.

Varela, F., and A. Coutinho. 1991. Second generation immune networks. *Immunol. Today* **12**, 159–166.

Varela, F., A. Andersson, G. Dietrich, A. Sundblad, D. Holmberg, M.D. Kazatchkine, and A. Coutinho. 1991. The population dynamics of antibodies in normal and autoimmune individuals. *Proc. Natl. Acad. Sci. USA* **88**, 5917–5921.

Vassilev, T., C. Gelin, S.V. Kaveri, M.T. Zilber, L. Boumsell, and M.D. Kazatchkine. 1993. Antibodies to the CD5 molecule in normal human immunoglobulins for therapeutic use (intravenous immunoglobulins, IVIg). *Clin. Exp. Immunol.* **92**, 369–72.

Vassilev, T., I. Bineva, G. Dietrich, S.V. Kaveri, and M.D. Kazatchkine. 1995. Variable region-connected, dimeric fraction of intravenous immunoglobulin enriched in natural autoantibodies. *J. Autoimmunity* **8**, 405–413.

Zouali, M., and A. Eyquem. 1983. Idiotypic/anti-idiotypic interactions in systemic lupus erythematosus: demonstration of oscillary levels of anti-DNA autoantibodies and reciprocal antiidiotypic activity in a single patient. *Ann. Inst. Pasteur Immunol.* **134C**, 377–391.

Chapter

SIX

Rheumatoid Factor Autoantibodies in Health and Disease

JACOB B. NATVIG, KEITH M. THOMPSON and MARIE BØRRETZEN

Institute of Immunology and Rheumatology and Oslo Sanitetsforenings
Rheumatism Hospital, The National Hospital, Fr.Qvams gt.1,
0172 Oslo, Norway

VINCENT BONAGURA

Division of Allergy and Immunology, Schneider Children's Hospital,
Long Island Jewish Medical Center, New York, USA

I. INTRODUCTION

The normal immune system maintains specific unresponsiveness to self antigens by tolerance mechanisms acting on both T-cells and B-cells; T-cells being rendered tolerant at much lower antigen concentrations than the B-cells (Chiller et al., 1970). Consequently, for many self antigens, tolerance exists only at the T-cell level. Autoreactive B-cells that escape deletion in the bone marrow (Nemazee and Buerki, 1989), may nevertheless be rendered anergic (Goodnow et al., 1988). Some self reactive B-cells seem to be totally "forbidden." Spontaneous autoimmunity involving autoantibodies to certain antigens, e.g., self A, B or H blood group antigens and self-MHC have not been described, and B-cell tolerance to these blood group antigens cannot be broken in vitro by potent B-cell activators (Rieben et al., 1992). In contrast, B-cells producing other self-reactive specificities (e.g., anti-IgG or Rheumatoid Factor, RF) occur in normal individuals, without any detrimental effects. In many autoimmune diseases it appears that such B-cells can become dominant, often with pathological effects.

Elevated levels of circulating RFs autoantibodies are found in a number of autoimmune diseases, particularly in Rheumatoid Arthritis (RA), where it is clear that they contribute to the pathogenesis of the disease by forming deposits of complement fixing complexes that cause tissue damage (Munthe and Natvig, 1972). RFs are frequently found as paraproteins or monoclonal components (MC) in lymphoproliferative diseases, such as Waldenström's Macroglobulinemia, where despite high circulating levels, they are rarely associated with symptoms typical of RA. RFs are also produced transiently in healthy animals and humans following immunization or infections (Welch et al., 1983; Stanley Jr. et al., 1987; Nemazee and Sato, 1983; Nemazee, 1985; Coulie and Van Snick, 1983). There is evidence that immune complexes are the triggering agents for RF production in normal immune responses (Nemazee, 1985) and that RFs, or RF-producing B-cells, have a role in clearing complexes, enhancing the avidity of IgG antibodies or presenting antigen (Van Snick et al., 1978; Roosnek and Lanzavecchia, 1991; Clarkson Jr. and Mellow, 1981). The lack of self-toxicity of RFs in healthy individuals implies that mechanisms exist to control the affinity and/or amounts of such autoantibodies, and so it is important to compare RF production and regulation in normals and patients with autoimmune disease in order to understand the disease pathology. The main aim of this presentation is to address whether there are any features of RFs produced in RA patients that can be identified as predisposing them to a pathological role.

II. THE GENETIC ORIGINS OF RF

Analysis of the structure and genetic origins of RFs has been approached in three ways; protein sequence determination of purified MC RFs, serological investigation with anti-V gene specific antisera and mAb, and nucleotide sequencing of RF genes isolated from immortalized cell lines. Serological investigations have the advantage of being able to determine the levels and proportions of different V-gene structures expressed by RFs in normals and patients. However, estimates based on such measures are vulnerable to V-gene epitopes being masked by RF binding to circulating IgG, or indeed being lost in extensively mutated V-genes. Whilst much more precise data on particular V-gene structures can be obtained from nucleotide sequences of RFs isolated as B-cell lines or hybridomas, it is extremely time consuming to generate large enough numbers of clones to be able to reliably ascertain relative frequencies.

In recent years there has been considerable progress in identifying the members of the human germline V-gene segment repertoire (Tomlinson et al., 1992; Matsuda and Honjo, 1996). Unfortunately, there still is no universally accepted nomenclature, and the same germline V-genes are often known by different names. Table 1 presents the germline gene segments mentioned in this article together with some of their alternative names, and references. For a complete, and updated record of human germline V-genes, readers are referred to the V Base of Tomlinson, Williams, Corbett, Cox and Winter, MRC Center for Protein Engineering, Cambridge, England.

Table 1. Nomenclature of Human Germline V-Gene Segments Referred to in this Presentation

Germline gene	Family	Alternative names
VH:		
DP-10 (Tomlinson et al. 1992)	1	hv1051 (Yang et al. 1993), 1M27 (Sasso et al. 1993), 5M27 (Sasso et al. 1993), HULGLVH1 (Crouzier et al. 1995), 57GTA8 (Ikematsu et al. 1992), DA-6 (Cook et al. 1994)
DP-75 (Tomlinson et al. 1992)	1	VI-2 (Shin et al. 1991), hv1L1 (Olee et al. 1992)
HG3 (Rechavi et al. 1983)	1	
hv1263 (Chen et al. 1989)	1	3M28 (Sasso et al. 1993), 9M28 (Sasso et al. 1993)
b18 (Olee et al. 1991)	3	hv3019b18 (Olee et al. 1991)
DP-31 (Tomlinson et al. 1992)	3	V3-9P (Matsuda et al. 1993)
DP-35 (Tomlinson et al. 1992)	3	V3-11 (Matsuda et al. 1993), 22-2B (Berman et al. 1988)
DP-42 (Tomlinson et al. 1992)	3	
DP-46 (Tomlinson et al. 1992)	3	3d216, GL-SJ2 (Pascual et al. 1990)
DP-47 (Tomlinson et al. 1992)	3	V3-23 (Matsuda et al. 1993), VH26 Chen (Chen et al. 1988)
DP-49 (Tomlinson et al. 1992)	3	1.9III (Berman et al. 1988)
DP-50 (Tomlinson et al. 1992)	3	hv3019b9 (Olee et al. 1991)
DP-53 (Tomlinson et al. 1992)	3	hvm148 (Fang et al. 1995), 13G12(57), VPVH (Denny et al. 1986), DA-8 (Cook et al. 1994)
DP-54 (Tomlinson et al. 1992)	3	V3-7 (Matsuda et al. 1993), HHG19 (Kuppers et al. 1992)
hv3019b13 (Olee et al. 1991)	3	
hv3005 (Chen, 1990)	3	b1 (Olee et al. 1991), b36e (Olee et al. 1991), b42 (Olee et al. 1991), 3d24(32)
V3-53 (Matsuda et al. 1993)	3	
VH4.22 (Sanz et al. 1989)	4	VHSP(19), VH-JA(20)
4.35 (Weng et al. 1992)	4	VIV-4 (Shin et al. 1991)
DP-71 (Tomlinson et al. 1992)	4	3d197d (van der Maarel et al. 1993), hv4c2 (Deftos et al. 1994), VH4.11 (Sanz et al. 1989), VH4.15 (Sanz et al. 1989), VH4-MC2 (Campbell et al. 1992), G411 (Ikematsu et al. 1993)
V2-1 (Sanz et al. 1989)	4	
V71-2 (Kodaira et al. 1986)	4	DP-66 (Tomlinson et al. 1992), H1 (van Es et al. 1992), VH4-MC3 (Campbell et al. 1992), VH4-MC3b (Campbell et al. 1992)
V71-4 (Kodaira et al. 1986)	4	
VH4.18 (Sanz et al. 1989)	4	DP-79(51), 4d154 (van der Maarel et al. 1993), MLH4-1 (Ikematsu et al. 1992), VH4-MC6 (Campbell et al. 1992), G418 (Ikematsu et al. 1993)
DP-21 (Tomlinson et al. 1992)	7	4d275a (van der Maarel et al. 1993)
VK:		
humkv325 (Radoux et al. 1986)	3b	DPK22 (Cox et al. 1994), A27 (Straubinger et al. 1988), humkv321 (Chen et al. 1986)
humkv328 (Liu et al. 1989)	3b	L16 (Huber et al. 1993), humkv31es (Chen et al. 1987)

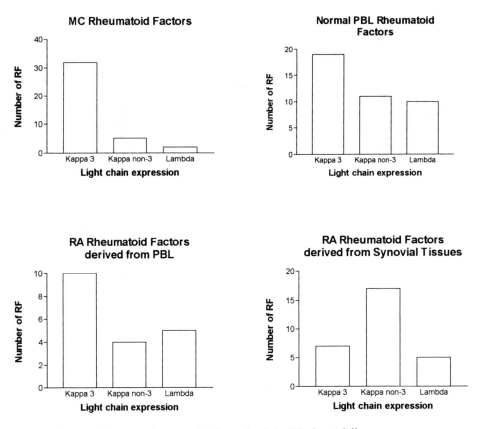

Figure 1. Expression of light chains by IgM RFs from different sources.

Monoclonal Component (MC) RF

RF activity is frequent among IgM MC produced by monoclonal B-cells in certain diseases such as mixed cryoglobulinemia, Waldenström's macroglobulinemia and chronic lymphocytic leukemia. Because of their availability in large quantities, the structure of MC RFs were the earliest RFs to be intensively studied, first using polyclonal anti-V-region and anti-idiotypic antibodies (Williams Jr. et al., 1968; Kunkel et al., 1973), and later using monoclonal antibodies (mAb) (Mageed et al., 1990; Silverman et al., 1988; Mageed et al., 1988; Mageed et al., 1986; Crowley et al., 1988; Carson and Fong, 1983). These data have been extensively reviewed and readers are referred to (Sasso, 1992; Randen et al., 1992a). MC RFs use a restricted set of variable region genes. The most striking restriction is seen in the predominant use of kappa light chains (~80% of all MC RF), with more than 90% utilizing gene segments of the Vκ3 gene family (Figure 1) (Randen et al., 1992a; Ledford et al., 1983). Studies using murine mAb 17.109 and 6B6.6 indicate that only two Vκ germline gene segments account for at least 60% of IgMκ MC RF; Kv325 (a Vκ3b family member recognized by 17.109) and Kv328 (a Vκ3a family member recognized by 6B6.6) (Radoux et al., 1986; Meindl et al., 1990; Liu et al., 1989; Crowley et al., 1988; Chen et al., 1987). Similarly, the V_H gene usage is shown in Figure 2 and Table 2.

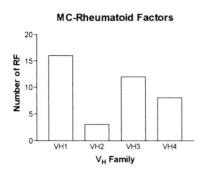

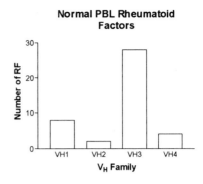

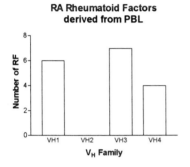

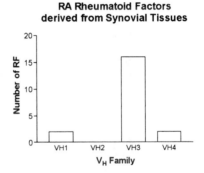

Figure 2. Expression of V_H families by IgM RFs from different sources.

When the V_H and V_L gene usage is considered together, MC RFs can be divided into three main groups (Figure 3). The largest group (~40%) consists of those expressing V_H1 gene segments almost always associated with Vκ3b gene segments (usually Kv325). This group is probably very closely related, if not identical, to the group of MC RFs expressing the Wa idiotype. All Wa positive MC IgM RFs appear to be constructed of Vκ3b light chains and V_H1 heavy chains (Newkirk et al., 1986; Newkirk et al., 1987; Ledford et al., 1983; Andrews and Capra, 1981). All of four sequenced Wa heavy chains use J_H4 segments (Andrews and Capra, 1981; Newkirk et al., 1987). Of 13 sequenced Wa light chains, all were found to use Jκ1 or Jκ2 segments, and the Vκ3b sequences were nearly identical, with only a few amino-acid substitutions in CDR1 and CDR3 (Goni et al., 1985; Newkirk et al., 1986; Newkirk et al., 1987; Ledford et al., 1983; Andrews and Capra, 1981) The V_H1 segments frequently express an epitope recognized by the mAb G6 (Mageed et al., 1986; Crowley et al., 1988). There is evidence that the germline V_H gene segment DP-10, or its alleles, may be responsible for encoding many of these antibodies (Kipps et al., 1989); G6 is known to recognize DP-10 and hv1263 germline gene segments (Kipps and Duffy, 1991) although it is still not certain how many other V_H1 gene segments G6 may recognize.

Table 2. Germline V_H Gene Segments Used by RFs

V_H	Germline	MC*	Normal PBL	RA PBL	ST**	All
1	DP-10	3	3	5	1	12
	DP-75	0	2	2	0	4
	HG3	0	0	0	1	1
	1-13	0	0	1	0	1
		3	5	8	2	18
3	DP-54	1	3	1	0	5
	DP-49	0	1	0	3	4
	DP-46	1	0	0	2	3
	hv3005	0	0	1	0	1
	b18	0	1	0	0	1
	DP-35	0	1	0	1	2
	DP-47	1	0	1	1	3
	DP-53	0	0	1	0	1
	DP-42	0	1	0	0	1
	V3-53	0	1	0	0	1
	DP-31	0	0	0	1	1
		3	8	4	8	23
4	4.18	0	0	2	1	3
	DP-71	0	1	1	0	2
	4.35	0	1	0	0	1
	DP-65	0	1	0	0	1
	4.22	0	0	1	0	1
	DP-66	0	0	0	1	1
		0	3	4	2	9
7	DP-21	0	0	0	1	1
Totals		6	16	16	13	51

*MC = monoclonal component. **ST = synovial tissue.

A second group (~20%) of MC RFs is characterized by the expression of the 6B6.6 epitope in conjunction with heavy chains using V_H gene segments recognized by the mAb LC1 (Silverman et al., 1990). The idiotope to which LC1 binds, maps to V_H FR1 (Potter et al., 1994), and binds antibodies derived from five VH4 family gene segments; V71-2, V71-4, VH4-18, VH72-1 and V2-1 (Potter et al., 1994; Pratt et al., 1991; Deane et al., 1993) (Figure 3). This group of RFs therefore all use Kv328-derived light chains, with a maximum of 5 different heavy chain variable region segments, and probably less.

The final group of MC RFs (~30%) use V_H3 heavy chain segments with a variety of light chain segments including lambda, κ1, κ3a, κ3b and perhaps others (Figure 3) (Randen et al., 1992a). Many of these antibodies express the V_H3 related epitope recognized by the mAb B6 (Crowley et al., 1990), and based on this, at least five members of the V_H3 family could be represented; DP-35 (22-2B), DP-46 (GL-SJ2),

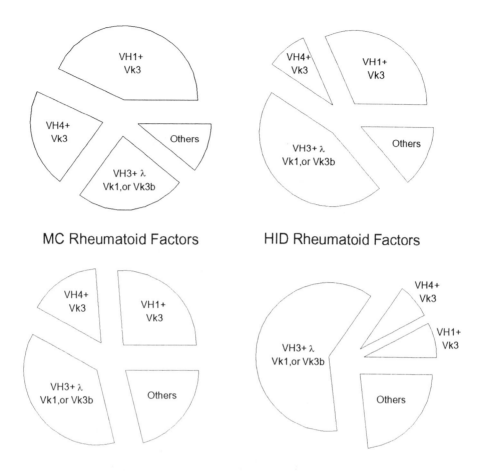

Figure 3. Major groups of IgM RFs based on V-gene family use.

DP-49 (1.9111), DP-50 (hv3019b9) and DP-54 (HHG19) (Suleyman et al., 1994). Three of these (DP-46, DP-49 and DP-50) are extremely homologous (98–99% similarity at the protein level) Table 3. Thus, there is effectively little diversity in the germline encoded structure of the V_H segments in this group.

Recently, two MC RFs have been sequenced at the nucleotide level, following isolation of cell lines from patients. The origins of both can be included in two of the groups described above; one, (HUL), was found to use a DP-10 V_H1-derived heavy chain combined with a Kv325-derived light chain (Crouzier et al., 1995), and the other (M7) uses a DP-54 V_H3-derived heavy chain combined with a Kv328-derived light chain (V. Agnello, personal communication).

RFs from Normals

Circulating IgM RFs have been studied in normal individuals using V-gene specific antibodies (Shokri et al., 1990; Kouri et al., 1990; Koopman et al., 1990; Crowley et al.,

Table 3. Nucleotide Similarity of V_H3 Germline Genes Used by RFs (germline genes with closer than 98% similarity are boxed; percent similarity in upper triangle, percent divergence in lower triangle)

	DP-31	DP-35	DP-46	DP-47	DP-49	DP-50	DP-53	DP-54	HV3005	DP-42	V3-53
DP-31	####	84.4	80.3	85.7	82.7	80.6	84.4	81.3	81	79.4	79.7
DP-35	13.3	####	85	89.1	85	83.7	87.1	87.4	85.4	88	88.3
DP-46	15.7	13.6	####	87.1	98	98	86.1	88.1	99.3	86.9	87.3
DP-47	12.3	10.2	11.2	####	88.4	84.7	87.4	85	87.8	89.7	90
DP-49	15	13.3	1.4	10.9	####	98	85.4	88.4	98	86.6	86.9
DP-50	18.6	16.3	2	14.4	2	####	86.7	87.8	98	82.5	82.7
DP-53	13	12.2	12.6	11.6	12.3	13.3	####	86.4	86.1	86.9	87.6
DP-54	15.7	10.9	10.5	12.9	9.6	12.2	11.9	####	88.1	82.8	83.2
HV3005	15.7	13.6	0.7	11.2	1.4	2	12.6	10.5	####	86.9	87.3
DP-42	15.5	10	11.3	7.2	11	15.8	11.3	13.1	11.3	####	99.7
V3-53	15.2	9.6	11	6.9	10.7	14.4	11	12.7	11	0.3	####
	DP-31	DP-35	DP-46	DP-47	DP-49	DP-50	DP-53	DP-54	HV3005	DP-42	V3-53

1990; Fong et al., 1986). IgM RFs purified from elderly, normal individuals, 29% was found to be inhibitable by the anti-idiotypic monoclonal antibody 17.109 (Fong et al., 1986), and thus using the Vκ3b gene segment Kv325. In normal individuals with elevated levels of RFs, 37% of the IgM RFs has been reported to express the V_H1 related epitope recognized by G6 (Shokri et al., 1990). RFs expressing both the 6B6.6 and B6 markers have been reported to represent very small fractions of RFs in normals (Koopman et al., 1990; Crowley et al., 1990; Crowley et al., 1988).

Monoclonal IgM RFs have also been isolated as hybridomas from healthy donors either following immunization, e.g., with mismatched RBC (Thompson et al., 1994; Børretzen et al., 1994), or without deliberate immunization (Stuber et al., 1992; Abderrazik et al., 1992). Analyses of these autoantibodies have shown that they share some similarities, and some differences compared with MC RFs. They predominantly use kappa light chains (>75%) and the majority of these use Vκ gene segments of the κ3 family (Figure 1). As found with the MC RFs, both the Kv325 and Kv328 gene segments are often used (Thompson et al., 1994; Børretzen et al., 1994). The three major groups identified in the MC RFs also account for the majority of the genetic structures making HID RFs (Figure 3). However, there is a difference in the contribution of different V_H families. In contrast to MC RFs, V_H1 is only half as frequently used (~20%) (Figure 3). Two V_H1 segments have so far been identified, DP-10 and DP-75 (Stuber et al., 1992; Abderrazik et al., 1992) Table 2, and as with MC RFs, these are almost always associated with kappa light chains using the Kv325 gene segment.

RFs encoded by V_H4 gene segments are also less frequent amongst normal RFs (~10%) (Figure 3b). Nucleotide sequencing of two of these suggests a similar structure to those found as MC; they use gene segments DP-71 and 4.35 and are coupled to Vκ3 light chains (Børretzen et al., unpublished data; Thompson et al., 1994).

The third group, characterized by expression of V_H3 heavy chains coupled to light chains of lambda, κ1, κ3a or κ3b origin, is well represented amongst normal RFs (~65%). Five different V_H gene segments have been identified including DP-54, DP-50, hv3019b, DP-35, DP-42.

RFs from RA Patients

Elevated levels of circulating RFs are found in the majority of RA patients. The central site of pathology is the synovial tissue which becomes chronically stimulated and may increase in weight 100 to 1000 fold. There is a proliferation of blood vessels in the tissues, and macrophages, dendritic cells and B and T lymphocytes accumulate, such that the majority of the tissue mass can be of lymphoid origin (Norton and Ziff, 1966). In synovial tissue, RFs and RF-secreting plasma cells can be found in considerable quantities secreting all major classes of immunoglobulin (Munthe and Natvig, 1972). The RFs are deposited as complexes in the synovial tissues, where they fix complement and generate inflammatory responses. The largest complexes are found in synovial tissues, but large, soluble complexes are found in the synovial fluid and these bind complement well. In the serum, complexes are usually smaller and non-complement binding (Natvig et al., 1989). It seems likely that the RFs produced locally in synovial tissue are the most relevant to the disease process, and there is evidence that they differ from those found in the circulation.

In order to determine the distribution of germline V genes in RFs from RA patients, human RF-producing hybridoma cells from the synovial tissues and blood of these patients were analyzed. At present we and others have identified about 30 RF-producing clones from RA patients, about half of them from synovial tissue. Their V gene family (Figures 1 and 2) and closest germline gene segments are shown in Table 2. About one-third of these RFs belong to the VH1 family and more than 50% of them used the germline DP10. However, only two of the VH1 RFs are from synovial tissues, one is from bone marrow and the rest from blood. Another third of the clones belongs to the VH3 family. Eight out of these are derived from three germline genes, DP-49, 47 and 46. The VH3 RFs are combined to light chains of the groups Vχ1, Vχ3a, Vχ3b and λ1. The VH4 family made up a third somewhat smaller group altogether representing about 20% of the RFs. These data fit well with previous idiotype studies (Thompson et al., 1994). As seen in Figures 1, 2 and 3 there are marked differences between V gene utilization of RFs in blood and synovial tissues in RA.

III. STRUCTURAL RESTRICTION IN THE HEAVY CHAIN CDR3 OF RF

Some striking structural restriction in the V regions of some IgM RFs have been reported (Andrews and Capra, 1981; Børretzen et al., 1995). Recently, 14 new IgM RFs produced in healthy immunized donors (HIDs) were analyzed and compared with RFs originating from RA patients and paraproteins or M-component (MC) RFs (Børretzen et al., 1995). Two groups with very restricted variable region structures were found (Table 4). Twelve RFs, 6 RA, 3 HID and 3 MC are encoded by V_H genes with closest homology to DP-10 all co-expressed Kv325 variable light chain germline genes. The same RFs have a remarkable restriction in CDR3 length, all between 12–14 amino acids and the CDR3 structures are also very homologous (Table 4, Figures 4 and 5). One HID RF had a CDR3 with only two amino acid differences from the CDR3 of an MC RF. Two sets of clonally related RFs, one from an RA patient and one from an HID, have CDR3s that differed by only three amino acids. The second group consisted of 5 RFs (1 RA, 3 HID and 1 MC) encoded by a V_H gene with closest homology to DP-54 all using the Kv328 V_L germline gene combined to Jk1 (Table 4, Figures 4 and 5). Four of these are rearranged to a D21/9 D segment in the same reading frame. The CDR3s are of very restricted length, compared to the CDR3 of other DP-54 antibodies (Figure 5), all of them of 16 to 17 amino acids, and showing great homology. Three RFs (1 from HID, 1 RA and 1 MC) have CDR3s differing by only three amino acids. The highly homologous V-regions in RFs from these two groups imply an initial selection to very similar, if not identical, epitopes. They appear to represent two important combinations of RFs expressed in normals during antigenic stimulation as part of the physiological RF processes, and do not represent RFs in the rheumatoid inflammatory tissues. In fact, only one of the 17 clones in these two groups originates from rheumatoid synovial tissue.

IV. DIFFERENCES IN THE ANTIGEN DRIVEN PROCESSES FOR RF   PRODUCTION IN RA AND NORMAL INDIVIDUALS

In typical antigen driven responses, the antibodies show evidence of somatic hypermutation and antigen selection. By analysis of the V genes encoding RFs we

Table 4. Similarities in the Structure of V Genes in Different RFs

Antibody	Origin	V_H	Length of CDR_H3	D-seg-ment	J_H	V_L	$J\kappa$
RF-TT9	HID PBL	DP-54	16	DLR1	3	Kv328	1
RF-MR5/41	HID PBL	DP-54	17	D21/9+D6	3	Kv328	1
RF-TT5	HID PBL	DP-54	16	D21/9	4	Kv328	1
M7	MC	DP-54	16	D21/9	3	Kv328	1
RA	PBL	DP-54	16	D21/9	3	Kv328	1
RF-MRc	HID PBL	DP-10	13	DA1 + nd	4	Kv325	1
RF-MR1	HID PBL	DP-10	12	nd*	4	Kv325	4
RF-TT1	HID PBL	DP-10	13	D1 + DxP4c	5	Kv325	1
BOR	MC	DP-10	12	nd*	4	Kv325	1
KAS	MC	DP-10	12	nd	4	Kv325	4
HUL	MC	DP-10	12	RC228	4	Kv325	4
mAB112/113	RA PBL	DP-10	13	DA1 + DN4	4	Kv325	4
Ro7	RA PBL	DP-10	14	DK4	4	Kv325	4
Ro45	RA PBL	DP-10	14	DK4	4	Kv325	2
Re12	RA PBL	DP-10	14	DN1 + DK4	4	Kv325	1
RF-TS1	RA ST	DP-10	13	DHFL16	3	Kv325	1
YES8c	RA BM	DP-10	13	DN1	4	Kv325	1

found evidence of somatic hypermutation in RFs from RA patients and from healthy immunized donors, both in IgM and IgG antibodies. Ten IgM RF-derived from synovial tissues of RA patients showed between 2 and 18 mutations per VH gene (Randen et al., 1992a,b). In addition, evidence of class switching were found in 3 IgG RFs with 2–11 mutations per VH gene (Randen et al., 1993a,b). RFs from immunized donors were also extensively mutated away from the VH germline with between 9 and 16 mutations. Somewhat fewer mutations were evident in the light chains (Børretzen et al., 1994).

Comparisons showed striking differences in the replacement (R) to silent (S) mutation ratio in the complimentarity determining regions(CDR) of RFs from RA synovial inflammation and normal immunized donors. In responses to exogenous antigens the hypermutation process is followed by both positive and negative selection pressures by which B-cells with high affinity receptors for antigens are selected positively. In contrast, B-cells with mutated receptors that have low affinity for antigen die by apoptosis. The increase in affinity can be accompanied by a characteristic evaluation of the R:S ratio in the CDR reflecting the selective process. Very surprisingly, RFs produced in healthy individuals following immunization showed a selection against replacement mutation in the CDRs. In the absence of selective pressures random mutations in CDR1 and 2 of the DP-10 gene segment would generate R:S ratios of 4.4. The overall R:S ratio of the CDR1 and 2 of RFs from one immunized donor (MR), particularly using this gene segment, is only 0.4, which is a significantly lower value than random ($p < 0.0027$, Fisher's exact test two-sided) (Børretzen et al., 1994). In contrast, 7 IgM RFs using the same DP-10 VH

(A)

RF using V$_H$ DP-54 :

```
RF-TT5  (Normal):       GDYYDSSGNY    H DAFDV JH4
mAb114  (RA PBL):       GDYYDYSGNY    I DAFDA JH3
M7  (MC):               GDYYDSGGDY    I DAFDI JH3
RF-MR5* (Normal):       GDYND--GSDSGFH DAFDL JH3
RF-MR41*(Normal):       GDYVD--GNYSGFH DAFDI JH3


RF-TT9  (Normal):       DPDMGRLERSVG    AFDI JH3
```

(B)

RF using V$_H$ DP-10 :

```
RF-MR1  (Normal):       EGRRMAA   NP YDY   JH4
BOR:    (MC):           EGRRMAI   NP FDY   JH4


mAb112/113  (RA PBL):   EGRSSDYS  NP FDY   JH4
RF-MRc  (Normal):       EGKAGDYS  NP FDY   JH4


RF-TT1  (Normal):       EGVSSKPS  NW FDP   JH5
KAS  (MC):              EGYGDYG   RP FDF   JH4
HUL  (MC):              EGARGPV   NP IDY   JH4
Re12  (RA PBL):         EGYPDTAMV NP FDY   JH4
Ro7  (RA PBL):          GSGEHTNMV VP FDY   JH4
Ro47  (RA PBL):         GWLDPSMAT TP FGF   JH4
Yes8c  (RA BM):         GIASAGTL  NY FFY   JH4
RF-TS1  (RA ST):        EDPYGDYVA NP FDI   JH3
```

Figure 4. A: The CDR$_H$3 amino acid sequences of five RFs using heavy chain germline combination DP-54/Kv328 are shown. **B:** Heavy chain CDR3 amino acid sequences of RFs using the germline combination DP-10/Kv325 are shown. RF-MRc represents a group of nine clonally related RFs having nearly the same CDR$_H$3 structures. BM = bone marrow; ST = synovial tissue. The J segments are underlined. Gaps are introduced to emphasize homologies. *Clonal pair.

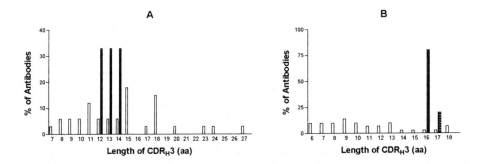

Figure 5. The percentage of DP-10 (A) and DP-54 (B) derived RFs are shown with filled bars and antibodies of other specificities having >90% homology with the same germline gene segments are shown according to the number of amino acids in the CDR3.

Table 5. Mean Number of Mutations away from Germline (GL) and Resulting Replacement (R): Silent (S) Ratios in IgM RFs Derived from Healthy Immunized Donors (HID), RA Synovial Tissue, and in IgM anti-Rh(D) Antibodies

Clones	Mutations from GL	Kd $\times 10^{-6}$ M	All FR			CDR1+2		
			R	S	R:S	R	S	R:S
10 HID RFs	12.0	2.00	17	16	1.1	7	16	0.4
7 RA RFs	16.1	0.30	30	34	0.9	33	14	2.4
7 Anti-RH(D)	4.3	0.07	8	12	0.7	8	1	8.0

segment as the immunized donor RFs, but derived from peripheral blood, synovial tissue and bone marrow of RA patients have an overall R:S ratio in the CDR1 and 2 of 2.4 (Table 5). Seven human monoclonal IgM antibodies directed to exogenous Rh (D) antigen have a higher R:S ratio in the CDR1 and 2 of 8.0.

As outlined above, there is clear evidence that that RFs in RA undergo both affinity maturation and class switching in contrast to RFs in healthy individuals. From one of the RA synovial tissues we obtained two clonally related IgM RFs (RFSJ1 and RFSJ2). RFSJ2 was only two nucleotide differences from its germline counterpart, whereas RFSJ1 had accumulated 18 nucleotide differences (Randen et al., 1992b). Similar differences were also seen in the light chains. In addition, functional affinity studies showed that the extensively mutated antibody had a hundred times higher affinity than the RFs closer to the germline. In addition, the isolation of IgG RFs demonstrated that class switching of RFs occurs in RA (Randen et al., 1993a,b; Olee et al., 1992). This evidence for affinity maturation and class switching contrasts with the evidence from normal immunized donors where there is little or no increase in affinity with the accumulation of mutations (Børretzen et al., 1994). This suggests that following hypermutation there is a tolerance mechanism operating on RFs producing B-cells in normals that constrains the affinity maturation process. RFs in RA do not appear to be subject to such control mechanisms.

V. ORIGIN OF RHEUMATOID FACTORS

The RFs found in rheumatoid synovial tissues and other inflammatory sites are to a large extent produced by local B lymphocytes and plasma cells, which behave differently from normal B lymphocytes in the circulation. They are in contrast to peripheral blood, highly activated as indicated by extensive spontaneous immuno-globulin and antibody synthesis. In line with this, they also have a restricted repertoire of antibody specificities, e.g., a considerable proportion of them produce autoantibodies, mostly RFs (Natvig et al., 1989). These local B lymphocytes develop into plasma cells and accumulate in the synovial tissues. The rheumatoid inflammatory tissues will in many situations have a morphology showing primary and secondary lymphoid follicles with typical germinal centers (Randen et al.,

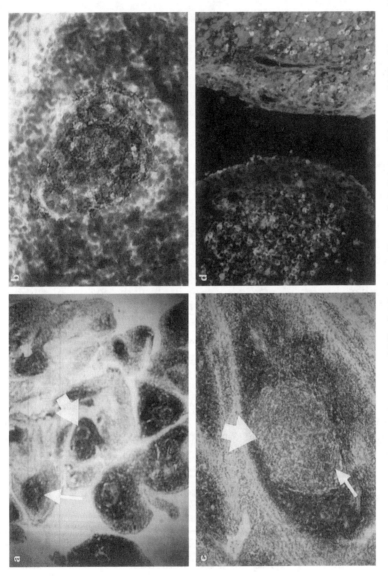

Figure 6 (see COLOR PLATE 5). Identification of germinal centers and follicular dendritic cell networks in RA synovial tissues. (a) The thin arrow identifies a primary follicle without a germinal center and the thick arrow identifies a secondary follicle containing a germinal center within the synovial tissue of an RA patient. The tissue is stained with anti-CD23 antibodies which recognize the follicular dendritic cell (FDC) network (brown) and is subsequently counterstained with hematoxylin (blue). (b) The network of dendrites typical of FCD identified with anti-CD23 antibodies in a rheumatoid synovium. (c) The classical dark (thin arrow) and light (thick arrow) zones of mature germinal center in rheumatoid synovial tissue identified with the Ki-67 antibody. Counterstained with haematolylin. (d) Example of clonal expansion in the synovial germinal centers. Staining with antibodies to kappa (green)- and lambda (red)-light chains. From Randen et al, 1995.

1995). The germinal centers are made up by interaction between B-cells, T-cells and follicular dendritic cells. The classical dark and light zones of the germinal centers can be identified by cell cycle associated nuclear antigen Ki-67.

In germinal centers the B-cells in the dark zones are dividing rapidly with little or no membrane Ig and are exposed to the hypermutation mechanisms. In the light zones centrocytes which express membrane Ig are selected for higher affinity Ig or die by apoptosis. Such a selection process apparently also occurs directly in the ectopic lymphoid tissues in synovial inflammation. Here primary and secondary lymphoid follicles are seen, partly with typical germinal centers staining positively for the CD23 antigen, the low affinity IgE receptor which shows the typical network of follicular dendritic cells in the secondary follicles (Figure 6). In our study we analyzed 24 patients and found 16 with lymphoid follicles and 4 of those with typical germinal centers. From one patient where several clones had been derived we found clear evidence of mutational processes both in heavy and light chains, and relatively high affinities that would indicate that these B-cells had been through typical germinal center reactions as described in normal lymphoid tissues (Liu and Banchereau, 1996; Pasqual et al., 1994). Similar findings have more recently been described by Schröder et al., 1996.

VI. PATHOGENETIC ROLE

In health, RFs have physiological roles whereas the roles in a variety of diseases are still under investigation. It is primarily in RA and some allied conditions such as Sjögrens Syndrome that high levels of RFs are found. There is now a series of evidence that RFs have pathogenic roles in RA. For example, seropositive RA is associated with poorer prognosis, presence of certain HLA DR 4 susceptibility genes and not infrequently rheumatoid nodules and vasculitis. Similar symptoms are also shown in Juvenile Rheumatoid Arthritis (JRA). In RA and probably also in JRA, the pathogenetic effect of RFs is primarily by being involved in immune complex formation which can activate complement and cause and sustain inflammation in effected joints (see Natvig et al., 1989). Thus, through the complement cascade and their mediators a series of inflammatory processes are activated. RF autoantibodies belong to different Ig classes, IgM and IgG predominate. However, a considerable amount of IgA RFs has also been demonstrated (Mellbye et al., 1990). IgA RFs may also be an indicator of disease activity together with IgM (Jonsson et al., 1995a,b). The RF autoantibodies bind to IgG and form complexes that can build up a considerable lattice in the synovial tissue. Large complement binding complexes are found in the tissues both in the intracellular spaces and inside the macrophages. Similarly, intracellular and soluble complement binding complexes are seen in the joint fluid and there is an inverse relation between the amount of complement and the amount of IgG complexes in the synovial fluid (Winchester et al., 1975). In contrast to the synovial tissues and fluid the complexes in the serum are small and mostly non complement binding. Apparently, there is a gradient from the largest complexes found in the synovial tissues to smaller complexes in the serum (Natvig et al., 1989). The immune complexes, particularly those containing IgG1 and IgG3 RFs are probably an important part of the pathogenetic mechanisms in RA because of their complement activation. There is also evidence that they are formed even in the plasma cells where the RF antibodies are produced, although the effect of this intracellular complexing of IgG RFs in plasma cells has not been extensively evaluated (Munthe and Natvig, 1972). Many IgG RFs producing cells have the unique property of producing antibodies directed towards determinants which are present in the constant region of the heavy chains of the same antibody population. This molecular self binding or self association was first proposed by Munthe and Natvig (1972) in rheumatoid synovial tissues and has also been extensively characterized in serum and joint fluids (Pope et al., 1975; Winchester et al., 1975). Some specific mechanisms may perpetuate the disease processes in RA. Firstly, RF antibodies produced by the plasma cells are immediately secreted in a complex form and the normal feedback mechanisms that are important for the downregulation of antibody responses may not function. Secondly, T-cells specific for Ig determinants have not been detected, probably because there is T-cell tolerance to Ig. Therefore another mechanism appears to work to give T-cell help for RF-production. By this system any immune complex taken up by B lymphocytes with RF autoantibody molecules as membrane Ig can stimulate T-cells to give help for further RF autoantibody production (Rosnek and Lanzavecchia, 1991). By this system, RF autoantibodies as membrane receptor molecules can bind any IgG immune complex, and peptides from antigens in this complex can stimulate T-cells. Thus, both the striking pathogenetic mechanisms of RFs through immune complex formation as well as T-cells stimulated partly through antigen presentation by RF B-cells adds to the pathogenetic mechanisms. Most of the T-cells in RA synovial fluid and tissues are proinflammatory Th1 cells which can also work as helper cells (Quayle et al., 1993).

VII.   STRUCTURE OF RFs THROUGH THREE-DIMENSIONAL MODELLING

In order to elucidate the three-dimensional structure, we have attempted to make a modelling of six different RFs from three patients (Randen et al., 1992a). The RFs also showed some differences in fine specificity. As mentioned above, the process of somatic mutation and antigen selection appears to be working on the RFs from RA patients. To assess this further it is important to obtain three-dimensional structures of the proteins. X-ray crystallography has demonstrated that recognition of epitopes on the antigen involves specific intraatomic contacts with the antibody molecules. Because no crystallographic data were available we decided to try to make a comparison on reasonable models. This can sometimes be obtained by comparison of primary structure with those of related highly resolved proteins. In the study by Randen et al. (1992a), modelling was performed in the following way: "Atomic ordinates for the V domains of highly resolved immunoglobulin fragments were obtained from the Brookhaven and Leeds Crystallographic Bases. The canonical forms which could best fit the RF CDR sequences were taken from the crystallographic structures and used to form the main chain of the RF CDRs which were placed onto the most homologous framework regions and energy minimized. Side chains were then positioned using the criteria of Ponder and Rickards and McGregor, and care taken to avoid collisions. The CDRs which did not fit canonical form were constructed by making deletions and additions to the nearest canonical structure using the conformational data given." The modelling is otherwise described in more detail earlier (Randen et al., 1992a). Figures 7A and 7B show

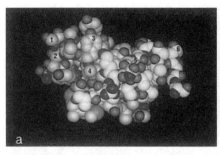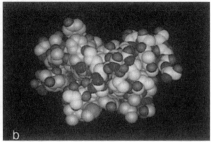

Figure 7 (see COLOR PLATE 6). Models of predicted binding regions of RF-SJ1 (a) and RF-SJ2 (b). Atoms are represented as spheres with the following colors: carbon atoms with the V_L are white, while the carbon atoms in the V_H chain are yellow. Nitrogen atoms are blue, oxygen atoms are red, and sulfur atoms are green. Amino acid sequence differences between RF-SJ2 and RF-SJ1 are numbered as follows: 1. Gly/Ser in V_H CDR3; 2. Gly/Ser in V_H CDR3; 3. Phe/Tyr in V_H CDR3; 4. Arg/Val in V_H CDR3; 5. Asn/Ser in V_L CDR2; 6. Ser/Thr in CDR1. Two other exposed substitutions: Ala/Gly in V_H CDR1 and Tyr/Asp in V_H CDR2 occur on the other side of the model to that shown. Antigen would be presented from the top of the picture. From Randen et al., 1992a.

models of the binding regions of RFSJ1 and RFSJ2, where 6 of the 8 exposed differences can be seen. The effect of these differences is changes in surface shape and polarity which would result in different epitope recognition.

In Figures 8A and 8B models of the potential binding regions of RFTS3 and RFKL1 in complex with the Cγ2–Cγ3 regions of IgG are shown. The 2 RFs are very different in shape and distribution of polar groups and also very different from RFSJ1 and RFSJ2. In all the RFs analyzed the interaction with the antigen involved contact points in all the CDR regions except CDR2 of the light chain.

Very recently, studies have now been made with crystals of one RF autoantibody RFAN (Sohi et al., 1996).

VIII. SPECIFICITIES OF RF

RF autoantibodies are directed against the Fc portion of the IgG molecules. The antigens are exposed in native IgG as indicated by inhibition studies with IgG in solution as well as binding studies. IgM RFs make 22 S complexes with one IgM RF molecule, with a valence of 5 (Metzger et al., 1970), and 5 IgG molecules. IgG RFs make intermediate complexes of 17–19 S (Mannik et al., 1988). RFs, however, react more strongly with IgG in immune complexes or in aggregated or denatured form, because this reaction is kinetically more favorable for crosslinking of many epitopes on IgG.

RFs can react with a variety of different antigenic sites in IgG Fc. These epitopes are found both in the CH2 and CH3 domains of the Fc fragment or in the

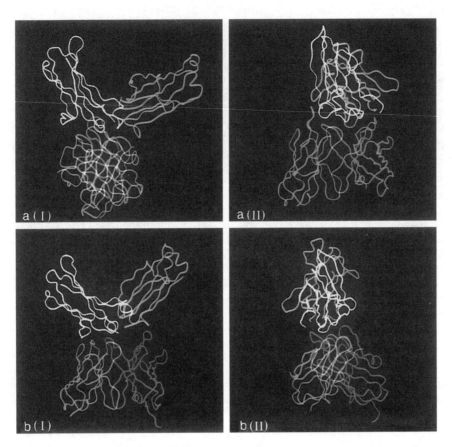

Figure 8 (see COLOR PLATE 7). Models of the RF V_L and V_H domains complexed with the target domains in the Fc part of IgG: (a) RF-TS3 and (b) RF-KL1. The models are shown with different orientations from each other so that the contact region can be seen more clearly. The predicted binding regions of the RFs and the domains of the Fc antigen were constructed as Connolly and van der Waals surfaces and searched for complementarity. These models show the main chain ribbon only. The variable heavy chain is blue, while the variable light chain is red. The $C\gamma2$ region is yellow; the $C\gamma3$ region is green. From Randen et al., 1992a.

interaction between these two domains and they are distributed among the 4 IgG subclasses in the human (Natvig et al., 1972; Artandi et al., 1991, 1992). The determinants that are recognized by RFs are mostly isotopic determinants present on all proteins of one or more IgG subclasses, but RFs can also recognize allotypic determinants present on genetic variants within a given IgG subclass. In fact, several new Gm allotypes in the human were first described by utilizing RFs (see Grubb, 1970). RFs can also detect so-called iso-allotypes (Gaarder and Natvig, 1970, 1972). In addition to their reaction with human IgG, RFs also frequently react with IgG from other species, particularly rabbit IgG which was used by Waaler in the original RF test (see Randen et al., 1989). Thus, RFs recognize a diverse range of antigenic determinants on human and other species' IgG.

Numerous reports describe in more detail the antigenic determinants for RFs within constant regions of the IgG subclasses (Allen and Kunkel 1966; Grubb, 1970; Gaarder and Natvig 1970, 1971; Sasso et al., 1988). Allen and Kunkel described a polyclonal IgM RF binding epitope on IgG; they called this non-allelic epitope ·'Ga". It is located within the heavy chain constant regions of human IgGl, 2, and 4 (Allen and Kunkel 1966; Sasso et al., 1988), the same IgG subclasses bound by *Staphylococcus aureus* protein A. RFs from RA patients differ from monoclonal IgM RFs derived from Waldenström disease in their binding patterns to IgG myeloma proteins of different subclasses (Sasso et al., 1988). The IgG1, 2 and 4 binding pattern predominates among RFs from RA patients, and monoclonal RFs from Waldenström patients (Capra et al., 1971). However, the ability to bind all 4 IgG subclasses is frequently found among RA–RFs compared with MC–RFs (Artandi et al., 1991; Bonagura et al., 1993). There is evidence that most RFs bind epitopes in the CH2–CH3 domains of human IgG (Natvig et al., 1972). Those studies used intact IgG myeloma proteins of different subclasses, or their pepsin or papain digested fragments, i.e., F(ab′)₂, Fc, pFc′ and F(acb′)₂, as RF binding substrates. Specific amino acids within the CH3 domain of IgG, (histidine 435 and tyrosine 436 in IgG1, 2, and 4), which are involved in *S. aureus* protein A binding, were reported to be important in RF binding (Sasso et al., 1988; Bonagura et al., 1993). This conclusion was derived from definitive X-ray diffraction studies, in which the B component of *S. aureus* protein A and the Fc fragment of IgG were co-crystallized (Deisenhofer, 1981), and from experiments in which binding of RFs to IgG was inhibited by specific chemical modifications of IgG (Sasso et al., 1988), or site-directed mutagenesis of residues in CH2 or CH3 domains of IgG (Bonagura et al., 1993).

Carbohydrate is also implicated in the immunologic perturbation that exists in RA (Parekh et al., 1985; Sumar et al., 1988; Schroenloher 1988). Carbohydrate at asparagine 297 within the CH2 domain of IgG may be a binding epitope, or it may modulate binding because of its effect on the tertiary structure of Fc (Parekh et al., 1985). Polyclonal IgG from RA patients contain an increased percentage of carbohydrate whose outer arms lack galactose and terminate in N-acetyl-glucosamine as compared to control IgG (Parekh et al., 1985; Sumar et al., 1988). This glycosylation variation is also found on polyclonal IgG from patients with tuberculosis and Crohn's disease who can express RF autoantibodies. Further studies with RF clones have shown different dependence on carbohydrate (Soltys et al., 1994). The precise evaluation of carbohydrate as an RF binding substrate will need further studies.

There is no consensus about the pattern of RF binding to IgG subclasses in various disease states. However, IgG3 has been reported to be bound more frequently by RFs from RA patient sera than previously thought (Robbins et al., 1986; Bonagura et al., 1993). Polyclonal RFs from RA patients uniformly bind IgG3, and a subgroup of monoclonal RFs from Waldenström's disease only bind IgG3 when clinical vasculitis is associated with monoclonal IgM RF expression. The discrepancy in these observations may be due to the methodologies used. In previous studies, identification of the determinants on IgG recognized by IgM RFs depended upon the use of myeloma IgG antibodies and their enzyme-cleaved fragments. Myeloma IgG obtained from peripheral blood can be contaminated with other IgG subclasses (Sasso et al., 1988); as a consequence, the results obtained in RF IgG binding assays can be misleading. Enzyme cleavage of IgG may create or destroy RF binding sites and yield misleading results.

Table 6. Comparison of RFs Produced in Various Situations

	RA patients	Proliferative diseases	Immunized normals
Predominant class	IgM frequently IgG, and IgA	IgM occasionally IgG	IgM
Clonality	Polyclonal	Monoclonal	Polyclonal
Deposition	Joints	No	No
Pathogenic effect in joints	Yes	No	No
Antigen driven	Yes	No	Yes
Hypermutation	Yes	Yes	Yes
Selective pressure on CDRs	Seen in IgG, not in IgM	?	Selection against replacement mutations
Affinity maturation	Yes	?	No

Recently the use of chimeric mouse/human antibodies to identify the specific amino acid sequences on human IgG constant regions bound by RFs has turned out to be valuable (Bonagura et al., 1993; Artandi et al., 1991, 1992). Variants of these antibodies can be genetically engineered to provide a greater flexibility in studying RF binding epitopes on IgG than was previously possible. The chimeric monoclonal antibodies are constructed by joining heavy and light chain mouse variable region segments, specific for the hapten dansyl (Bonagura et al., 1993), to respective γ or κ human constant regions. The genetically engineered genes are expressed in mouse myeloma cells by gene transfection. The resulting antibodies are used as binding substrates in a modified RF ELISA. By switching or mutagenizing constant regions of the various IgG subclasses, and then producing the modified antibodies using gene transfection, it is possible to identify and compare the IgG binding sites bound by RFs. These chimeric IgG antibodies of the four different subclasses have been shown to be identical in all functional analyses that are dependant on tertiary molecular structure compared to their naturally occurring counterparts (Bruggemann et al., 1987). Most recently it has been shown that specificty of RFs derived from healhty immunized donors differs from some RA-derived RFs. However, HID-derived RFs show similar reactivity with chimeric IgG subclass antibodies compared with monoclonal component RFs (Bonagura et al., 1995). These studies show that gentically engineered IgG antibodies are valuable tools for further studies on RFs and their specificities.

IX. CONCLUSION

RFs produced in RA patients have a number of differences when compared to RFs produced in healthy immunized donors (Table 6). They display a different preferential use of V_L and V_H gene families. Although RFs accumulate mutations in the variable regions in both health and disease, there is a striking difference in the patterns of mutation. RFs from normals are characterized by a very low R:S ratio in the CDR1+2, considerably lower than seen amongst the RFs from RA patients. It is possible that this reflects the fact that RF specificity is encoded in the germline, and mutations resulting in replacement amino acids will result in the loss of specificity. Although this possibility can only be definitely addressed by site directed mutagenesis experiments, our data suggests an alternative explanation. The fact that there is little increase in affinity with increasing numbers of mutations in the group of clonally related RFs from an immunized normal suggests that there is a normal controlling mechanism to limit the affinity of RF autoantibodies. The situation in patients with RA seems to be different. Here there is evidence of both affinity maturation and class switching. The higher affinity of the RA-derived RFs may contribute to the pathogenesis of the disease.

ACKNOWLEDGMENTS

This work was supported by the Norwegian Women's Health Organization and the Norwegian Research Council.

REFERENCES

Abderrazik, M., M. Moynier, R. Jefferis, R.A. Mageed, B. Combe, J. Sany, and J. Brochier. 1992. Analysis of monoclonal rheumatoid factors obtained from the B-cell repertoire in rheumatoid arthritis. *Scand. J. Immunol.* **35**, 149.

Allen J.C., and H.G. Kunkel. 1966. Hidden rheumatoid factors with specificity for native gamma globulins. *Arthritis and Rheum.* **9**, 758.

Andrews, D.W., and J.D. Capra. 1981. Complete amino acid sequence of variable domains from two monoclonal human anti-gamma globulins of the Wa cross-idiotypic group: suggestion that the J segments are involved in the structural correlate of the idiotype. *Proc. Natl. Acad. Sci. USA* **78**, 3799.

Artandi, S., S.M. Canfield, N.H. Tao, K.I. Calame, S.L. Morrison, and V.R. Bonagura. 1991. Molecular analysis of IgN rheumatoid factor binding to chimeric IgG. *J. Immunol.* **146**, 603.

Artandi, S.E., K.L. Calame, S.L. Morrison, and V.R. Bonagura. 1992. Monoclonal IgM rheumatoid factors bind IgG at a discontinuous epitope comprised of amino acid loops from heavy-chain constant region domains 2 and 3. *Proc. Natl. Acad. Sci. USA* **89**, 94–98.

Berman, J.E., S.J. Mellis, R. Pollock, C.L. Smith, H. Suh, B. Heinke, C. Kowal, U. Surti, L. Chess, and C.R. Cantor. 1988. Content and organization of the human Ig VH locus: definition of three new VH families and linkage to the Ig CH locus. *EMBO J.* **7**, 727.

Bonagura, V.R., S.E. Artandi, A. Davidson, I. Randen, N. Agostion, K. Thompson, J.B. Natvig, and S.L. Morrison. 1993. Mapping studies reveal unique epitopes on igg recognized by rheumatoid arthritis-derived monoclonal rheumatoid factors. *J. Immunol.* **151**, 3840–3852.

Bonagura, V.R., N. Agostino, T. Kwong, M. Børretzen, K.M. Thompson, J.B. Natvig, and S.L. Morrison. 1995. Healthy immunized donors (HIDs) and rheumatoid arthritis patients produce IgM rheumatoid factors (RFs) that react differently with genetically engineered, chimeric IgG antibodies (cIgG). *Arthritis Rheum.* **38** (No. 9 Supplement), S166 (Abstract).

Børretzen, M., I. Randen, E. Zdarsky, O. Forre, J.B. Natvig, and K.M. Thompson. 1994. Control of autoantibody affinity by selection against amino acid replacements in the complementarity determining regions. *Proc. Natl. Acad. Sci. USA* **26**, 12917.

Børretzen, M., I. Randen, J.B. Natvig, and K.M. Thompson. 1995. Structural restriction in the heavy chain CDR3 of human rheumatoid factors. *J. Immunol.* **155**, 3630–3637.

Bruggemann, M., G.T. Williams, C.I. Bindon, M.R. Clark, M.R. Walker, R. Jefferis, H. Waldmann, and M.S. Neuberger. 1987. Comparison of the effector functions of human immunoglobulins using a matched set of chimeric antibodies. *J. Exp. Med.* **166**, 1351.

Campbell, M.J., A.D. Zelenetz, S. Levy, and R. Levy. 1992. Use of family specific leader region primers for PCR amplification of the human heavy chain variable region gene repertoire. *Mol. Immunol.* **29**, 193.

Capra, J.D., and J.M. Kehoe. 1975. Hypervariable regions, idiotypy, and the antibody-combining site. *Adv. Immunol.* **20**, 1–40.

Capra, J.D., and D.G. Klapper. 1976. Complete amino acid sequence of the variable domains of two human IgM anti-gamma globulins (Lay/Pom) with shared idiotypic specificities. *Scand. J. Immunol.* **5**, 677.

Capra, J.D., J.M. Kehoe, R.J. Winchester, and H.G. Kunkel. 1971. Structure–function relationships among anti-gamma globulin antibodies. *Ann. N.Y. Acad. Sci.* **90**, 371.

Carson, D.A., and S. Fong. 1983. A common idiotope on human rheumatoid factors identified by a hybridoma antibody. *Mol. Immunol.* **20**, 1081.

Chen, P.P. 1990. Structural analyses of human developmentally regulated Vh3 genes. *Scand. J. Immunol.* **31**, 257.

Chen, P.P., K. Albrandt, N.K. Orida, V. Radoux, E.Y. Chen, R. Schrantz, F.T. Liu, and D.A. Carson. 1986. Genetic basis for the cross-reactive idiotypes on the light chains of human IgM anti-IgG autoantibodies. *Proc. Natl. Acad. Sci. USA* **83**, 8318.

Chen, P.P., K. Albrandt, T.J. Kipps, V. Radoux, F.T. Liu, and D.A. Carson. 1987. Isolation and characterization of human VkIII germ-line genes. Implications for the molecular basis of human VkIII light chain diversity. *J. Immunol.* **139**, 1727.

Chen, P.P., M.F. Liu, S. Sinha, and D.A. Carson. 1988. A 16/6 idiotype-positive anti-DNA antibody is encoded by a conserved VH gene with no somatic mutation. *Arthritis Rheum.* **31**, 1429.

Chen, P.P., M.F. Liu, C.A. Glass, S. Sinha, T.J. Kipps, and D.A. Carson. 1989. Characterization of two immunoglobulin VH genes that are homologous to human rheumatoid factors. *Arthritis Rheum.* **32**, 72.

Chiller, J.M., G.S. Habicht, and W.O. Weigle. 1970. Cellular sites of immunologic unresponsiveness. *Proc. Natl. Acad. Sci. USA* **65**, 551.

Clarkson, A.B. Jr., and G.H. Mellow. 1981. Rheumatoid factor-like immunoglobulin M protects previously uninfected rat pups and dams from *Trypanosoma lewisi*. *Science* **214**, 186.

Cook, G.P., I.M. Tomlinson, G. Walter, H. Riethman, N.P. Carter, L. Buluwela, G. Winter, and T.H. Rabbitts. 1994. A map of the human immunoglobulin V–H locus completed by analysis of the telomeric region of chromosome 14q. *Nature Genet.* **7**, 162.

Coulie, P., and J. Van Snick. 1983. Rheumatoid factors and secondary immune responses in the mouse. II. Incidence, kinetics and induction mechanisms. *Eur. J. Immunol.* **13**, 895.

Cox, J.P.L., I.M. Tomlinson, and G. Winter. 1994. A directory of human germ-line V-kappa segments reveals a strong bias in their usage. *Eur. J. Immunol.* **24**, 827.

Crouzier, R., T. Martin, and J.L. Pasquali. 1995. Monoclonal IgM rheumatoid factor secreted by CD5-negative B cells during mixed cryoglobulinemia. Evidence for somatic mutations and intraclonal diversity of the expressed VH region gene. *J. Immunol.* **154**, 413.

Crowley, J.J., R.D. Goldfien, R.E. Schrohenloher, H.L. Spiegelberg, G.J. Silverman, R.A. Mageed, R. Jefferis, W.J. Koopman, D.A. Carson, and S. Fong. 1988. Incidence of three cross-reactive idiotypes on human rheumatoid factor paraproteins. *J. Immunol.* **140**, 3411.

Crowley, J.J., R.A. Mageed, G.J. Silverman, P.P. Chen, F. Kozin, R.A. Erger, R. Jefferis, and D.A. Carson. 1990. The incidence of a new human cross-reactive idiotype linked to subgroup VHIII heavy chains. *Mol. Immunol.* **27**, 87.

Deane, M., L.E. MacKenzie, F.K. Stevenson, P.Y. Youinou, P.M. Lydyard, and R.A. Mageed. 1993. The genetic basis of human V(H)4 gene family-associated cross-reactive idiotype expression in CD5+ and CD5- cord blood B-lymphocyte clones. *Scand. J. Immunol.* **38**, 348.

Deftos, M., T. Olee, D.A. Carson, and P.P. Chen. 1994. Defining the genetic origins of three rheumatoid synovium-derived IgG rheumatoid factors. *J. Clin. Invest.* **93**, 2545.

Deisenhofer, J. 1981. Crystallographic refinement and atomic models of a human Fc fragment and its complex with fragment B of protein A from Staphylococcus aureus at 2.9- and 2.8-Å resolution. *Biochem.* **20**, 2361.

Denny, C.T., Y. Yoshikai, T.W. Mak, S.D. Smith, G.F. Hollis, and I.R. Kirsch. 1986. A chromosome 14 inversion in a T-cell lymphoma is caused by site-specific recombination between immunoglobulin and T-cell receptor loci. *Nature* **320**, 549.

Fang, Q., C.C. Kannapell, S.M. Fu, S.H. Xu, and F. Gaskin. 1995. V-H and V-L gene usage by anti-beta-amyloid autoantibodies in Alzheimer's disease: Detection of highly mutated V regions in both heavy and light chains. *Clin. Immunol. Immunopathol.* **75**, 159.

Fong, S., P.P. Chen, T.A. Gilbertson, J.R. Weber, R.I. Fox, and D.A. Carson. 1986. Expression of three cross-reactive idiotypes on rheumatoid factor autoantibodies from patients with autoimmune diseases and seropositive adults. *J. Immunol.* **137**, 122.

Gaarder, P.I., and J.B. Natvig. 1970. Hidden rheumatoid factors reacting with "non a" and other antigens of native autologous IgG. *J. Immunol.* **105**, 928.

Gaarder, P.I., and J.B. Natvig. 1972. Two new antigens of human IgG "non bo" and "non b1" related to the Gm system. *J. Immunol.* **108**, 617.

Goni, F., P.P. Chen, B., Pons Estel, D.A. Carson, and B. Frangione. 1985. Sequence similarities and cross-idiotypic specificity of L chains among human monoclonal IgM kappa with anti-gamma-globulin activity. *J. Immunol.* **135**, 4073.

Goodnow, C.C., J. Crosbie, S. Adelstein, T.B. Lavoie, S.J. Smith Gill, R.A. Brink, H. Pritchard Briscoe, J.S. Wotherspoon, R.H. Loblay, K. Raphael, et al. 1988. Altered immunoglobulin expression and functional silencing of self-reactive B lymphocytes in transgenic mice. *Nature* **334**, 676.

Grubb, R. 1970. *The Genetic Markers of Human Immunoglobulins.* Springer-Verlag, Berlin, p. 152.

Huber, C., K.F. Schable, E. Huber, R. Klein, A. Meindl, R. Thiebe, R. Lamm, and H.G. Zachau. 1993. The V kappa genes of the L regions and the repertoire of V kappa gene sequences in the human germ line. *Eur. J. Immunol.* **23**, 2868.

Ikematsu, H., N. Harindranath, and P. Casali. 1992. Somatic mutations in the VH genes of high-affinity antibodies to self and foreign antigens produced by human CD5+ and CD5- B lymphocytes. *Ann. N. Y. Acad. Sci.* **651**, 319.

Ikematsu, H., M.T. Kasaian, E.W. Schettino, and P. Casali. 1993. Structural analysis of the VH–D–JH segments of human polyreactive IgG mAb. Evidence for somatic selection. *J. Immunol.* **151**, 3604.

Jonsson, T., S. Arinbjarnarson, J. Thorsteinsson, K. Steinsson, A.J. Geirsson, H. Jonsson, and H. Valdimarsson. 1995a. Raised IgA rheumatoid factor (RF) but not IgM RF or IgG RF is associated with extra-articular manifestations in rheumatoid arthritis. *Scand. J. Rheumatol.* **24**, 372–375.

Jonsson, T., H. Thorsteinsson, S. Arinbjarnarson, J. Thorsteinsson, and H. Valdimarsson. 1995b. Clinical implications of IgA rheumatoid factor subclasses. *Ann. Rheum. Dis.* **54**, 578–581.

Kipps, T.J., and S.F. Duffy. 1991. Relationship of the CD5 B cell to human tonsillar lymphocytes that express autoantibody-associated cross-reactive idiotypes. *J. Clin. Invest.* **87**, 2087.

Kipps, T.J., E. Tomhave, L.F. Pratt, S. Duffy, P.P. Chen, and D.A. Carson. 1989. Developmentally restricted immunoglobulin heavy chain variable region gene expressed at high frequency in chronic lymphocytic leukemia. *Proc. Natl. Acad. Sci. USA* **86**, 5913.

Kodaira, M., T. Kinashi, I. Umemura, F. Matsuda, T. Noma, Y. Ono, and T. Honjo. 1986. Organization and evolution of variable region genes of the human immunoglobulin heavy chain. *J. Mol. Biol.* **190**, 529.

Koopman, W.J., R.E. Schrohenloher, and D.A. Carson. 1990. Dissociation of expression of two rheumatoid factor cross-reactive kappa L chain idiotopes in rheumatoid arthritis. *J. Immunol.* **144**, 3468.

Kouri, T., J. Crowley, K. Aho, T. Palosuo, H. Isomaki, R. Von Essen, M. Heliovaara, D. Carson, and J.H. Vaughan. 1990. Occurrence of two germline-related rheumatoid factor idiotypes in rheumatoid arthritis and in non-rheumatoid seropositive individuals. *Clin. Exp. Immunol.* **82**, 250.

Kunkel, H.G., V. Agnello, F.G. Joslin, R. Winchester, and J.D. Capra. 1973. Cross idiotypic specificity among monoclonal IgM proteins with anti-gamma-globulin activity. *J. Exp. Med.* **137**, 331.

Kuppers, R., U. Fischer, K. Rajewsky, and A. Gause. 1992. Immunoglobulin heavy and light chain gene sequences of a human CD5 positive immunocytoma and sequences of 4 novel VHIII germline genes. *Immunol. Lett.* **34**, 57.

Ledford, D.K., F. Goni, M. Pizzolato, E.C. Franklin, A. Solomon, and B. Frangione. 1983. Preferential association of kappa IIIb light chains with monoclonal human IgM kappa autoantibodies. *J. Immunol.* **131**, 1322.

Liu, M.F., D.L. Robbins, J.J. Crowley, S. Sinha, F. Kozin, T.J. Kipps, D.A. Carson, and P.P. Chen. 1989. Characterization of four homologous L chain variable region genes that are related to 6B6.6 idiotype positive human rheumatoid factor L chains. *J. Immunol.* **142**, 688.

Liu, Y.-J., and J. Banchereau. 1996. The pathway and regulation of peripheral B cells development. *Immunologist* **4**, 55–69.

Mageed, R.A., M. Dearlove, D.M. Goodall, and R. Jefferis. 1986. Immunogenic and antigenic epitopes of immunoglobulins. XVII. Monoclonal antibodies reactive with common and restricted idiotopes to the heavy chain of human rheumatoid factors. *Rheumatol. Int.* **6**, 179.

Mageed, R.A., D.A. Carson, and R. Jefferis. 1988. Immunogenic and antigenic epitopes of immunoglobulins. XXIII. Idiotypy and molecular specificity of human rheumatoid factors: analysis of cross-reactive idiotype of rheumatoid factor paraproteins from the Wa idiotype group in relation to their IgG subclass specificity. *Scand. J. Immunol.* **28**, 233.

Mageed, R.A., D.M. Goodall, and R. Jefferis. 1990. A highly conserved conformational idiotope on human IgM rheumatoid factor paraproteins of the Wa cross-reactive idiotype family defined by a monoclonal antibody. *Rheumatol. Int.* **10**, 57.

Mannik, F., F.A. Nardella, and E.H. Sasso. 1988. Rheumatoid factors in immune complexes of patients with rheumatoid arthritis. *Springer Semin. in Immunopathol.* **10**(2/3), 215–230.

Matsuda, F., and T. Honjo. 1996. Organization of the human immunoglobulin heavy-chain locus. *Adv. Immunol.* **62**, 1–29.

Matsuda, F., E.K. Shin, H. Nagaoka, R. Matsumura, M. Haino, Y. Fukita, S. Takaishi, T. Imai, J.H. Riley, R. Anand, E. Soeda, and T. Honjo. 1993. Structure and physical map of 64 variable segments in the 3(I)0.8-megabase region of the human immunoglobulin heavy-chain locus. *Nature Genet.* **3**, 88.

Meindl, A., H.G. Klobeck, R. Ohnheiser, and H.G. Zachau. 1990. The V kappa gene repertoire in the human germ line. *Eur. J. Immunol.* **20**, 1855.

Mellbye, O.J., F. Vartdal, J. Pahle, and T.E. Mollnes. 1990. IgG and IgA subclass distribution of total immunoglobulin and rheumatoid factors in rheumatoid tissue plasma cells. *Scand. J. Rheumatol.* **19**, 333–340.

Metzger, H. 1970. Structure and function of γM macroglobulins. *Adv. Immunol.* **12**, 57–116.

Munthe, E., and J.B. Natvig. 1972. Immunoglobulin classes, subclasses and complexes of IgG rheumatoid factor in rheumatoid plasma cells. *Clin. Exp. Immunol.* **12**, 55.

Natvig, J.B., and M.W. Turner. 1970. Rheumatoid anti-Gm factors with specificity for the pFc' subfragment of human immunoglobulin G. *Nature* **225**, 855.

Natvig, J.B., N.W.I Turner, and P.I. Gaarder. 1972. IgG antigens of the C-gamma-2 and C-gamma-3 homology regions interacting with rheumatoid factors. *Clin. Exp. Immunol.* **12**, 177.

Natvig, J.B., I. Randen, K.M. Thompson, O. Forre, and E. Munthe. 1989. The B cell system in the rheumatoid inflammation. New insights into the pathogenesis of rheumatoid arthritis using synovial B cell hybridoma clones. *Springer Semin. Immunopathol.* **11**, 301.

Nemazee, D.A. 1985. Immune complexes can trigger specific, T cell-dependent, autoanti-IgG antibody production in mice. *J. Exp. Med.* **161**, 242.

Nemazee, D., and K. Buerki. 1989. Clonal deletion of autoreactive B lymphocytes in bone marrow chimeras. *Proc. Natl. Acad. Sci. USA* **86**, 8039.

Nemazee, D.A., and V.L. Sato. 1983. Induction of rheumatoid antibodies in the mouse. Regulated production of autoantibody in the secondary humoral response. *J. Exp. Med.* **158**, 529.

Newkirk, M., P.P. Chen, D. Carson, D. Posnett, and J.D. Capra. 1986. Amino acid sequence of a light chain variable region of a human rheumatoid factor of the Wa idiotypic group, in part predicted by its reactivity with antipeptide antibodies. *Mol. Immunol.* **23**, 239.

Newkirk, M.M., R.A. Mageed, R. Jefferis, P.P. Chen, and J.D. Capra. 1987. Complete amino acid sequences of variable regions of two human IgM rheumatoid factors, BOR and KAS of the Wa idiotypic family, reveal restricted use of heavy and light chain variable and joining region gene segments. *J. Exp. Med.* **166**, 550.

Norton, W.L., and M. Ziff. 1966. Electron microscopic observations on the rheumatoid synovial membrane. *Arthritis Rheum.* **9**, 589.

Olee, T., P.M. Yang, K.A. Siminovitch, N.J. Olsen, J. Hillson, J. Wu, F. Kozin, D.A. Carson, and P.P. Chen. 1991. Molecular basis of an autoantibody-associated restriction fragment length polymorphism that confers susceptibility to autoimmune diseases. *J. Clin. Invest.* **88**, 193.

Olee, T., E.W. Lu, D.F. Huang, R.W. Gil Soto, M. Deftos, F. Kozin, D.A. Carson, and P.P. Chen. 1992. Genetic analysis of self-associating immunoglobulin G rheumatoid factors from two rheumatoid synovia implicates an antigen-driven response. *J. Exp. Med.* **175**, 831.

Parekh, R.B., R.A. Dwek, B.J. Sutton, D.L. Fernandes, A. Leung, D. Stanworth, and T.W. Rademacher. 1985. Association of rheumatoid arthritis and primary osteoarthritis with changes in glycosylation pattern of total serum IgG. *Nature* **316**, 452.

Pascual, V., I. Randen, K.M. Thompson, M. Sioud, O. Forre, J. Natvig, and J.D. Capra. 1990. The complete nucleotide sequences of the heavy chain variable regions of six monospecific rheumatoid factors derived from Epstein–Barr virus-transformed B cells isolated from the synovial tissue of patients with rheumatoid arthritis. Further evidence that some autoantibodies are unmutated copies of germ line genes. *J. Clin. Invest.* **86**, 1320.

Pascual, V., Y.-J. Liu, A. Magalski, O. de Bouteiller, J. Banchereau, and J.D. Capra. 1994. Analysis of somatic mutation in five B cell subsets of human tonsil. *J. Exp. Med.* **180**, 329–339.

Potter, K.N., Y.C. Li, and J.D. Capra. 1994. The cross-reactive idiotopes recognized by the monoclonal antibodies 9G4 and LC1 are located in framework region 1 of two non-overlapping subsets of human V(H)4 family encoded antibodies. *Scand. J. Immunol.* **40**, 43.

Pratt, L.F., R. Szubin, D.A. Carson, and T.J. Kipps. 1991. Molecular characterization of a supratypic cross-reactive idiotype associated with IgM autoantibodies. *J. Immunol.* **147**, 2041.

Quayle, A.J., P. Chomarat, P. Miossec, J. Kjeldsen-Kragh, O. Forre, and J.B. Natvig. 1993. Rheumatoid inflammatory T cell clones express mostly TH_1, but also TH_2 and mixed (TH_0-like) cytokine patterns. *Scand. J. Immunol.* **38**, 75–82.

Radoux, V., P.P. Chen, J.A. Sorge, and D.A. Carson. 1986. A conserved human germline V kappa gene directly encodes rheumatoid factor light chains. *J. Exp. Med.* **164**, 2119.

Randen, F.M., K.M. Thompson, J.B. Natvig, 0. Forre, and K. Wallen. 1989. Human monoclonal rheumatoid factors derived from the polyclonal repertoire of rheumatoid synovial tissue: production and characterization. *Clin. Exp. Immunol.* **78**, 13.

Randen, I., K.M. Thompson, V. Pascual, K. Victor, D. Beale, J. Coadwell, O. Forre, J.D. Capra, and J.B. Natvig. 1992a. Rheumatoid factor V genes from patients with rheumatoid arthritis are diverse and show evidence of an antigen driven response. *Immunol. Rev.* **128**, 49.

Randen, I., D. Brown, K.M. Thompson, N. Hughes-Jones, V. Pascual, K. Victor, J.D. Capra, Ø. Førre, and J.B. Natvig. 1992b. Clonally related IgM rheumatoid factors undergo affinity maturation in the rheumatoid synovial tissue. *J. Immunol.* **148**, 3296–3301.

Randen, I., V. Pascual, K. Victor, K.M. Thompson, Ø. Førre, J.D. Capra, and J.B. Natvig. 1993a. Synovial IgG rheumatoid factors show evidence of an antigen-driven immune response and a shift in the V gene repertoire compared to IgM rheumatoid factors. *Eur. J. Immunol.* **23**, 1220–1225.

Randen, I., K.M. Thompson, S.J. Thorpe, Ø. Førre, and J.B. Natvig. 1993b. Human monoclonal IgG rheumatoid factors from the synovial tissue of patients with rheumatoid arthritis. *Scand. J. Immunol.* **37**, 668–672.

Randen, I., O.J. Mellbye, Ø. Førre, and J.B. Natvig. 1995. The identification of germinal centres and follicular dendritic cell network in rheumatoid synovial tissue. *Scand. J. Immunol.* **41**, 481–486.

Rechavi, G., D. Ram, L. Glazer, R. Zakut, and D. Givol. 1983. Evolutionary aspects of immunoglobulin heavy chain variable region (VH) gene subgroups. *Proc. Natl. Acad. Sci. USA* **80**, 855.

Rieben, R., A. Tucci, U.E. Nydegger, and R.H. Zubler. 1992. Self tolerance to human A and B histo-blood group antigens exists at the B cell level and cannot be broken by potent polyclonal B cell activation in vitro. *Eur. J. Immunol.* **22**, 2713.

Robbins, D.L., J. Skilling, W.F. Benisek, and R. Wistar. 1986. Estimation of the relative avidity of 19 IgM rheumatoid factor secreted by rheumatoid synovial cells for human IgG subclasses. *Arth. Rheum.* **29**, 122.

Roosnek, E., and A. Lanzavecchia. 1991. Efficient and selective presentation of antigen–antibody complexes by rheumatoid factor B cells. *J. Exp. Med.* **173**, 487.

Sanz, I., P. Kelly, C. Williams, S. Scholl, P. Tucker, and J.D. Capra. 1989. The smaller human VH gene families display remarkably little polymorphism. *EMBO J.* **8**, 3741.

Sasso, E.H. 1992. Immunoglobulin V genes in rheumatoid arthritis. *Rheum. Dis. Clin. North Am.* **18**, 1.

Sasso, E.H., C.V. Barber, F.A. Nardella, W.J. Yount, and M. Mannik. 1988. Antigen specificities of human monoclonal and polyclonal IgM rheumatoid factors. *J. Immunol.* **140**, 3098–3107.

Sasso, E.H., K. Willems van Dijk, A.P. Bull, and E.C. Milner. 1993. A fetally expressed immunoglobulin VH1 gene belongs to a complex set of alleles. *J. Clin. Invest.* **91**, 2358.

Schröder, A.E., A. Greiner, C. Seyfert, and C. Berek. 1996. Differentiation of B cells in the nonlymphoid tissue of the synovial membrane of patients with rheumatoid arthritis. *Proc. Natl. Acad. Sci. USA* **93**, 221–225.

Schronenloher, R.E. 1988. IgG as antigen in human rheumatic disease. *Scand. J. Rheum.* **75S**, 133.

Shin, E.K., F. Matsuda, H. Nagaoka, Y. Fukita, T. Imai, K. Yokoyama, E. Soeda, and T. Honjo. 1991. Physical map of the 3' region of the human immunoglobulin heavy chain locus: clustering of autoantibody-related variable segments in one haplotype. *EMBO J.* **10**, 3641.

Shokri, F., R.A. Mageed, E. Tunn, P.A. Bacon, and R. Jefferis. 1990. Qualitative and quantitative expression of VHI associated cross reactive idiotopes within IgM rheumatoid factor from patients with early synovitis. *Ann. Rheum. Dis.* **49**, 150.

Silverman, G.J., R.D. Goldfien, P. Chen, R.A. Mageed, R. Jefferis, F. Goni, B. Frangione, S. Fong, and D.A. Carson. 1988. Idiotypic and subgroup analysis of human monoclonal rheumatoid factors. Implications for structural and genetic basis of autoantibodies in humans. *J. Clin. Invest.* **82**, 469.

Silverman, G.J., R.E. Schrohenloher, M.A. Accavitti, W.J. Koopman, and D.A. Carson. 1990. Structural characterization of the second major cross-reactive idiotype group of human rheumatoid factors. Association with the VH4 gene family. *Arthritis Rheum.* **33**, 1347.

Sohi, M.K., A.L. Corper, T. Wan, M. Steinitz, R. Jefferis, D. Beale, M. He, A. Feinstein, B.J. Sutton, and M.M. Taussig. 1996. Crystallization of a complex between the Fab fragment of a human immunoglobulin M (IgM) rheumatoid factor (RF–AN) and the Fc fragment of human IgG4. *Immunology* **88**, 636–641.

Soltys, A.J., F.C. Hay, J.S. Axford, M.G. Jones, I. Randen, K.M. Thompson, and J.B. Natvig. 1994. The binding of synovial tissue-derived human monoclonal immunoglobulin M rheumatoid factor to immunoglobulin G preparations of differing galactose content. *Scand. J. Immunol.* **40**, 135–143.

Stanley, S.L. Jr., J.K. Bischoff, and J.M. Davie. 1987. Antigen-induced rheumatoid factors. Protein and carbohydrate antigens induce different rheumatoid factor responses. *J. Immunol.* **139**, 2936.

Straubinger, B., E. Huber, W. Lorenz, E. Osterholzer, W. Pargent, M. Pech, H.D. Pohlenz, F.J. Zimmer, and H.G. Zachau. 1988. The human VK locus. Characterization of a duplicated region encoding 28 different immunoglobulin genes. *J. Mol. Biol.* **199**, 23.

Stuber, F., S.K. Lee, S.L. Bridges Jr., W.J. Koopman, H.W. Schroeder Jr., F. Gaskin, and S.M. Fu. 1992. A rheumatoid factor from a normal individual encoded by VH2 and V kappa II gene segments. *Arthritis Rheum.* **35**, 900.

Suleyman, S., K.M. Thompson, O. Forre, M. Sioud, I. Randen, R.A. Mageed, and J.B. Natvig. 1994. Three new cross-reacting idiotopes as markers for the products of two distinct human V_H3 genes expressed in the early repertoire. *Scand. J. Immunol.* **40**, 681.

Sumar, N., I.M. Roitt, K.B. Bodman, D.A. Isenberg, F.C. Hay, J.S. Axford, C.B. Colaco, R.B. Parekh, T.W. Rademacher, and R.A. Owek. 1988. Reduced N-glycosylation of serum IgG is disease restricted. *Arth. Rheum.* **31**, 593.

Thompson, K.M., I. Randen, M. Børretzen, O. Forre, and J.B. Natvig. 1994. Variable region gene usage of human monoclonal rheumatoid factors derived from healthy donors following immunization. *Eur. J. Immunol.* **24**, 1771.

Thompson, K.M., M. Børretzen, and J.B. Natvig. 1995. New data on rheumatoid factors in health and disease. *Rheumatology in Europe* **24** (Supplement 2), 165–167.

Thompson, K.M., M. Børretzen, I. Randen, O. Forre, and J.B. Natvig. 1995. V-gene repertoire and hypermutation of rheumatoid factors produced in rheumatoid synovial inflammation and immunized healthy donors. *Ann. N.Y. Acad. Sci.* **764**, 440–450.

Thompson, N., I. Randen, J.B. Natvig, E.A. Mageed, R. Jefferis, O.A. Carson, M.H. Tighe, and O. Forre. 1990. Human monoclonal rheumatoid factors derived from the polyclonal repertoire of rheumatoid synovial tissue: incidence of cross-reactive idiotypes and expression of VH and Vk subgroups. *Eur. J. Immunol.* **20**, 863.

Tomlinson, I.M., G. Walter, J.D. Marks, M.B. Llewelyn, and G. Winter. 1992. The repertoire of human germline V(H) sequences reveals about 50 groups of V(H) segments with different hypervariable loops. *J. Mol. Biol.* **227**, 776.

Van der Maarel, S., K.W. van Dijk, C.M. Alexander, E.H. Sasso, A. Bull, and E.C. Milner. 1993. Chromosomal organization of the human VH4 gene family. Location of individual gene segments. *J. Immunol.* **150**, 2858.

Van Es, J.H., M. Heutink, H. Aanstoot, and T. Logtenberg. 1992. Sequence analysis of members of the human Ig VH4 gene family derived from a single VH locus. Identification of novel germ-line members. *J. Immunol.* **149**, 492.

Van Snick, J.L., E. Van Roost, B. Markowetz, C.L. Cambiaso, and P.L. Masson. 1978. Enhancement by IgM rheumatoid factor of in vitro ingestion by macrophages and in vivo clearance of aggregated IgG or antigen–antibody complexes. *Eur. J. Immunol.* **8**, 279.

Welch, M.J., S. Fong, J. Vaughan, and D. Carson. 1983. Increased frequency of rheumatoid factor precursor B lymphocytes after immunization of normal adults with tetanus toxoid. *Clin. Exp. Immunol.* **51**, 299.

Weng, N.P., J.G. Snyder, L.Y. Yu Lee, and D.M. Marcus. 1992. Polymorphism of human immunoglobulin VH4 germ-line genes. *Eur. J. Immunol.* **22**, 1075.

Williams, R.C. Jr., H.G. Kunkel, and J.D. Capra. 1968. Antigenic specificities related to the cold agglutinin activity of gamma M globulins. *Science* **161**, 379.

Yang, P.M., T. Olee, D.A. Carson, and P.P. Chen. 1993. Characterization of two highly homologous autoantibody-related VH1 genes in humans. *Scand. J. Immunol.* **37**, 504.

Zachau, H.G. 1996. The human immunoglobulin κ genes. *Immunologist* **4**, 49–54.

INDEX

INDEX

Volume 1

INDEX

Volume 2

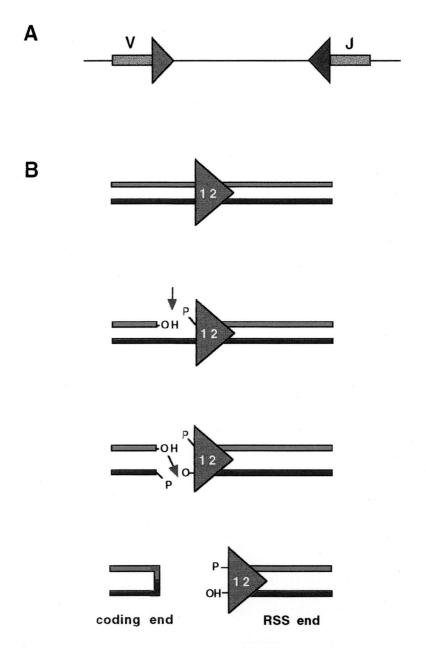

coding end   **RSS end**

Plate 1 (see Chapter 1, Figure 1). Model for the V(D)J recombination cleavage steps. **A:** DNA substrates for V(D)J recombination are pairs of Recombination Signal Sequences (RSS, blue and red triangles) containing opposite spacer lengths of 12 and 23 bp. Ig and T cell receptor coding sequences are adjoined to these RSS. **B:** The cleavage reactions of V(D)J recombination initiation. A two step reaction has been formulated for this process (McBlane et al., 1995; van Gent et al., 1996). Single-strand cleavage of the phosphodiester bond flanking the RSS element (top strand in the orientation shown, XXX'CACAGTG) is followed by hairpin generation by intramolecular nucleophilic attack. Red arrows denote cleavage positions on both strands. Both steps require RAG1 and RAG2. Coordination of the cleavage reactions between RSS(12) and RSS(23) elements obeys the 12/23 spacer rule (Eastman et al., 1996).

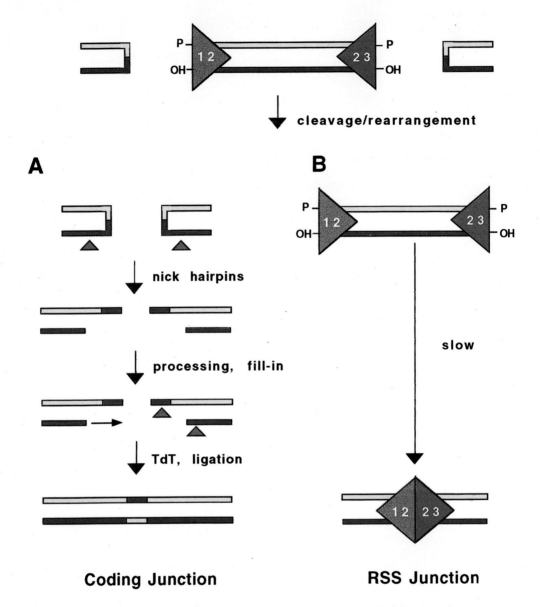

cleavage/rearrangement

A

B

nick hairpins

processing, fill-in

slow

TdT, ligation

Coding Junction

RSS Junction

Plate 2 (see Chapter 1, Figure 2). Model for the rearrangement and joining steps of V(D)J recombination. The products of the initiation steps of V(D)J recombination are two covalently sealed coding DNA ends (hairpins) and two blunt-ended RSS elements displayed in the linear array consistent with a chromosomal deletional event. Gene rearrangement involves the rejoining of strands from the two cleavages as shown in Part A and B. The relationship between cleavages and rearrangement strand selection are poorly understood. **A:** Coding end joining may be viewed as being started by the terminal endonucleolytic scission of hairpins (red arrows), generating a variety of DNA overlaps. Processing of these structures includes the deletion and addition of nucleotides in the novel junctions formed. P nucleotides arise from asymmetric cleavage of hairpins (indicated by portions of the bottom strand appended to top strand ends) and filling in. Additional red arrows denote mismatch correction of coding ends prior to ligation. N nucleotides are added in an untemplated fashion. **B:** Blunt-end cleaved RSS ends are joined in a separable reaction, producing RSS-RSS fusions that are precise.

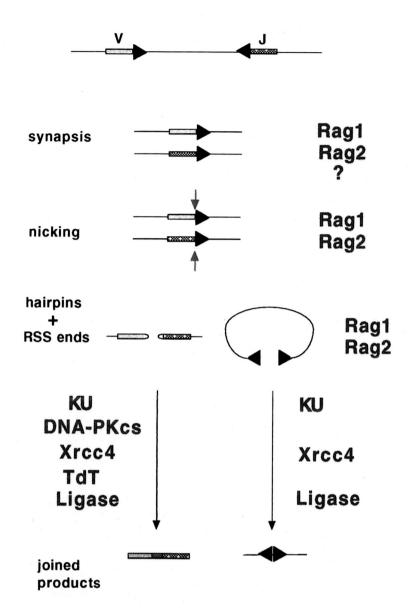

Plate 3 (see Chapter 1, Figure 3). Protein requirements for V(D)J recombination. Two lymphoid specific proteins, RAG1 and RAG2, are essential for the initiation reactions of V(D)J recombination. Both proteins are needed for the two steps involved in making double strand breaks at each RSS. A group of DNA repair proteins are important for the product formation steps of V(D)J recombination as shown. The Ku heterodimer and Xrcc4 protein are necessary for both RSS and coding end joining. In contrast, the DNA-dependent protein kinase catalytic subunit, which associates with Ku, is primarily needed only for coding end joining. Processing enzymes, including factors that cleave hairpins, fill-in or excise DNA ends, and ligate products have not been identified.

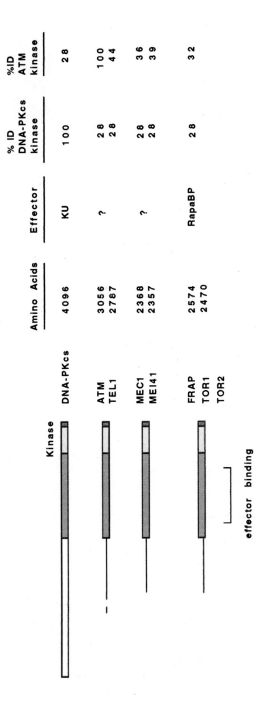

Kinase	Amino Acids	Effector	% ID DNA-PKcs kinase	%ID ATM kinase
DNA-PKcs	4096	KU	100	28
ATM	3056	?	28	100
TEL1	2787		28	44
MEC1	2368	?	28	36
MEI41	2357		28	39
FRAP	2574	RapaBP	28	32
TOR1	2470			
TOR2				

effector binding

Plate 4 (see Chapter 1, Figure 6). Homology between DNA-PK$_{cs}$-related gene products. The DNA-dependent protein kinase catalytic subunit is a member of the PI-3 type kinase family. The other related protein kinases in this group also have C-terminal protein kinase domains as shown. Identity relative to DNA-PK$_{cs}$ and ATM kinase domains are illustrated, and the homology groups are ordered as previously (Hartley et al., 1995; Jackson, 1996; Keith et al., 1995). DNA-PK$_{cs}$ and FRAP are the only members of this group for which protein cofactors (the Ku heterodimer and Rapamycin binding protein) have been identified. Yellow = kinase homology; green = family-specific homology in the COOH terminus; blue = homology regions that may mediate effector binding.

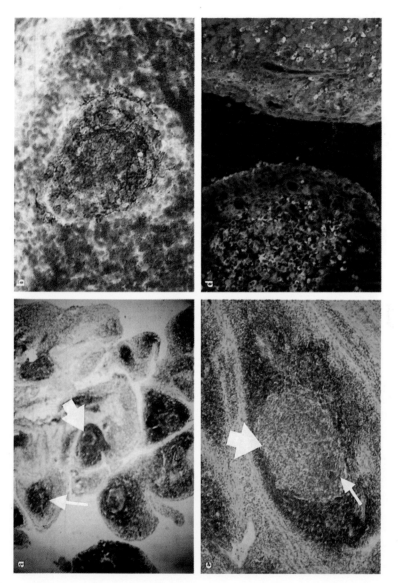

Plate 5 (see Chapter 6, Figure 6). Identification of germinal centers and follicular dendritic cell networks in RA synovial tissues. (a) The thin arrow identifies a primary follicle without a germinal center and the thick arrow identifies a secondary follicle containing a germinal center within the synovial tissue of a rheumatoid arthritis patient. The tissue is stained with anti-CD23 antibodies which recognize the follicular dendritic cell (FDC) network (brown) and is subsequently counterstained with hematoxylin (blue). (b) The network of dendrites typical of FCD identified with anti-CD23 antibodies in a rheumatoid synovium. (c) The classical dark (thin arrow) and light (thick arrow) zones of mature germinal center in rheumatoid synovial tissue identified with the Ki-67 antibody. Counterstained with haematolylin. (d) Example of clonal expansion in the synovial germinal centers. Staining with antibodies to kappa (green)- and lambda (red)-light chains.

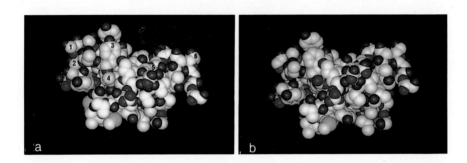

Plate 6 (see Chapter 6, Figure 7). Models of predicted binding regions of RF-SJ1 (a) and RF-SJ2 (b). Atoms are represented as spheres with the following colors: carbon atoms with the V_L are white, while the carbon atoms in the V_H chain are yellow. Nitrogen atoms are blue, oxygen atoms are red, and sulfur atoms are green. Amino acid sequence differences between RF-SJ2 and RF-SJ1 are numbered as follows: 1. Gly/Ser in V_H CDR3; 2. Gly/Ser in V_H CDR3; 3. Phe/Tyr in V_H CDR3; 4. Arg/Val in V_H CDR3; 5. Asn/Ser in V_L CDR2; 6. Ser/Thr in CDR1. Two other exposed substitutions: Ala/Gly in V_H CDR1 and Tyr/Asp in V_H CDR2 occur on the other side of the model to that shown. Antigen would be presented from the top of the picture.

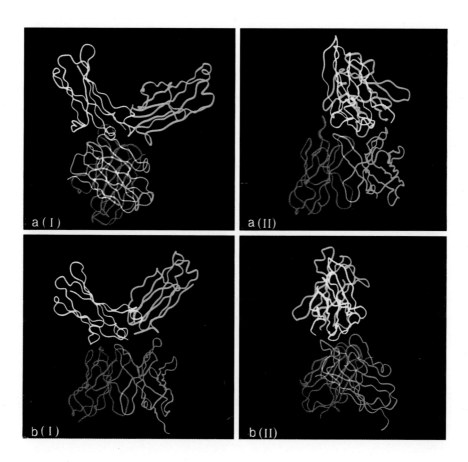

Plate 7 (see Chapter 6, Figure 8). Models of the RF V_L and V_H domains complexed with the target domains in the Fc part of IgG: (a) RF-TS3 and (b) RF-KL1. The models are shown with different orientations from each other so that the contact region can be seen more clearly. The predicted binding regions of the RF and the domains of the Fc antigen were constructed as Connolly and van der Waals surfaces and searched for complementarity. These models show the main chain ribbon only. The variable heavy chain is blue, while the variable light chain is red. The Cγ2 region is yellow; the Cγ3 region is green.